Informatik aktuell

AF148223

Herausgeber: Wilfried Brauer
im Auftrag der Gesellschaft für Informatik (GI)

Weitere Bände in dieser Reihe:
http://www.springer.com/series/2872

Hans-Peter Meinzer · Thomas Martin Deserno
Heinz Handels · Thomas Tolxdorff
Herausgeber

Bildverarbeitung
für die Medizin 2013

Algorithmen – Systeme – Anwendungen

Proceedings des Workshops
vom 3. bis 5. März 2013 in Heidelberg

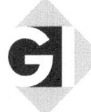

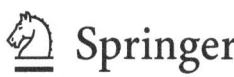

Herausgeber
Hans-Peter Meinzer
Abteilung für Medizinische und Biologische
  Informatik H0100
Deutsches Krebsforschungszentrum
Heidelberg, Deutschland

Thomas Martin Deserno, geb. Lehmann
Institut für Medizinische Informatik
Rheinisch-Westfälische Technische
  Hochschule Aachen
Aachen, Deutschland

Heinz Handels
Institut für Medizinische Informatik
Universität zu Lübeck
Lübeck, Deutschland

Thomas Tolxdorff
Charité – Universitätsmedizin Berlin
Institut für Medizinische Informatik
Berlin, Deutschland

ISSN 1431-472X
ISBN 978-3-642-36479-2   ISBN 978-3-642-36480-8   (eBook)
DOI 10.1007/978-3-642-36480-8

CR Subject Classification (1998): A.0, H.3, I.4, I.5, J.3, H.3.1, I.2.10, I.3.5, I.3.7, I.3.8, I.6.3

Die Deutsche Nationalbibliothek verzeichnet diese Publikation in der Deutschen Nationalbibliografie; detaillierte bibliografische Daten sind im Internet über http://dnb.d-nb.de abrufbar.

Springer ist Teil der Fachverlagsgruppe Springer Science+Business Media (www.springer.com)

Bildverarbeitung für die Medizin 2013

Veranstalter

MBI   Medizinische und Biologische Informatik
Deutsches Krebsforschungszentrum (DKFZ) Heidelberg
mit Unterstützung durch die Fachgesellschaften:

BVMI   Berufsverband Medizinischer Informatiker
CURAC   Deutsche Gesellschaft für Computer- und Roboterassistierte Chirurgie
DGBMT   Fachgruppe Medizinische Informatik
der Deutschen Gesellschaft für Biomedizinische Technik im VDE
GMDS   Arbeitsgruppe Medizinische Bild- und Signalverarbeitung
der Deutschen Gesellschaft für Medizinische Informatik,
Biometrie und Epidemiologie
IEEE   Joint Chapter Engineering in Medicine and Biology, German Section

Tagungsvorsitz

Prof. Dr. Hans-Peter Meinzer

Medizinische und Biologische Informatik – Deutsches Krebsforschungszentrum (DKFZ) Heidelberg

Lokale Organisation

Hans-Peter Meinzer
Peter Neher
Alexander Seitel
Janina Dunning
Beatrice Bartik
u.v.m.

Medizinische und Biologische Informatik – Deutsches Krebsforschungszentrum (DKFZ) Heidelberg

Verteilte BVM-Organisation

Prof. Dr. Thomas M. Deserno, Christoph Classen, Jan Dovermann
Rheinisch-Westfälische Technische Hochschule Aachen (Tagungsband)

Prof. Dr. Heinz Handels, Dr. Jan-Hinrich Wrage
Universität zu Lübeck (Begutachtung)

Prof. Dr. Hans-Peter Meinzer, Dr. Alexander Seitel
Deutsches Krebsforschungszentrum Heidelberg (Anmeldung)

Prof. Dr. Thomas Tolxdorff, Dr. Thorsten Schaaf
Charité – Universitätsmedizin Berlin (Internetpräsenz)

Programmkomitee

Industrieaussteller und Sponsoren

STRYKER	Stryker Leibinger GmbH & Co. KG Bötzinger Strasse 41, 79111 Freiburg
HDE	Heidelberg Engineering GmbH Tiergartenstrasse 15, 69121 Heidelberg
NDI	NDI Europe GmbH Fritz Reichle-Ring 2, 78315 Radolfzell
IEEE	IEEE Joint Chapter Engineering in Medicine and Biology German Section 3 Park Avenue, 17th Floor, New York, YN, 10016-5995 USA
DGBMT	Deutsche Gesellschaft für Biomedizinische Technik im VDE Stresemannallee 15, 60596 Frankfurt
CURAC	Computer- und Roboterassistierte Chirurgie e.V. Postfach 70 01 49, 70571 Stuttgart
GMDS	Deutsche Gesellschaft für Medizinische Informatik, Biometrie und Epidemiologie e.V. Industriestraße 154, 50996 Köln
BVMI	Berufsverband Medizinischer Informatiker e.V. Scheidt 1, 41812 Erkelenz

Preisträger des BVM-Workshops 2012 in Berlin

Der BVM-Award für eine herausragende Diplom-, Bachelor-, Master- oder Doktorarbeit aus dem Bereich der Medizinischen Bildverarbeitung ist mit 1.000 € dotiert und wurde im Jahre 2012 geteilt. Die je mit einem Preisgeld von 250 € dotierten BVM-Preise zeichnen besonders hervorragende Arbeiten aus, die auf dem Workshop präsentiert wurden.

BVM-Award 2012 für eine herausragende Dissertation

Dr.-Ing. Andreas Fieselmann (Lehrstuhl für Mustererkennung, Friedrich-Alexander Universität, Erlangen-Nürnberg)
Interventional Perfusion Imaging Using C-arm Computed Tomography: Algorithms and Clinical Evaluation

BVM-Award 2012 für eine herausragende Bachelor-Arbeit

Benjamin Köhler (Institut für Simulation und Grafik/Lehrstuhl für Visualiserung, Otto-von-Guericke-Universität Magdeburg)
Rekonstruktion neuronaler Faserbündel mittels globalem Fiber-Tracking ausgehend von einem aus HARDI-Daten erzeugten ODF-Feld

BVM-Preis 2012 für die beste wissenschaftliche Arbeit

Lars Ruthotto mit *Fabian Gigengack, Martin Burger, Carsten H. Wolters, Xiaoyi Jiang, Klaus P. Schäfers, Jan Modersitzki* (Universität zu Lübeck)
A Simplified Pipeline for Motion Correction in Dual Gated Cardiac PET

BVM-Preis 2012 für die zweitbeste wissenschaftliche Arbeit

Astha Jaiswal mit *William J. Godinez, Roland Eils, Maik J. Lehmann, Karl Rohr* (BIOQUANT, Universität Heidelberg)
Tracking Virus Particles in Microscopy Images Using Multi-Frame Association

BVM-Preis 2012 für die drittbeste wissenschaftliche Arbeit

Sebastian Gollmer mit *Thorsten M. Buzug* (Universität zu Lübeck)
Formmodellbasierte Segmentierung des Unterkiefers aus Dental-CT-Aufnahmen. Ein vollautomatischer Ansatz

BVM-Preis 2012 für den besten Vortrag

Marlit Erbe mit *Mandy Grüttner, Timo F. Sattel, Thorsten M. Buzug* (Universität zu Lübeck)
Experimentelle Realisierungen einer vollständigen Trajektorie für die magnetische Partikel-Bildgebung mit einer feldfreien Linie

BVM-Preis 2012 für die beste Posterpräsentation

Alina Toma mit *Anne Régnier-Vigouroux, Andreas Mang, Tina A. Schütz, Stefan Becker, Thorsten M. Buzug* (Universität zu Lübeck)
In-silico Modellierung der Immunantwort auf Hirntumorwachstum

Vorwort

Die Analyse und Verarbeitung medizinischer Bilddaten hat sich im Laufe der letzten Jahrzehnte zu einem nicht mehr wegzudenkenden Baustein moderner Diagnose- und Therapiesysteme entwickelt. Computer-basierte Operationsplanung hat genauso den Weg in die klinische Routine gefunden wie Computer-Assistenzsysteme zur exakten Platzierung von Instrumenten. Hierbei steht stets das Ziel im Vordergrund, die Behandlung des Patienten sicherer und effizienter zu gestalten, um somit zu dessen bestmöglicher Genesung beizutragen. Herausfordernd ist dabei insbesondere, dass neben der Entwicklung neuer und der Verbesserung bestehender Bildverarbeitungsalgorithmen auch deren Relevanz im klinischen Alltag ständig kritisch hinterfragt werden muss.

Der Workshop „Bildverarbeitung für die Medizin" bietet genau für diese Art von Diskussion eine ideale Plattform, da sich dort nun schon im 20. Jahr Experten aus dem interdisziplinären Umfeld der medizinischen Bildverarbeitung versammeln, um neue Ideen zu diskutieren und zukünftige Ziele festzulegen. Auch für junge Nachwuchswissenschaftler stellt der Workshop ein hervorragendes Podium dar, um über ihre Bachelor-, Master-, Promotions- oder Habilitationsprojekte berichten zu können.

Der diesjährige Workshop findet zum nunmehr vierten Mal in Heidelberg statt und vereint in diesem Jahr insbesondere wissenschaftlich hochaktuelle Themen mit dem klinischen Alltag. Hierfür konnten zwei renommierte Gastredner gewonnen werden:

- *Prof. Dr. Daniel Elson*, Imperial College London, wird über das Thema „Biophotonics" referieren.
- *Prof. Dr. Ron Kikinis*, Harvard Medical School, Boston, wird den Aspekt der Forschungstranslation in seinem Vortrag „Medical Image Computing for Translational Biomedical Research" näher erläutern und mit Experten aus Industrie, Forschung und Medizin über dieses wichtige Thema diskutieren.

Des Weiteren findet dieses Jahr zum ersten Mal eine Session statt, in der Abteilungsleiter aus dem Gebiet der medizinischen Bildverarbeitung über Zukunftsperspektiven des Forschungszweiges referieren und diskutieren werden. Erstmalig wird es auch ein Diskussionsforum geben, in dem junge Wissenschaftler mit Vertretern aus Industrie und Forschung über mögliche Karrierewege diskutieren können.

Die verteilte Organisation des Workshops, durchgeführt von Einrichtungen aus Aachen, Berlin, Heidelberg und Lübeck, erwies sich ein weiteres Mal als vorteilhaft für die Durchführung der Veranstaltung. Nach Begutachtung aller eingereichten Beiträge durch jeweils drei unabhängige Gutachter – organisiert von den Kollegen aus Lübeck – wurden insgesamt 61 Beiträge angenommen, wobei hiervon 40 als Vorträge, 19 als Poster und 2 als Softwaredemonstrationen auf dem Workshop präsentiert werden. Eine schriftliche Langfassung aller Beiträge (bis zu 6 Seiten) wird im Tagungsband erscheinen, der von den Aachener

Kollegen aufbereitet und vom Springer-Verlag in der bewährten Reihe „Informatik Aktuell" der Gesellschaft für Informatik (GI) elektronisch publiziert wird. Weitere Informationen zum Workshop sind auf der von den Berliner Kollegen gepflegten Internetpräsenz http://www.bvm-workshop.org zu finden.

Als zusätzliches Rahmenprogramm werden am Tag vor dem wissenschaftlichen Programm drei Tutorien angeboten:

– *Dipl. Inform. med. Marco Nolden* und *Dipl. Phys. Sascha Zelzer*, Abteilung Medizinische und Biologische Informatik, Deutsches Krebsforschungszentrum Heidelberg, geben eine Einführung in die Erstellung interaktiver medizinischer Bildverarbeitungssysteme auf Basis des Open-Source Medical Imaging Interaction Toolkits (MITK) und dessen zugrundeliegenden Bibliotheken. Anhand der Entwicklung einer Beispielanwendung mit MITK werden Datenmanagements- und GUI-Komponenten vorgestellt sowie die Nutzung der wichtigsten ITK-Komponenten zur Segmentierung und Registrierung und der wichtigsten VTK-Komponenten zur Visualisierung gezeigt. Ferner wird die Anbindung weiterer Toolkits und eigener Anwendungen mit den Konzepten und Schnittstellentechnologien der Common Toolkit (CTK) Initiative demonstriert.

– *PD Dr. med. Beat Müller* und *Felix Nickel*, Klinik für Allgemein-, Viszeral- und Transplantationschirurgie, Universität Heidelberg, bieten den Teilnehmern Einblick in die laparoskopischen Techniken der minimal-invasiven Chirurgie. Es werden Übungen zur Kameraführung und zum Umgang mit den Instrumenten durchgeführt um insbesondere die Eigenheiten der speziellen räumlichen Wahrnehmung beim Operieren mit indirekter Sicht über die Kamera kennenzulernen.

– *Dr. Jakob Valvoda*, Anwaltssozietät Boehmert und Boehmert, München, gibt eine Einführung in den Themenkomplex der Patentierung von Erfindungen und richtet insbesondere den Fokus auf computer-implementierte Erfindungen (Software) im Bereich der medizinischen Bildverarbeitung. Nach einer Einführung in die grundlegenden Begriffe der Patentierbarkeit, der Technizität und der Patentfähigkeit von Erfindungen werden an konkreten Fallbeispielen zusammen mit den Tutoriums-Teilnehmern Patentansprüche entworfen und analysiert.

An dieser Stelle möchten wir allen, die bei den umfangreichen Vorbereitungen und der Durchführung des Workshops beteiligt waren und sind, unseren herzlichen Dank für ihr Engagement bei der Organisation aussprechen: den Referenten der Gastvorträge, den Autoren der Beiträge, den Referenten der Tutorien, den Industrierepräsentanten, dem Programmkomitee, den Fachgesellschaften, den Mitgliedern des BVM-Organisationsteams und allen Mitarbeitern der Abteilung Medizinische und Biologische Informatik des Deutschen Krebsforschungszentrums Heidelberg.

Wir wünschen allen Teilnehmerinnen und Teilnehmern des Workshops BVM 2013 lehrreiche Tutorien, viele interessante Vorträge, Gespräche an den Postern, bei den Softwaredemonstrationen und bei der Industrieausstellung sowie spannende neue Kontakte zu Kolleginnen und Kollegen aus dem Bereich der medizinischen Bildverarbeitung.

Januar 2013

Hans-Peter Meinzer (Heidelberg)
Thomas Deserno (Aachen)
Heinz Handels (Lübeck)
Thomas Tolxdorff (Berlin)

Inhaltsverzeichnis

Die fortlaufende Nummer am linken Seitenrand entspricht den Beitragsnummern, wie sie im endgültigen Programm des Workshops zu finden sind. Dabei steht V für Vortrag, P für Poster und S für Softwaredemonstration.

Eingeladene Vorträge

V1   *Kikinis R:* Medical Image Computing for Translational Biomedical Research 1

V2   *Elson DS:* Surgical Imaging and Biophotonics 2

Navigation

V3   *Mastmeyer A, Hecht T, Fortmeier D, Handels H:* Ray-Casting-Based Evaluation Framework for Needle Insertion Force Feedback Algorithms 3

V4   *Hecht T, Mastmeyer A, Fortmeier D, Handels H:* 4D-Planung von Nadelpfaden für Punktionseingriffe mit der Ray-Casting-Methode .. 9

V5   *März K, Franz AM, Stieltjes B, Zahn A, Seitel A, Iszatt J, Radeleff B, Meinzer H-P, Maier-Hein L:* Navigierte ultraschallgeführte Leberpunktion mit integriertem EM Feldgenerator 15

V6   *Wetzl J, Taubmann O, Haase S, Köhler T, Kraus M, Hornegger J:* GPU-Accelerated Time-of-Flight Super-Resolution for Image-Guided Surgery 21

V7   *Magaraggia J, Egli A, Kleinszig G, Graumann R, Angelopoulou E, Hornegger J:* Calibration of a Camera-Based Guidance Solution for Orthopedic and Trauma Surgery 27

XVI

Bildanalyse 1

V8   *Richter M, Merhof D:* Optimized Cortical Subdivision for
Classification of Alzheimer's Disease With Cortical Thickness   33

V9   *Dinse J, Martin P, Schäfer A, Geyer S, Turner R, Bazin P-L:*
Quantifying Differences Between Primary Cortical Areas in Humans
Based on Laminar Profiles in In-Vivo MRI Data   39

V10   *Glaßer S, Niemann U, Preim U, Preim B, Spiliopoulou M:*
Classification of Benign and Malignant DCE-MRI Breast Tumors by
Analyzing the Most Suspect Region   45

V11   *Goch CJ, Stieltjes B, Henze R, Hering J, Meinzer H-P,
Fritzsche KH:* Quantification of Changes in Language-Related Brain
Areas in Autism Spectrum Disorders Using Large-Scale Network
Analysis   51

V12   *Mang A, Stritzel J, Toma A, Becker S, Schuetz TA, Buzug TM:*
Personalisierte Modellierung der Progression primärer Hirntumoren
als Optimierungsproblem mit Differentialgleichungsnebenbedingung   57

Segmentierung 1

V13   *Pohle-Fröhlich R, Brandt C, Koy T:* Segmentierung der lumbalen
Bandscheiben in MRT-Bilddaten   63

V14   *Schwarzenberg R, Freisleben B, Kikinis R, Nimsky C, Egger J:* Ein
kubusbasierter Ansatz zur Segmentierung von Wirbeln in
MRT-Aufnahmen   69

V15   *Graser B, Seitel M, Al-Maisary S, Grossgasteiger M, Heye T,
Meinzer H-P, Wald D, de Simone R, Wolf I:* Computer-Assisted
Analysis of Annuloplasty Rings   75

V16   *König T, Rak M, Steffen J, Neumann G, von Rohden L,
Tönnies KD:* Texture-Based Detection of Myositis in
Ultrasonographies   81

V17   *Morariu CA, Gross S, Pauli J, Aach T:* Segmentierung von
Kolonpolypen in NBI-Bildmaterial mittels gaborfilterbasierten
Multikanal-Level-Sets   87

Methoden

V18 *Kiencke S, Levakhina YM, Buzug TM:* Greedy Projection Access
Order for SART 93

V19 *Lempe G, Zaunseder S, Wirthgen T, Zipser S, Malberg H:* ROI
Selection for Remote Photoplethysmography 99

V20 *Xia Y, Maier A, Dennerlein F, Hofmann HG, Hornegger J:* Scaling
Calibration in the ATRACT Algorithm 104

V21 *Pilz T, Fried E, van Waasen S, Wagenknecht G:* Improvement of an
Active Surface Model by Adaptive External Forces 110

V22 *Scherf N, Kunze M, Thierbach K, Zerjatke T, Burek P, Herre H,
Glauche I, Roeder I:* Assisting the Machine 116

Registrierung & Simulation

V23 *Berkels B, Cabrilo I, Haller S, Rumpf M, Schaller C:*
Co-Registration of Intra-Operative Photographs and Pre-Operative
MR Images 122

V24 *Wang J, Borsdorf A, Hornegger J:* Depth-Layer-Based Patient
Motion Compensation for the Overlay of 3D Volumes onto X-Ray
Sequences 128

V25 *Marx M, Ehrhardt J, Werner R, Schlemmer H-P, Handels H:*
4D-MRT-basierte Simulation der Lungenbewegung in statischen
CT-Daten 134

V26 *Fortmeier D, Mastmeyer A, Handels H:* Image-Based Palpation
Simulation With Soft Tissue Deformations Using Chainmail on the
GPU 140

V27 *Krüger J, Ehrhardt J, Bischof A, Handels H:* Simulation
mammographischer Brustkompression zur Generierung von
MRT-Projektionsbildern 146

Bildanalyse 2

V28 *Shen M, Zimmer B, Leist M, Merhof D:* Automated Image
Processing to Quantify Cell Migration 152

V29 *Gerner B, Töpfer D, Museyko O, Engelke K:* Impact of
     Segmentation in Quantitative Computed Tomography 158

V30 *Haak D, Simon H, Yu J, Harmsen M, Deserno TM:* Bone Age
     Assessment Using Support Vector Machine Regression 164

V31 *Mualla F, Schöll S, Sommerfeldt B, Hornegger J:* Using the
     Monogenic Signal for Cell-Background Classification in Bright-Field
     Microscope Images 170

V32 *Gayetskyy S, Museyko O, Hess A, Schett G, Engelke K:* Bildgebende
     Charakterisierung und Quantifizierung der Vaskulogenese bei
     Arthritis 175

Poster Bildanalyse

P1   *Pener I, Schmidt M, Hahn HK:* Towards Fully Automated Tracking
     of Carotid and Vertebral Arteries in CT Angiography 181

P2   *Lawonn K, Gasteiger R, Preim B:* Qualitative Evaluation of Feature
     Lines on Anatomical Surfaces 187

P3   *Duygu Özmen :* Bestimmung der Lage der Papilla Duodeni Major
     im Bild eines Duodenoskops 193

P4   *Chitiboi T, Homeyer A, Linsen L, Hahn H:* Object-Based Image
     Analysis With Boundary Properties 199

P5   *Nowack S, Wittenberg T, Paulus D, Bergen T:* Merkmalsverfolgung
     für die Panoramaendoskopie 205

P6   *Friedrich D, Cobos AL, Biesterfeld S, Böcking A, Meyer-Ebrecht D:*
     Konturverfeinerung über Fourierdeskriptoren 211

Poster Bildgebung

P7   *Schönmeyer R, Schmidt G, Meding S, Walch A, Binnig G:*
     Automated Co-Analysis of MALDI and H&E Images of Retinal
     Tissue for an Improved Spatial MALDI Resolution 217

P8   *Thiering B, Nagarajah J, Lipinski H-G:* Fusion von Szintigrafie und
     CT für die Schilddrüsendiagnostik 223

P9   *Wu H, Maier A, Hornegger J:* Iterative CT Reconstruction Using
      Curvelet-Based Regularization 229

Poster Registrierung & Simulation

P10   *Kislinskiy S, Golembiovský T, Duriez C, Riesenkampff E,*
      Kuehne T, Meinzer H-P, Wald D: Simulationsgestützte
      Operationsplanung bei angeborenen Herzfehlern 235

P11   *Hoffmann M, Bourier F, Strobel N, Hornegger J:*
      Structure-Enhanced Visualization for Manual Registration in
      Fluoroscopy 241

P12   *Friedl S, König S, Weyand M, Wittenberg T, Kondruweit M:*
      Dynamic Heart Valve Cusp Bending Deformation Analysis 247

Poster Segmentierung

P13   *Nzegne PMK, Faltin P, Kraus T, Chaisaowong K:* 3D Lung Surface
      Analysis Towards Segmentation of Pleural Thickenings 253

P14   *Surup T, Hänler A, Homeier A, Petersik A, von Oldenburg G,*
      Burgkart R: Verfahren zur Referenzmodellerstellung für die
      Evaluierung CT-basierter Segmentierung des
      Kortikalis-Spongiosa-Überganges im Femur 259

P15   *Burmester FS, Gollmer ST, Buzug TM:* Untersuchung der
      Normalverteilungsannahme bei der statistischen Formmodellierung . 265

P16   *Al-Zubaidi A, Chen L, Hagenah J, Mertins A:* Robust Feature for
      Transcranial Sonography Image Classification Using
      Rotation-Invariant Gabor Filter 271

P17   *Tian M, Yang Q, Maier A, Schasiepen I, Maass N, Elter M:*
      Automatic Histogram-Based Initialization of K-Means Clustering in
      CT 277

P18   *Fried E, Pilz T, van Waasen S, Wagenknecht G:* Extraction of
      Partial Skeletons for Semi-Automatic Segmentation of Cortical
      Structures 283

P19   Bista SR, Dogan S, Astvatsatourov A, Mösges R, Deserno TM:
      Automatic Conjunctival Provocation Test Using Hough Transform
      of Extended Canny Edge Maps 290

Softwaredemos

S1   Hachmann H, Faltin P, Kraus T, Chaisaowong K:
      3D-Segmentierungskorrektur unter Berücksichtigung von
      Bildinformationen für die effiziente und objektive Erfassung
      pleuraler Verdickungen 296

S2   Franz AM, März K, Seitel A, Müller M, Zelzer S, Nodeln M,
      Meinzer H-P, Maier-Hein L: MITK-US: Echtzeitverarbeitung von
      Ultraschallbildern in MITK 302

Segmentierung 2

V33   Eck S, Wörz S, Biesdorf A, Müller-Ott K, Rippe K, Rohr K:
      Segmentation of Heterochromatin Foci Using a 3D Spherical
      Harmonics Intensity Model 308

V34   Fränzle A, Bretschi M, Bäuerle T, Bendl R: Automatic Detection of
      Osteolytic Lesions in Rat Femur With Bone Metastases 314

V35   Jung F, Kirschner M, Wesarg S: A Generic Approach to Organ
      Detection Using 3D Haar-Like Features 320

V36   Libuschewski P, Siedhoff D, Timm C, Weichert F: Mobile Detektion
      viraler Pathogene durch echtzeitfähige
      GPGPU-Fuzzy-Segmentierung 326

V37   Koch M, Bauer S, Hornegger J, Strobel N: Towards Deformable
      Shape Modeling of the Left Atrium Using Non-Rigid Coherent Point
      Drift Registration 332

Bildgebung

V38   Bier B, Schwemmer C, Maier A, Hofmann HG, Xia Y,
      Hornegger J, Struffert T: Convolution-Based Truncation Correction
      for C-Arm CT Using Scattered Radiation 338

V39 *Ruthotto L, Mohammadi S, Heck C, Modersitzki J, Weiskopf N:*
Hyperelastic Susceptibility Artifact Correction of DTI in SPM 344

V40 *Blendowski M, Wilms M, Werner R, Handels H:* Simulation und
Evaluation tiefenbildgebender Verfahren zur Prädiktion
atmungsbedingter Organ- und Tumorbewegungen 350

V41 *Fränkel S, Wunder K, Heil U, Groß D, Schulze R, Schwanecke U,
Düber C, Schömer E, Weinheimer O:* Total Variation
Regularization in Digital Breast Tomosynthesis 356

V42 *Okur A, Shakir DI, Matthies P, Hartl A, Ziegler SI, Essler M,
Lasser T, Navab N:* Freehand Tomographic Nuclear Imaging Using
Tracked High-Energy Gamma Probes 362

Kategorisierung der Beiträge 369

Autorenverzeichnis 371

Stichwortverzeichnis 375

Medical Image Computing for Translational Biomedical Research

Ron Kikinis

Surgical Planning Laboratory, Brigham and Women's Hospital,
Harvard Medical School
kikinis@bwh.harvard.edu

Medical Image Computing (MIC) is an emerging interdisciplinary field at the intersection of computer science, electrical engineering, physics, mathematics and medicine. The field develops computational and mathematical methods for solving problems pertaining to medical images and their use for biomedical research and clinical care. The main goal of Medical Image Computing is to extract clinically relevant information or knowledge from medical images (from Wikipedia). MIC research is traditionally performed in academic settings and results in working prototypes and demos. There is an increasing need for converting such prototypes into tools that can be used for translational biomedical research. Creating such tools requires modular software architecture and effective interdisciplinary teams. Open source platforms are emerging as an effective solution to translation in MIC.

H.-P. Meinzer et al. (Hrsg.), *Bildverarbeitung für die Medizin 2013*, Informatik aktuell,
DOI: 10.1007/978-3-642-36480-8_1, © Springer-Verlag Berlin Heidelberg 2013

Surgical Imaging and Biophotonics

Daniel S. Elson

Imperial College London
daniel.elson@imperial.ac.uk

Surgical imaging describes the application of a broad range of imaging, vision and optical techniques to assist surgeons for intrasurgical decision making. Some of these techniques aim to replace current technology such as the xenon lamp with new ergonomic and functional light sources that are able to enhance the surgeon's view. During this presentation a number of surgical imaging and biophotonics devices that are currently in development will be reviewed. Some of these are able to distinguish between healthy and diseased tissue non-invasively and without the use of external biomarkers, while others can be used for general illumination using spectrally flexible broadband lasers or LED illumination. Another area where surgical imaging may find an important role is in robotic-assisted minimally invasive surgery. Devices that are capable of precise motion have led to the possibility of careful movement of spectroscopic instruments across the tissue surface and improved mosaicing of microscopic image fields. Furthermore, the use of a da Vinci rigid endoscope will be described with 3D stereoscopic reconstruction and alignment of multimodal optical images. This registration allows the extraction of tissue oxygenation and perfusion in bowel and womb tissue, which could potentially be used to image changes in tissue blood supply during a surgery. Finally a new endoscopic method for detecting the 3D surface profile of different tissues has been developed based on the projection of spectrally encoded spots onto the tissue surface together with a method of triangulation. This technology has been assessed in vitro and results suggest that it could be used to align and register pre-operative medical images onto the live endoscopic view for surgical guidance.

H.-P. Meinzer et al. (Hrsg.), *Bildverarbeitung für die Medizin 2013*, Informatik aktuell,
DOI: 10.1007/978-3-642-36480-8_2, © Springer-Verlag Berlin Heidelberg 2013

Ray-Casting-Based Evaluation Framework for Needle Insertion Force Feedback Algorithms

Andre Mastmeyer[1], Tobias Hecht[1], Dirk Fortmeier[1,2], Heinz Handels[1]

[1]Institute of Medical Informatics, University of Lübeck
[2]Graduate School for Computing in Medicine and Life Sciences, University of Lübeck
mastmeyer@imi.uni-luebeck.de

Abstract. Segmentation of patient data often is a mandatory step for surgical simulations featuring haptic rendering. To alleviate the burden of manual segmentation we chose direct haptic volume rendering based on CT gray values and partially segmented patient data. In this study, the fields of application are lumbar puncture and spinal anesthesia. We focus on a new evaluation method driven by ray-casting to define paths from the skin to the spinal canal. In a comparison of our reference system AcusVR to a newer algorithm, force outputs are found to be similar in 99% of the tested paths.

1 Introduction

Surgical training systems let surgeons improve skills effectively without any risk. Among others, preoperative planning, anatomic education and training of surgical procedures are the focus of these systems. Technically, the real-time performance for volume visualization, tissue deformation and haptic feedback are of major interest. Regarding the necessary virtual patients, the manual preparation mainly comprises the tedious contouring of organs and structures in CT patient data.

In [1] needle insertion simulation is presented as a challenging field of research with many aspects ranging from mimicking stiffness, cutting and friction forces at the needle tip and shaft to needle bending in real-time.

Haptic feedback in virtual environments has been qualitatively evaluated by [2], the techniques presented there are of key importance for regional anesthesia simulation [3]. However, quantitative evaluation of the proposed algorithms still remains a gap to be filled.

Previously from our group, AcusVR [4, 5] has been published being a realistic and valuable tool for the simulation of needle punctures using a Sensable Phantom 6DOF (Fig. 1). Its major bottleneck is the complete expert segmentation of patient image data. Alternatively, we propose direct haptic volume rendering using partially segmented data [6]. Haptic transfer functions and the segmentation of only a few structures try to provide a mock-up of a complete segmentation, where voxel classification based on a heuristical transfer function set-up fills the gaps between the delineated structures.

H.-P. Meinzer et al. (Hrsg.), *Bildverarbeitung für die Medizin 2013*, Informatik aktuell,
DOI: 10.1007/978-3-642-36480-8_3, © Springer-Verlag Berlin Heidelberg 2013

Here, we focus on the thorough evaluation of the latter approach by automatically generating a large number of plausible puncture paths.

The paper is organized as follows: First, we describe the data used. Force calculation is briefly reviewed as presented in [6, 7]. Afterwards, we describe the ray-casting method used to evaluate force outputs. Evaluation is done quantitatively by comparing force output from the (modified) reference system AcusVR and the new (modified) approach.

2   Methods

One standard abdominal CT patient scan with isotropic voxel size 1.0 mm and 240 slices is used (Fig. 4(a)). The complete segmentation of the virtual patient including bone, ligaments, spinal canal, inter-vertebral disks, fat, muscle, skin and liver is available and used for haptic rendering [4, 5]. The AcusVR system [5] is our gold standard to which we compare force output. The system used here only needs a subset of the segmentations for force output.

In proxy based haptic rendering [6, 7], the device tip x_t is attached to a virtual spring with stiffness parameter k. On the other end the spring is held back by a proxy x_p that sticks to an organ surface. The force between tip and proxy is depended on their Euclidean distance and is given by Hookes law. The calculation for haptic feedback runs at 1000 Hz (Fig. 3).

2.1   Direct haptic volume rendering

In the method proposed by [6], transfer functions are used to obtain the haptic parameters, if missing a segmented structure at the needle tip. An axial slice

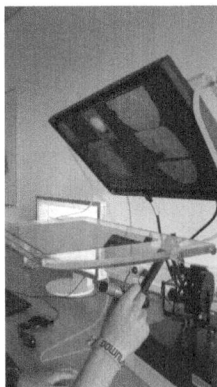
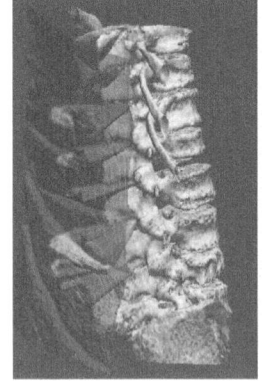
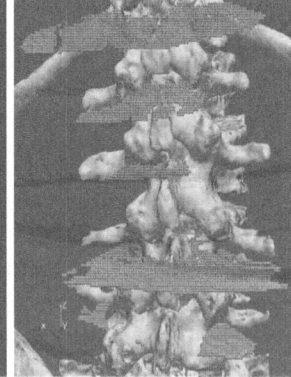

Fig. 1. The haptic device and workbench.

Fig. 2. Reference paths (green), skin (tan) and bone (white). In lumbar puncture only the lower groups of paths are relevant, while in spinal anesthesia the upper three groups are also interesting. Left: paths targeting the spinal canal. Right: path starting points on the skin.

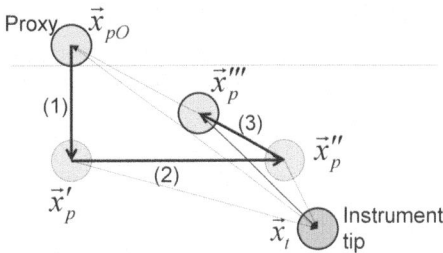

Fig. 3. Proxy-based haptic rendering recapitulated: (1) The proxy position x_p' for the surface penetrability along the normal vector of a virtual surface is determined. (2) The position x_p'' tangentially to the surface is calculated. (3) A viscosity term retracts the proxy to the position x_p'''.

(see axial slice in Fig. 4(b)) shows plausible tissue classifications between large volume structure such as skin (orange), fat (yellow), muscle (red) and bone (white). In these classes different haptic parameters are valid. However, the small volume and key structures spinal canal and inter-vertebral disk as well as the flavum ligaments fall falsely into the domain of the large volume structures. Consequently, manual segmentations are still provided for these structures.

2.2   Evaluation method framework

In our new evaluation framework we define a large number of plausible puncture paths automatically, which are used to steer the needle tip back and forth ("reference paths") assuming constant velocity (Fig. 2). Hence, absolutely reproducible force outputs are obtained for comparing different haptic force calculation algorithms. A high number of paths consisting of two points are automatically defined to reflect successful user experience.

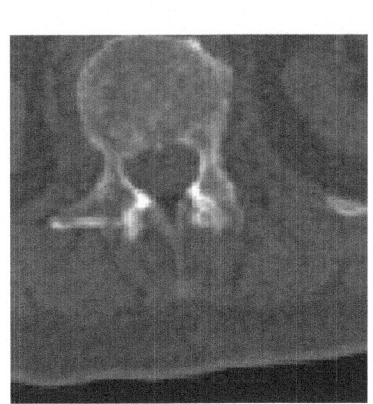
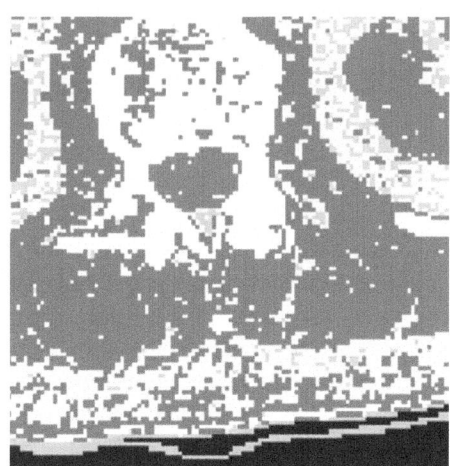

Fig. 4. An axial slice of the reference data: (a) original gray values, (b) visual transfer function applied with tissue classes air (black), skin (orange), muscle (red) and bone (white).

For this aim, ray-casting is used to determine the visibility of the spinal canal from the perspective of the source structure, i.e. the skin. The algorithm checks whether a direct line to the spinal canal can be drawn without touching impenetrable structures such as bone. In other words, we apply the ray-casting technique driven by the 3D-Bresenham algorithm [8]. The Bresenham algorithm features integer arithmetic operations to draw a line from source to target voxels. In our implementation, line-of-sight connections from each skin voxel line to each spinal canal voxel are drawn. For all rays starting from a skin voxel, the shortest path shorter than our needle length (75 mm) is selected as a "reference path". Taking into account not only one shortest path at a source voxel would exponentially increase the computational burden with little insight gain for the study. The ray-casting algorithm is implemented in CUDA-C and runs in parallel on NVIDIA graphics hardware.

In this study, we end up with 4038 automatically defined paths (Fig. 2) that reflect trainee experience with the system, i.e. starting from the skin they reach the spinal canal target within needle length and do not collide with bony structures. Force rendering of bone has been changed in the newer haptic algorithm due to a new force feedback device, thus comparison results would systematically be biased on bone touching paths. With our new Sensable 6DOF HighForce device much higher forces can be exerted as in the original AcusVR set-up (22 N vs. 7 N).

At every position of the reference path at the needle tip two force outputs are calculated:

1. by the algorithm used in AcusVR and
2. by the method using a partial segmentation and gray values based transfer functions.

As measures to compare the force output values we show the "mean of squared errors" (MSE) and "maximum absolute error" (MAE). For statistical assessment of the errors found the p-value from two-sided t-tests is used.

3   Results

In Tab. 1 the errors for the force ouputs along the paths are shown for the two error measures, MSE and MAE. Due to the large amount of errors, we show tail and head of sorted error lists. In the left resp. right half of the table the worst resp. best case paths of this study are given.

For MSE the worst case paths show small but significantly different force feedback from the reference system AcusVR (Fig. 4(a)). In these cases, closer investigation shows air gaps in the assumed complete segmentation, which the original AcusVR algorithm is sensitive to while the newer algorithm is not affected. These flaws can be easily corrected by filling the spurious gaps in the segmentation. The worst maximum absolute errors are not significant (Figs. 5, 4(b), 4(c)).

Significant errors concentrate in a certain area in the lower right part of the back of the patient. This was exactly the area from where paths collide with unexpected air cavities (Fig. 4(a)).

Table 1. Comparison of force output values calculated by AcusVR to new algorithm variant. Asterisks indicate significantly different force feedback ($p < 0.05$). Plus signs mark paths where air holes are present in the segmentation. MSE means "mean squared error", MAE denotes the "maximum absolute error".

Worst Paths			Best Paths		
Rank in Metric	MSE [N^2]	MAE [N]	Rank in Metric	MSE [N^2]	MAE [N]
4038	0.5403*+	4.4955	9	0.0044+	0.535
4037	0.5364*+	4.4932+	...	...	...
4036	0.5349*+	4.4926	6	0.0042	0.5262
4035	0.5239*+	4.4871	5	0.0041	0.5233
4034	0.5135*+	4.4846+	4	0.0041	0.5116
4033	0.5103*+	4.4785	3	0.0040	0.5116+
...	...*+	...	2	0.0036	0.5004
4021	0.4337	4.4495	1	0.0032	0.5+

Using CUDA for path calculations takes only 3 minutes of time instead of over 15 minutes in a CPU implementation.

On average we found MSE resp. MAE to be 0.053 ± 0.077 N^2 resp. 1.7817 ± 1.293 N. Statistically significant errors are present in only 0.6% of all paths.

4   Discussion

In [6] a new approach has been presented that considerably reduces the segmentation preparation workload from days to hours.

Evaluation there was only carried out on 12 manually selected paths. In this paper, an evaluation framework producing a large number (4038) of automatically generated, densely packed paths is used. This new tool even stronger underlines direct haptic rendering to be a valuable method. Important structures such as ligaments are clearly reproduced by the simulation and for unsegmented structures errors are small. As shown the high number of test paths helps to further prove the validity in comparison to the reference system AcusVR. Generally speaking, the ray-casting based quality check is a good concept for the

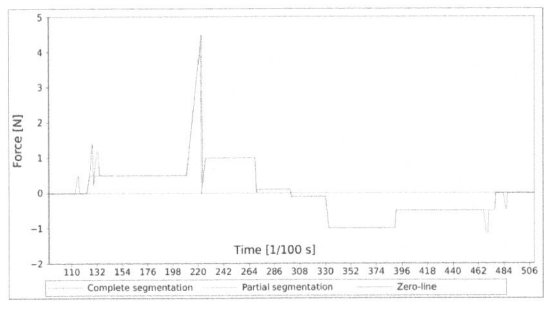

Fig. 5. Force curves for erroneous path with high maximum absolute error: AcusVR calculated force (blue) vs. newer algorithm (magenta): The force outputs for the paths are very similar despite of outlier errors near the skin and at the ligamentum peak.

Fig. 6. Color coded errors of reference paths: (a) MSE, note that the maximum errors hide on the very right in a fold of the skin marked with a red circle (b) MAE and (c) p-value.

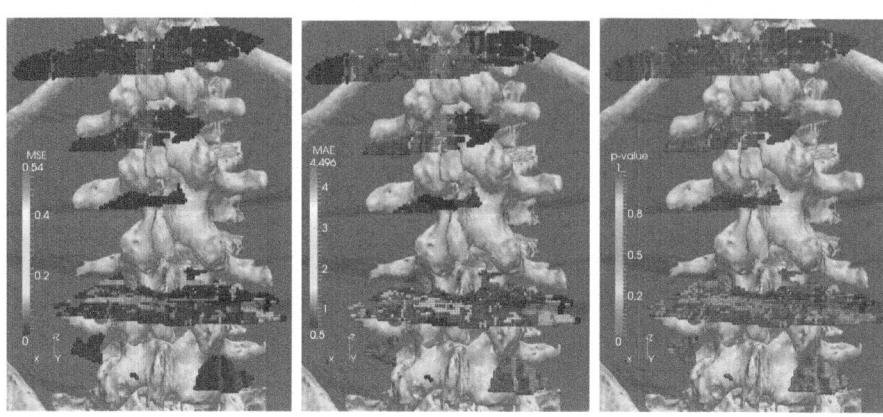

development of haptic algorithms in general. In future, we will use the proposed evaluation methodology to further improve the algorithms, check quality at other surgical sites and test for inter-patient applicability of the used heuristics.

Acknowledgement. This work is supported by the German Research Foundation (DFG, HA 2355/10-1).

References

1. Abolhassani N, Patel R, Moallem M. Needle insertion into soft tissue: a survey. Med Eng Phys. 2007;29(4):413–31.
2. Ullrich S, Kuhlen T. Haptic palpation for medical simulation in virtual environments. IEEE Trans Vis Comput Graph. 2012;18(4):617–25.
3. Ullrich S, Grottke O, Fried E, et al. An intersubject variable regional anesthesia simulator with a virtual patient architecture. Int J CARS. 2009;4(6):561–70.
4. Färber M, Hoeborn E, Dalek D, et al. Training and evaluation of lumbar punctures in a VR-environment using a 6DOF haptic device. Stud Health Technol Inform. 2008;132:112–4.
5. Färber M, Hummel F, Gerloff C, et al. Virtual reality simulator for the training of lumbar punctures. Methods Inf Med. 2009;48(5):493–501.
6. Mastmeyer A, Fortmeier D, Handels H. Direct haptic volume rendering in lumbar puncture simulation. IOS Press; 2012.
7. Lundin K, Ynnerman A, Gudmundsson B. Proxy-based haptic feedback from volumetric density data. Eurohaptics Conference. 2002; p. 104–9.
8. Bresenham JE. Algorithm for computer control of a digital plotter. IBM Syst J. 1965;4(1):25–30.

4D-Planung von Nadelpfaden für Punktionseingriffe mit der Ray-Casting-Methode

Tobias Hecht[1], Andre Mastmeyer[1], Dirk Fortmeier[1,2], Heinz Handels[1]

[1]Institut für Medizinische Informatik, Universität zu Lübeck
[2]Graduate School of Computing in Medicine and Life Sciences, Universität zu Lübeck
hecht@informatik.uni-luebeck.de

Kurzfassung. Die Nadelpunktion ist ein etabliertes Verfahren für die minimal-invasive Behandlung von Läsionen in der Leber. Nadelpunktionen werden präzise anhand von CT-Daten des Patienten geplant, um das Risiko einer Komplikation zu minimieren. Die vorliegende Arbeit hat die Planung von Nadelpfaden anhand von 4D-Bilddaten bei Punktionseingriffen unter Berücksichtigung der durch die Atmung hervorgerufenen Bewegungen zum Ziel. In allen Phasen des Atemzyklus berechnet ein Ray-Casting-Verfahren Verbindungspfade von der Haut zu der Läsion unter Berücksichtigung undurchdringlicher Strukturen. Ein Bewertungssystem bewertet jeden Pfad in allen Phasen. Schließlich wird der beste Pfad mit einem Zwei-Stufen-Min-Max-Schema gewählt. Die Planungsergebnisse werden anhand von 6 Patientendatensätzen getestet. Die einfache Planung anhand einer Phase wird mit der Planung unter Berücksichtigung der Atmung verglichen. In einer Studie konnte eine tendenzielle Verbesserung der Planung mit 4D-Bilddaten gegenüber der Planung mit 3D-Bilddaten erreicht werden.

1 Einleitung

Die Leber ist nach den Lymphknoten der zweithäufigste Ort für metastasierte Erkrankungen. In 80% der Fälle kommt ein chirurgischer Eingriff nicht in Frage und es muss auf alternative Methoden zugegriffen werden [1]. Eine dieser Methoden ist die Nadelpunktion. Nadelpunktionseingriffe müssen akkurat geplant werden, da die Genauigkeit sich positiv auf die Qualität der Ergebnisse dieser Eingriffe auswirkt [2].

Die Planung erfolgt anhand von 3D-Bilddaten des Patienten, so dass keine Atmung oder sonstige Bewegungen berücksichtigt werden. Jedoch wird die Behandlung von Lebertumoren, die sich oft dicht unter der Lunge befinden, durch die Atembewegung stark beeinflusst.

Baegert et al. [3] hat ein Konzept vorgestellt, bei dem die Berechnung eines optimalen Pfades in zwei Phasen aufgeteilt ist. In der ersten Phase werden die Pfade berechnet, die keine kritische Struktur beschädigen oder durch die Nadellänge gänzlich ausgeschlossen werden. In der zweiten Phase werden dann die übrigen Pfade mit Hilfe weiterer Kriterien bewertet.

H.-P. Meinzer et al. (Hrsg.), *Bildverarbeitung für die Medizin 2013*, Informatik aktuell,
DOI: 10.1007/978-3-642-36480-8_4, © Springer-Verlag Berlin Heidelberg 2013

Seitel et al. [4] und Engel et al. [5] haben dieses Konzept aufgegriffen und eine Implementierung vorgestellt, die einen optimalen Pfad nach dem Pareto-Prinzip auswählt. Ein Nadelpfad gilt als pareto-optimal, wenn er in keinem Kriterium verbessert werden kann, ohne in einem anderen Kriterium schlechter zu werden. In einer retrospektiven Evaluation wurden Testdaten verwendet, bei denen es im OP zu Komplikationen kam. In vier der zehn getesteten Datensätze hätte der von dem Arzt gewählte Pfad zu keiner Komplikation führen dürfen. Dennoch kam es in allen vier Fällen zum Pneumothorax. Als mögliche Ursache wurde die Bewegung durch die Atmung der Patienten genannt, welche in der statischen 3D-Planung nicht berücksichtigt wird [4]. Die berechneten Pfade beziehen sich nur auf eine einzige Atemphase.

Da die Leber sich unmittelbar unter der Lunge befindet, werden die Positionen von Lebertumoren von der Atmung beeinflusst. Die vorliegende Arbeit stellt eine Erweiterung der Planung von Nadelpfaden vor, welche einen optimalen Punktionspfad unter Berücksichtigung der Atmung des Patienten ermittelt. Hierbei wird mit Hilfe von segmentierten 4D-Daten eine Menge von Pfaden errechnet, welche in allen Atemphasen als mögliche Pfade in Frage kommen und anschließend unter Berücksichtigung aller Atemphasen bewertet werden.

2 Material und Methoden

In unserem Ansatz wurde das Konzept von Baegert et al. [3] verwendet. Es werden sogenannte Ausschlusskriterien (hard constraints) definiert. Jeder Pfad, der von mindestens einem dieser Ausschlusskriterien betroffen ist, wird aus der Menge der möglichen Pfade genommen und für die weiteren Berechnungen ignoriert. Alle übrigen Pfade werden mit Hilfe definierter Bewertungskriterien (soft constraints) bewertet (Seitel et al. [4]). In der vorliegenden Arbeit werden zwei Kriterien beispielhaft vorgestellt.

Das Verdeckungskriterium (Abb. 1(d)) schließt alle Pfade aus, die auf ihrem Weg von der Haut zum Tumor durch eine Risikostruktur blockiert werden. Der Tumor wird anschaulich von der Risikostruktur auf diesem Pfad verdeckt.

Der kritische Abstand (Abb. 1(e)) bewertet den Pfad P nach dem kleinsten Abstand zu einer Risikostruktur in Abhängigkeit vom Minimum $d_{r,min}$ und dem Maximum $d_{r,max}$ aller Pfade

$$w_1(P) = \frac{d_r(P) - d_{r,min}}{d_{r,max} - d_{r,min}} \qquad (1)$$

2.1 4D-Erweiterung der Planung

Die Berücksichtigung der Atmung wird durch die Verwendung eines 4D-Bilddatensatzes des Patienten ermöglicht. In jedem 3D-Bild, im folgenden Atemphase genannt, erfolgt die Nadelpfadplanung nach dem erwähnten Konzept mittels

Ausschluss- und Bewertungskriterien. Eine Atemphase wird als Referenzbild gewählt. Für jeden Pfad werden die korrespondierenden Pfade in allen Atemphasen, ggf. mittels Interpolation, ermittelt und mit dem Minimum der Bewertungen aller gefundenen korrespondierenden Pfade bewertet. Der optimale Pfad der 4D-Planung ist somit derjenige, der unter Berücksichtigung der Atmung des Patienten am besten bewertet ist. Er wird am Ende am Referenzbild visualisiert.

2.2 Evaluation

Ziel der 4D-Planung ist es, die Planung von Nadelpfaden durch Berücksichtigung der Atembewegung des Patienten zu verbessern.

Hierzu wird bei allen Patienten in jeder Atemphase der optimale Pfad ermittelt und in den Bilddaten der übrigen Atemphasen eingesetzt. Die Bewertungen aller Pfade in allen Atemphasen wird ermittelt und die durchschnittliche Bewertung und das Minimum der Bewertungen der Pfade mit der Bewertung des optimalen Pfades aus der 4D-Planung verglichen. Beim Vergleich des Minimums wird bei der Einzelphasenplanung das Maximum der Minima aller Pfade in allen Atemphasen gewählt. Für den statistischen Vergleich der durchschnittlichen Bewertungen wird der Holm-Sidak-Test verwendet und alle besten Pfade aus der Einzelphasenplanung mit dem besten Pfad aus der Mehrphasenplanung verglichen. Als Ausgangslage wurden alle Bewertungskriterien gleich gewichtet. Die Nadellänge wurde auf 150 mm festgelegt. Als Referenzbild wurde eine Phase mit mittlerem Atemvolumen gewählt.

Zusätzlich zur Bewertung der Pfade wurde noch überprüft, ob ein einzelner, in einer Atemphase ermittelter Pfad in den Bilddaten der übrigen Atemphasen den Tumor treffen würden. Eine Bewertung mit dem Wert 0 wird dabei als

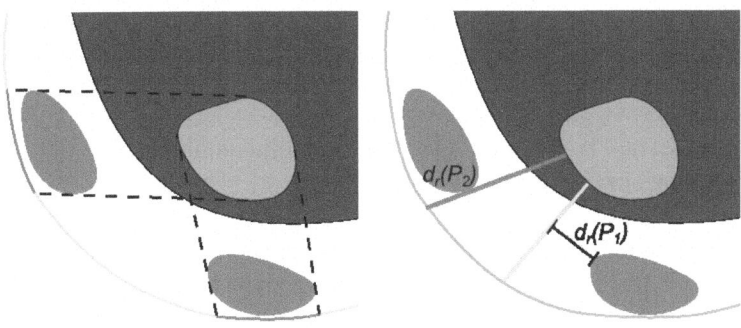

(d) Verdeckungskriterium   (e) Kritischer Abstand

Abb. 1. Schematische Darstellung ausgewählter Kriterien zur Bestimmung des optimalen Pfades. Der Tumor ist in rosa, die Leber in dunkelrot, die Risikostrukturen in grau und die Haut in orange dargestellt. In (d) wird die abgeschirmte Haut in rot dargestellt. In (e), wird ein guter Pfad (P_1) mit einem schlechten Pfad (P_2) verglichen.

„Ziel verfehlt" definiert. Zur Normierung wird die Anzahl der Tumorgewebetreffer durch die Anzahl der Atemphasen dividiert und im folgenden als Trefferquote bezeichnet.

Die verwendeten 4D-CT-Testdaten kommen von der Washington University School of Medicine in St. Louis, USA [6]. Für die Studie wurden sechs Patienten mit 9-14 Atemphasen ausgewählt. Für jeden Patienten wurden in einer Atemphase die Haut, die Knochen, die Lungen und der Körper segmentiert. In jeder dieser Segmentierungen wurde ein kleiner, kugelförmiger Tumor künstlich unmittelbar unter die Lunge gesetzt. Die Segmentierung wurde durch eine nicht-lineare Registrierung [7] auf die Bilddaten zu den übrigen Atemphasen transferiert, da diese zur Bestimmung und Bewertung der Pfade in diesen Atemphasen benötigt werden. Hierbei wird beginnend von einer Atemphase auf die benachbarten Atemphasen des Zyklus registriert und die segmentierte Atemphase deformiert (Abb. 2).

3 Ergebnisse

In Abb. 3 sind qualitative Ergebnisse von Patient 3 beispielhaft dargestellt. Es ist deutlich zu sehen, wie der rote Bereich (schlechte Pfade) im Ergebnis der Mehrphasenplanung 3(c) größer ist. Teile des roten Bereichs wären bei der Einzelphasenplanung nicht beachtet worden.

Tab. 1 stellt die quantitativen Ergebnisse in einer Tabelle dar und zeigt einen direkten Vergleich zwischen der Einzelphasenplanung und der Mehrphasenplanung. In allen Fällen ist das Minimum der optimalen Pfade der Einzelphasenplanung höchstens so groß, wie das Minimum des optimalen Pfades der Mehrphasenplanung. Für das Maximum gilt dies für vier Fälle. In fünf Fällen ist das Minimum des optimalen Pfades der Mehrphasenplanung sogar größer. Der Pfad der Mehrphasenplanung ist tendenziell besser, als die durchschnittliche Bewertung der Pfade der Einzelphasenplanung. In vier Fällen ist die Trefferquote der Mehrphasenplanung genauso hoch, wie die Trefferquote der Einzelphasenplanung. Bei zwei Fällen ist die Trefferquote der Mehrphasenplanung höher. In vier Fällen ist die Trefferquote der Mehrphasenplanung 100%. Bei der Einzelphasenplanung sind es drei Fälle.

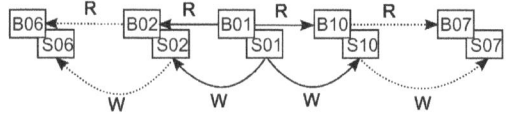

Abb. 2. Beginnend von Atemphase 1 wird in beide Richtungen des Atemzyklus von Atemphase zu Atemphase eine nicht-lineare Registrierung (R) auf die Bilddaten (B) vorgenommen und die Segmentierungen (S) verformt (W). Der Vorgang endet, sobald die mittlere Atemphase erreicht ist.

Tabelle 1. Diese Tabelle stellt den Mittelwert (MW) aller Bewertungen der Einzelphasenplanung (EP), des schlechtesten Pfades der EP (EP_{min}), des besten Pfades der EP (EP_{max}) und der Mehrphasenplanung (MP) jedes Patienten dar. Ein einseitiger Holm-Sidak-Test (HS) prüft den Anteil der Pfade der EP, die sich signifikant dem Pfad der MP unterscheiden. Außerdem werden die Minima (Min) und die Trefferquoten (TQ) der EP und der MP jedes Patienten verglichen.

	Pat. 1	Pat. 2	Pat. 3	Pat. 4	Pat. 5	Pat. 6
MW:						
EP_{min}	$0,82 \pm 0,12$	$0,82 \pm 0,08$	$0,57 \pm 0,26$	$0,79 \pm 0,08$	$0,63 \pm 0,29$	$0,78 \pm 0,06$
EP_{max}	$0,90 \pm 0,03$	$0,86 \pm 0,01$	$0,75 \pm 0,02$	$0,86 \pm 0,04$	$0,82 \pm 0,07$	$0,90 \pm 0,03$
EP	$0,86 \pm 0,07$	$0,85 \pm 0,04$	$0,72 \pm 0,09$	$0,83 \pm 0,06$	$0,79 \pm 0,11$	$0,84 \pm 0,08$
MP	$0,90 \pm 0,01$	$0,86 \pm 0,01$	$0,76 \pm 0,02$	$0,84 \pm 0,02$	$0,82 \pm 0,02$	$0,89 \pm 0,01$
HS:						
Anteil	0,00%	0,00%	0.07%	0.00%	0.07%	0.35%
Min:						
EP	0,83	0,84	0,72	0,74	0,71	0,83
MP	0,89	0,84	0,74	0,82	0,79	0,87
TQ:						
EP	100,00%	100,00%	100,00%	92,58%	69,23%	85,71%
MP	100,00%	100,00%	100,00%	92,58%	84,61%	100,00%

4 Diskussion

Die Planung unter Berücksichtigung der Atmung ist tendenziell besser, als die Planung anhand einer einzigen Atemphase. Die Trefferquote hat sich im Schnitt ebenfalls verbessert. Die Tumoren wurden künstlich an eine Position nahe der Lunge gesetzt, um eine relativ starke Bewegung der Tumoren durch Atembewegungen zu erzeugen. Durch die Bewegung des Tumors werden mehr Pfade

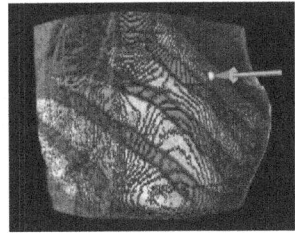
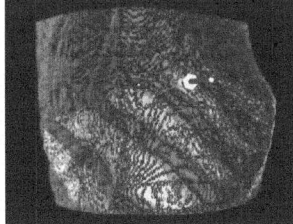
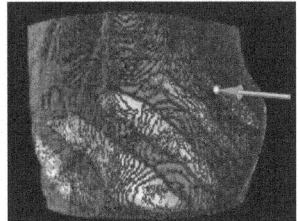

(a) Max. Ausatmung   (b) Max. Einatmung   (c) MP Ergebnis

Abb. 3. Beispielhafte Darstellung des Ergebnisses von Pat. 3. Es werden die Phasen der maximalen Ein- und der Ausatmung gezeigt und das Ergebnis der Mehrphasenplanung. In den grünen Bereichen liegen die Pfade mit einer guten und in den roten Bereichen die Pfade mit einer schlechten Bewertung. Ein Pfeil visualisiert den besten Pfad.

von Risikostrukturen verdeckt, als bei der Planung anhand einer einzigen Atemphase. Die Mehrphasenplanung ergibt im jeweils schlechtesten Fall eine bessere Bewertung als die Einzelphasenplanung. Auch diese Beobachtung unterstützt die Verbesserung der Planung unter Berücksichtigung der Atmung. Damit zeigen sich insgesamt viele Hinweise für die Verbesserung der Planung von Nadelpfaden unter Berücksichtigung der Atembewegung des Patienten. Dieses Verfahren lässt sich auch auf andere Organe anwenden. Für weitere Evaluationen sollten reale Fälle mit nicht kugelförmigen Tumoren und detailliertere Segmentierungen, u.a. von Gefäßen, verwendet werden. Es empfiehlt sich andere Gewichtungen für die Bewertungskriterien zu testen.

Literaturverzeichnis

1. Pereira PL. Actual role of radiofrequency ablation of liver metastases. Eur Radiol. 2007;17(8):2062–70.
2. Nath S, Chen Z, Yue N, et al. Dosimetric effects of needle divergence in prostate seed implant using 125l and 103Pd radioactive seeds. Med Phys. 2000;27(5):1058–66.
3. Baegert C, Villard C, Schreck P, et al. Multi-criteria trajectory planning for hepatic radiofrequency ablation. Proc MICCAI. 2007; p. 676–84.
4. Seitel A, Engel M, Sommer CM, et al. Computer-assisted trajectory planning for percutaneous needle insertions. Med Phys. 2011;38(6):3246–59.
5. Engel M, Seitel A, Fangerau M, et al. Schnelle Zugangsplanung für die perkutane Punktion der Leber. Proc BVM. 2010; p. 216–20.
6. Ehrhardt J, Werner R, Säring D, et al. An optical based method for improved reconstruction of 4D CT data sets acquired during free breathing. Med Phys. 2007;34(2):711–21.
7. Schmidt-Richberg A, Ehrhardt J, Werner R, et al. Diffeomorphic diffusion registration of lung CT images. Proc MICCAI. 2010; p. 55–62.

Navigierte ultraschallgeführte Leberpunktion mit integriertem EM Feldgenerator

Keno März[1], Alfred Michael Franz[1], Bram Stieltjes[2], Alexandra Zahn[3], Alexander Seitel[1], Justin Iszatt[1], Boris Radeleff[4], Hans-Peter Meinzer[1], Lena Maier-Hein[1]

[1]Juniorgruppe Computer-Assistierte Interventionen
Abteilung Medizinische und Biologische Informatik, DKFZ Heidelberg.
[2]Quantitative Bild-basierte Krankheitscharakterisierung, DKFZ Heidelberg
[3]Gastroenterologie, Innere Medizin, Medizinische Klinik Heidelberg
[4]Diagnostische und Interventionelle Radiologie, Radiologische Klinik Heidelberg
k.maerz@dkfz-heidelberg.de

Kurzfassung. Leberpunktionen sind ein elementares Werkzeug zur Diagnosesicherung von Raumforderungen. Zentrale Erfolgsfaktoren sind neben dem Treffen der Zielregion die Vermeidung von Risikostrukturen sowie eine geringe Eingriffsdauer. Es wurden bereits Navigationslösungen für Ultraschall vorgeschlagen, welche aber aufgrund ihrer Komplexität keine weite Verbreitung in der klinischen Praxis fanden. Wir stellen das erste Verfahren vor, welches eine Ultraschallsonde und einen neuen kompakten elektromagnetischen Feldgenerator zu einer einzigen mobilen Modalität verbindet, mit welcher Patientenanatomie und Instrumente relativ zueinander erfasst werden können. In einer Phantomstudie zeigen wir, dass sich das neue Konzept für eine akkurate Nadelinsertion ohne Verletzung von Risikostrukturen eignet.

1 Einleitung

Leberpunktionen werden bisher vor allem unter Ultraschall (US)- oder Computertomographie (CT)-Führung vorgenommen. US hat in diesem Kontext gegenüber der CT einige Vorteile: Die Untersuchung ist günstig, schnell durchführbar, in Echtzeit und frei von Strahlenbelastung [1]. Die Bildqualität leidet jedoch bei erschwerenden Umständen beträchtlich. Zum Beispiel verringert Adipositas des Patienten den Bildkontrast in der Zielregion stark und beeinträchtigt die sichere Identifikation des Tumors, während Leberverhärtungen (z.B. bei Leberzirrhose) die Sichtbarkeit der Punktionsnadel im Gewebe verschlechtern. Konventionelle Eingriffe werden zudem meist innerhalb der Schallebene (engl: *in-plane*) durchgeführt: Eine spezielle Nadelführung wird an der Ultraschallsonde befestigt und führt die Nadel genau entlang der Bildebene. Dies ist zwar problematisch, da die Beweglichkeit der Sonde während des Eingriffes eingeschränkt wird, aber nötig, weil die dünne Nadel im Bild sonst nur schwer zu erkennen ist bzw. der Nadelweg nur schlecht vorhergesagt werden kann. Liegen Risikostrukturen nahe der Zielregion, wird der Eingriff weiter verkompliziert. Ist eine US-Punktion

H.-P. Meinzer et al. (Hrsg.), *Bildverarbeitung für die Medizin 2013*, Informatik aktuell,
DOI: 10.1007/978-3-642-36480-8_5, © Springer-Verlag Berlin Heidelberg 2013

schließlich zu riskant, wird die Punktion unter CT-Führung durchgeführt. Dies bedeutet neben einem höheren Kosten- und Zeitaufwand auch eine hohe Strahlenbelastung durch mehrfach durchgeführte CT-Scans.

Deshalb wurden von verschiedener Seite Navigationslösungen vorgestellt, jedoch haben diese nicht den Weg in den klinischen Alltag gefunden. Bisherige Ansätze erlauben u.a. die Registrierung mit CT-Aufnahmen [2], Volumensegmentierung [3], 3D-Rekonstruktion [4] und Ablationsvisualisierung [5], benötigen aber auch eine Vorverarbeitung der Daten oder Integration weiterer Modalitäten. Dies verkompliziert jedoch den eigentlich einfachen Ansatz der US-geführten Punktion und erschwert somit die Integration in den klinischen Workflow.

Ein elementarer Teil aller Navigationslösungen ist die Lokalisation (Tracking) von Patient und Instrument. Elektromagnetische (EM) Trackingsysteme bieten hierbei den Vorteil, dass sie keine Sichtverbindung zum getrackten Objekt benötigen. Sie sind aber anfällig gegenüber Störungen durch Metallobjekte in der Nähe des Trackvolumens, was die Positionierung des Generators schwierig macht. Mit einem neuen, kompakten elektromagnetischen Feldgenerator (FG) werden diese Probleme vermeidbar, gleichzeitig haben Messungen die hohe Genauigkeit des FG bestätigt [6, 7]. Eine Kombination von FG und US Sonde liegt angesichts der kompakten Bauart des FG auf der Hand [7]. Dies bedeutet u.a. eine hohe Präzision und Genauigkeit des Trackings, da sich die interessante Region automatisch im Zentrum des Feldes befindet. Durch das kleine Trackingvolumen wird der Abstand zu Metall im Arbeitsbereich größer und damit das Trackingsystem unanfälliger gegenüber Störungen. In dieser Arbeit binden wir die kombinierte Modalität aus US-Sonde und FG erstmals in ein Navigationsystem für Nadelpunktionen ein und testen es im Phantom.

2 Material und Methoden

Als Feldgenerator verwenden wir einen neuen, kompakten und mobilen Prototypen (NDI Aurora® *Compact FG 7-10*). Dieser FG wurde mit der US-Sonde zu einer kombinierten Modalität verbunden. Kürzlich vorgestellte Studien zeigen eine hohe Präzision und Genauigkeit des Systems [6], wobei die US-Sonden das Tracking nur vernachlässigbar stören [7]. Zur Kalibrierung von Sonde zu FG wurde eine einfache punktbasierte Registrierung mit getrackten Nadeln durchgeführt, welche keine zusätzliche Hardware benötigt und von einer Person in Kürze durchgeführt werden kann. Der schematische Aufbau ist in Abb. 1 (links) dargestellt. Ein Hautmarker, welcher zur Lokalisation des Patienten dient, wird läsionsnah auf der Haut befestigt.

2.1 Markierung der Risikostrukturen (Zoning)

Zunächst untersucht der Arzt die Umgebung der Zielstruktur mit dem Ultraschallgerät. Findet er eine Risikostruktur, markiert er diese auf der Bildebene. Eine Kugel um die Struktur erscheint und markiert diesen Bereich als Risikozone. Obwohl andere Formen optional zugelassen werden können, beschränken wir uns für diese Evaluation nach dem Prinzip der Effizienz bewusst auf Kugeln, da sie vom Benutzer leicht zu handhaben sind und andersartige Strukturen (z.B. die Pfortader) schnell durch Setzen mehrerer Zonen angenähert werden können. Die Positionen der Zonen werden während des Eingriffs kontinuierlich relativ zum Hautmarker berechnet. So ist die Einschätzung der räumlichen Lage der Zonen zum Ultraschallbild jederzeit möglich. Wenn der Arzt mit dem Ergebnis des Zoning zufrieden ist, setzt er die Nadel an und startet die Navigation.

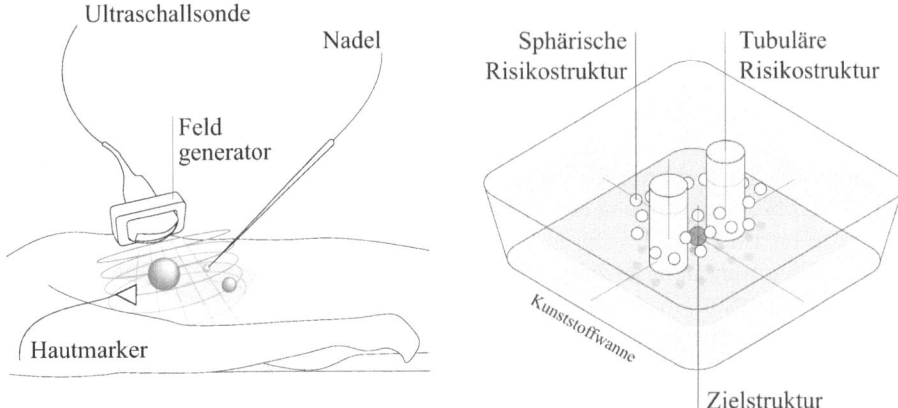

Abb. 1. Schematischer Aufbau des Navigationssystems (links) and Schema der verwendeten Phantome (rechts). Die Zielstruktur liegt zwischen tubulären Risikostrukturen.

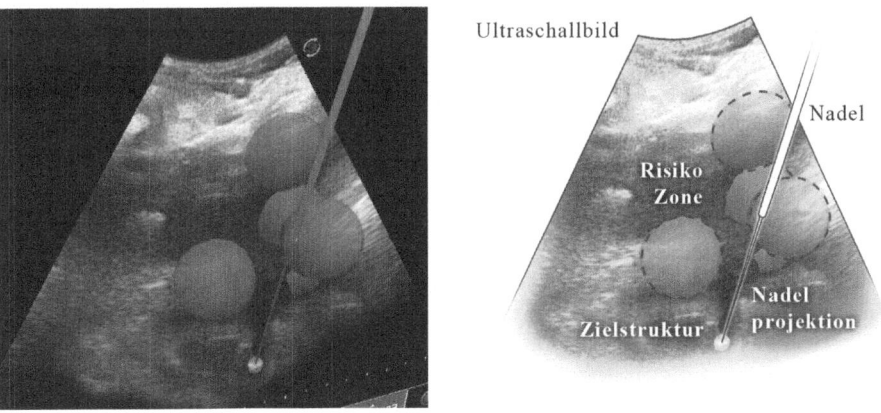

Abb. 2. Ausschnitt aus der Nadelnavigation am Phantom mit Risikostrukturen. Screenshot (links) und Diagramm mit Erläuterungen (rechts).

2.2 Navigation

Das System führt den Arzt mit einer Navigationsvisualisierung zum Ziel. Diese projiziert den Pfad der Nadel auf die Bildebene (Abb. 2). Zusätzlich wird eine 3D-Szene angezeigt, in welcher das Ultraschallbild, die Nadel und weitere Strukturen außerhalb der Bildebene zu sehen sind (Abb. 1). Insgesamt ist so eine genaue Einschätzung des Nadelpfades möglich.

2.3 Evaluation

Zur Umsetzung der Evaluationssoftware wurde das Medical Imaging Interaction Toolkit (MITK, *www.mitk.org*) [8] verwendet. Zur Kalibrierung wurde eine getrackte Nadel anhand eines vorgegebenen Musters 13 mal in die Bildebene eingeführt und die Nadelspitze manuell markiert. Das Muster deckt die Ultraschallebene möglichst komplett ab. Die Software führt eine punktbasierte Registrierung durch und gibt den Fiducial Registration Error (FRE) aus. Um die Genauigkeit der Kalibrierung zu überprüfen, wurde ein Target Registration Error (TRE) bestimmt, indem der Fehler der Punktkoordinaten zu neun bekannten Punkten im Phantom bestimmt wurde. Die Genauigkeit des Verfahrens wurde vor der Phantomstudie in zehn Durchgängen quantifiziert.

Zur Evaluation unseres Ansatzes wurden neun baugleiche Gelphantome aus ballistischer Gelatine angefertigt, welche jeweils eine Hochrisikosituation darstellen. Die Zielstruktur war nur schwierig ohne Verletzung der Risikostrukturen erreichbar (Abb. 1b). 14 Punktionen wurden durch einen Arzt mit US-Erfahrung, 14 weitere durch einen Techniker durchgeführt, wobei die ersten beiden Punktionen als nicht gewerteter Testlauf fungierten.

Die gemessenen Parameter waren: Dauer des Punktionsvorgangs (Eingriffsdauer), wie oft die Nadel ganz oder teilweise zurückgezogen wurde (Rückführbewegungen), Anteil der getroffenen Zielstrukturen (Trefferrate), Abstand der Nadelspitze zum Mittelpunkt der Zielstruktur (Genauigkeit), minimaler Abstand zu jeder Risikozone während des Eingriffs (Sicherheitsabstand) und die Zahl der verletzten Risikostrukturen. Die letzten drei Parameter wurden durch ein Kontroll-CT, das jeweils nach der Punktion eines Phantoms angefertigt wurde, ermittelt.

3   Ergebnisse

Unsere Kalibrierungsmethodik erreichte einen TRE von $1,3\pm0,3$ mm(n=10). Für die Gelphantomversuche wurden nur Kalibrierungen zugelassen, welche einen TRE kleiner oder gleich dem Mittelwert aufwiesen.

Tab. 1 zeigt die Ergebnisse der Phantomversuche. Es wurden zwei Risikostrukturen verletzt, welche in beiden Fällen nicht markiert wurden. Arzt und Techniker erreichten Punktionsgenauigkeiten von $2,8$ mm respektive $3,4$ mm und verfehlten beide jeweils einmal die Zielstruktur, was einer Trefferquote von 92% entspricht. Der punktierende Arzt gab an, dass die verfehlte Punktion auf einem eigenen Korrekturversuch beruhte. Die Software zeigte in diesem Fall an, dass die Zielstruktur verfehlt wurde.

Tabelle 1. Ergebnisse der Punktionsversuche.

	Arzt	Techniker	Gesamt
n	12	12	24
Trefferrate	92%	92%	92%
Genauigkeit	$2,8 \pm 1,1$ mm	$3,4 \pm 1,23$ mm	$3,1 \pm 1,2$ mm
Verletzungen	2	0	2
Sicherheitsabstand	$4,6 \pm 3,3$ mm	$9,0 \pm 4,5$ mm	$4,6 \pm 3,9$ mm
Rückführbewegungen	$0,8 \pm 0,6$	$0,9 \pm 0,8$	$0,9 \pm 0,7$
Dauer	82 ± 39 s	42 ± 21 s	62 ± 30 s

4 Diskussion

Die Integration bisheriger Ansätze für Ultraschallnavigation in den klinischen Alltag scheitert häufig an der Komplexität der Navigation, welche den Workflow des Arztes behindert. Unserer Kenntnis nach ist dies der erste Ansatz zur Integration eines mobilen Feldgenerators in ein Navigationssystem und die Ergebnisse sind vielversprechend. Gerade bei ultraschallbasierten Eingriffen, für welche die Geschwindigkeit und Einfachheit der Bildgebung auch den Grund für ihre weite Verbreitung darstellt, ist diese Entwicklung wünschenswert. Unser Ansatz ermöglicht es dem Arzt, seinen Workflow weitestgehend beizubehalten und stützt ihn je nach Komplexität der Punktion. Schwer sicht- oder erreichbare Läsionen können durch Markierung der Risikostrukturen sicherer punktiert werden. Das im Vergleich zu üblichen Feldgeneratoren kleine Feld deckt das Eingriffsvolumen ab und wird dabei dank des Abstands zu metallischen oder ferromagnetischen Gegenständen, wie der Patientenliege nicht anfällig für Störungen.

In der Literatur wurden verschiedene Kalibrierungsverfahren für US-Sonden mit Trackingsystemen vorgestellt. Neben einfachen punktbasierten Ansätzen sind vor allem Cross-Wire und N-Wire Phantome erwähnenswert [9]. Der von uns gewählte Ansatz ist zwar einfach, erreichte aber dennoch einen vielversprechenden TRE von $1,31$ mm. Das wir in unserem Fall auch mit einem punktbasieren Ansatz gute Ergebnisse erreichten, erklären wir uns durch die rigide Verbindung von Feldgenerator und Ultraschallsonde, die den Trackingfehler minimiert. Ob die Kalibrierung durch Einsatz anderer Verfahren weiter verbessert werden kann, muss in künftigen Studien untersucht werden.

Die Punktionsergebnisse zeigen, dass Risikostrukturen sicher umgangen werden können, wenn der Arzt sie markiert. Beide der verletzten Strukturen wurden getroffen, weil sie nicht markiert wurden. Die Trefferquote ist mit jeweils einem Fehlversuch bei Arzt und Techniker als gut zu bewerten. In einem Fall hat das System den Fehler korrekt vorhergesagt. Während der Versuche stellte sich heraus, dass sich 21G-Nadeln in ballistischer Gelatine stark verbiegen, was Korrekturen der Nadeltrajektorie nötig machte. Sowohl Arzt als auch Techniker zogen die Nadel im Schnitt weniger als ein mal pro Versuch zurück, wobei diese Zahl aufgrund der sehr dünnen Nadeln nur bedingt aussagekräftig ist. Mit dickeren Nadeln könnte sie u.U. weiter verringert werden. Zukünftige Arbeiten am System umfassen z.b. semiautomatische Segmentierungsverfahren, welche das Zoning erleichtern könnten, sowie Bewegungskompensationsmechanismen [10] und Pfadplanungsanwendungen für schwierige Situationen. Da schon ein Hautmarker an der Hautoberfläche angebracht ist, könnte es möglich sein, die Atembewegung zu quantifizieren und so strukturelle Verschiebungen im Zielorgan auszugleichen. Ultraschallgeführte Punktionen werden im Allgemeinen unter Atemstillststand („Luft anhalten") durchgeführt, dennoch sollte das System nach dieser Studie auch in realistischeren Szenarien mit Einbeziehung der Atembewegung getestet werden.

Abschließend können wir anhand der Ergebnisse sagen, dass die Methode einen vielversprechenden Ansatz darstellt. Die Verwendung des mobilen FGs in Verbindung mit der Ultraschallsonde löst eine Reihe von Problemen wie die der Positionierung und Störanfälligkeit elegant, ohne den Arzt zusätzlich zu belasten.

Danksagung. Dieses Projekt wurde im Rahmen des DFG-geförderten Graduiertenkollegs 1126: Intelligente Chirurgie durchgeführt. Die Autoren bedanken sich des Weiteren bei Sigmar Fröhlich, Gina Jackson, Stefan Kirsch und Nina Stecker (NDI Europe GmbH) für die Bereitstellung des Compact FG sowie weiterer Versuchs-Materialien wie Sensoren und Punktionsnadeln.

Literaturverzeichnis

1. Khati NJ, Gorodenker J, Hill M. Ultrasound-guided biopsies of the abdomen. Ultrasound Q. 2011;27(4):255–68.
2. Clevert DA, Paprottka PM, Helck A, et al. Image fusion in the management of thermal tumor ablation of the liver. Clin Hemorheol Microcirc. 2012;52(2):205–16.
3. Noble JA, Boukerroui D. Ultrasound image segmentation: a survey. IEEE Trans Med Imaging. 2006;25(8):987–1010.
4. Solberg OV, Lindseth F, Torp H, et al. Freehand 3D ultrasound reconstruction algorithms: a review. Ultrasound Med Biol. 2007;33(7):991–1009.
5. Sindram D, Swan RZ, Lau KN, et al. Real-time three-dimensional guided ultrasound targeting system for microwave ablation of liver tumours: a human pilot study. HPB. 2011;13(3):185–91.
6. Maier-Hein L, Franz AM, Birkfellner W, et al. Standardized assessment of new electromagnetic field generators in an interventional radiology setting. Med Phys. 2012;39(6):3424–34.
7. Franz AM, März K, Hummel J, et al. Electromagnetic tracking for US-guided interventions: standardized assessment of a new compact field generator. J Comput Ass Radiol Surg. 2012;7(6):813–8.
8. Wolf I, Vetter M, Wegner I, et al. The medical imaging interaction toolkit. Med Image Anal. 2005;9(6):594–604.
9. Mercier L, Lango T, Lindseth F, et al. A review of calibration techniques for freehand 3-D ultrasound systems. Ultrasound Med Biol. 2005;31(4):449–71.
10. McClelland JR, Hawkes DJ, Schaeffter T, et al. Respiratory motion models: a review. Med Image Anal. 2013;17(1):19–42.

GPU-Accelerated Time-of-Flight Super-Resolution for Image-Guided Surgery

Jens Wetzl[1,*], Oliver Taubmann[1,*], Sven Haase[1], Thomas Köhler[1,2],
Martin Kraus[1,2], Joachim Hornegger[1,2]

[1]Pattern Recognition Lab, FAU Erlangen-Nuremberg
[2]Erlangen Graduate School in Advanced Optical Technologies (SAOT)
*These authors contributed equally to this work
jens.wetzl@fau.de

Abstract. In the field of image-guided surgery, Time-of-Flight (ToF) sensors are of interest due to their fast acquisition of 3-D surfaces. However, the poor signal-to-noise ratio and low spatial resolution of today's ToF sensors require preprocessing of the acquired range data. Super-resolution is a technique for image restoration and resolution enhancement by utilizing information from successive raw frames of an image sequence. We propose a super-resolution framework using the graphics processing unit. Our framework enables interactive frame rates, computing an upsampled image from 10 noisy frames of 200×200 px with an upsampling factor of 2 in 109 ms. The root-mean-square error of the super-resolved surface with respect to ground truth data is improved by more than 20% relative to a single raw frame.

1 Introduction

Image-guided surgery provides physicians with helpful information and thus speeds up and improves medical interventions. One pertinent example is enhanced surface representations for augmented reality applications [1]. Time-of-Flight (ToF) sensors hold great potential for acquiring 3-D surfaces during an intervention due to their fast and dense acquisition technique. However, these sensors still suffer from low spatial resolution compared to state-of-the-art color sensors. Furthermore, high temporal and spatial noise in the range data is a major issue. To compensate for this, various preprocessing and calibration techniques have been proposed [2, 3]. Besides these approaches, super-resolution techniques present a promising alternative with the capability to improve noisy range data while increasing their spatial resolution. The goal of multi-frame super-resolution is to fuse several low-resolution (LR) frames into one high-resolution (HR) image while preserving edges and suppressing noise [4]. Each LR frame shows the scene from a slightly different viewpoint. The motion between successive frames is utilized to obtain a finer sampling compared to a single image.

As shown by Schuon et al. [5], the quality of range images can be improved significantly by super-resolution. However, their approach uses a simplified imaging

H.-P. Meinzer et al. (Hrsg.), *Bildverarbeitung für die Medizin 2013*, Informatik aktuell,
DOI: 10.1007/978-3-642-36480-8_6, © Springer-Verlag Berlin Heidelberg 2013

model where the point spread function (PSF) to model sampling of a camera is not taken into account and only translational motion between successive frames is assumed. The application of this method to image-guided surgery at interactive frame rates is infeasible due to prohibitive computational effort. General purpose super-resolution in real time has been demonstrated in [6], proposing an interpolation-based scheme with no appropriate physical model for image generation and a restriction to translational motion.

In this paper, we present a framework capable of recovering HR images from a series of preregistered LR images at interactive frame rates for intraoperative image restoration. Our method is based on a generative image model and formulated as a nonlinear optimization problem. The imaging model used for super-resolution covers affine motion and a Gaussian PSF. All steps of the algorithm are accelerated using the graphics processing unit (GPU) with Nvidia's CUDA platform to enable image-guided surgery at interactive frame rates.

2   Materials and methods

The super-resolution framework presented in this paper is based on a maximum a posteriori (MAP) estimate of the desired HR image. We use a limited-memory Broyden-Fletcher-Goldfarb-Shanno (L-BFGS) optimizer for minimization of the MAP cost function (Fig. 1).

2.1   Maximum a posteriori super-resolution

Our method is based on a forward model that describes the generation of LR frames from the ideal HR image that should be recovered. Let $x \in \mathbb{R}^N$ be an HR image where the pixels are arranged in linear order. The kth LR frame $y^{(k)} \in \mathbb{R}^M$, $M < N$, out of a sequence of K frames $y^{(1)}, \ldots, y^{(K)}$ is related to x according to

$$y^{(k)} = W^{(k)}x + \varepsilon^{(k)} \tag{1}$$

where $W^{(k)}$ denotes the system matrix which models warping, blur and decimation of the HR image and $\varepsilon^{(k)}$ is zero-mean Gaussian noise corrupting the kth LR

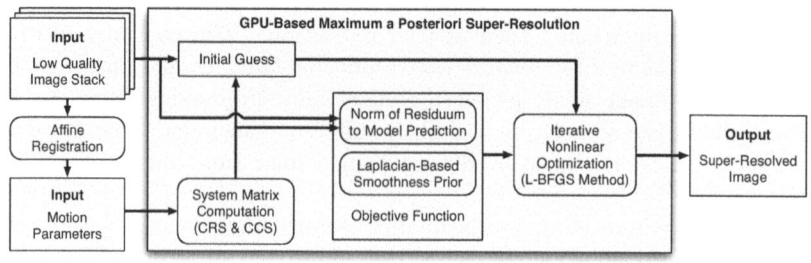

Fig. 1. System overview of our super-resolution framework.

image. Each LR frame $\boldsymbol{y}^{(k)}$ for $k \geq 2$ is related to $\boldsymbol{y}^{(1)}$ by an affine homography $\boldsymbol{H}^{(k)} \in \mathbb{R}^{3 \times 3}$ such that $\boldsymbol{u}' = \boldsymbol{H}^{(k)}\boldsymbol{u}$, where $\boldsymbol{u}$ and $\boldsymbol{u}'$ are homogeneous pixel coordinates in $\boldsymbol{y}^{(k)}$ and $\boldsymbol{y}^{(1)}$ respectively. Modeling blur caused by the camera with a Gaussian PSF, the elements of the system matrix are given by

$$W_{\mathrm{mn}} = \exp\left(-\frac{(\boldsymbol{v}_{\mathrm{n}} - \boldsymbol{u}'_{\mathrm{m}})^T \, \nabla \boldsymbol{H} (\nabla \boldsymbol{H})^T \, (\boldsymbol{v}_{\mathrm{n}} - \boldsymbol{u}'_{\mathrm{m}})}{2\sigma^2}\right) \tag{2}$$

where σ specifies the width of the PSF, $\nabla \boldsymbol{H}$ denotes the Jacobian of the affine transform $\boldsymbol{H}\boldsymbol{u}$ with respect to $\boldsymbol{u} = (u_1, u_2, 1)$, $\boldsymbol{v}_n$ is the position of the nth HR pixel and $\boldsymbol{u}'_{\mathrm{m}}$ is the position of the mth LR pixel transformed into the HR coordinate system [4]. The rows of the system matrix are normalized to unity.

The super-resolved image $\boldsymbol{x}^*$ is the minimum of the objective function

$$\boldsymbol{x}^* = \mathrm{argmin}_{\mathrm{x}} \left(\|\boldsymbol{W}\boldsymbol{x} - \boldsymbol{y}\|_2^2 + \lambda \cdot \|\boldsymbol{h}_\delta\left(\boldsymbol{D}\boldsymbol{x}\right)\|_1\right) \tag{3}$$

where $\boldsymbol{y}$ and $\boldsymbol{W}$ are the stacked LR images and system matrices respectively. For regularization, we use the pseudo-Huber loss function $\boldsymbol{h}_\delta(\cdot)$ applied element-wise as $h_\delta(a) = \delta^2(\sqrt{1 + (a/\delta)^2} - 1)$ on the Laplacian $\boldsymbol{D}\boldsymbol{x}$ of the HR image $\boldsymbol{x}$, with λ controlling the strength of the prior. This imposes smoothness on the super-resolved image and prevents our estimation from converging to undesirable solutions where noise is amplified. The minimum of the objective function is a MAP estimate for the desired HR image [4]. Minimization is performed by the Quasi-Newton optimizer described in section 2.2.

We note that all system matrix elements can be computed independently according to (2). For better load-balancing, one GPU thread per matrix row is used. To reduce the memory footprint, W_{mn} is set to zero beyond 3 standard deviations of the point spread function, enabling us to store $\boldsymbol{W}$ efficiently in a sparse matrix format. Furthermore, the Laplacian filtered image and the pseudo-Huber prior are calculated pixel-wise in parallel.

2.2 L-BFGS optimizer

As the gradient of the objective function given in (3) is nonlinear in the pixels of the HR image, we use an iterative L-BFGS optimizer [7] for nonlinear minimization. This algorithm is one of the most popular members of the family of Quasi-Newton methods and does not store a dense approximation of the Hessian, making it well-suited for a GPU implementation with limited memory. Despite relying on a low-rank representation, it is known to converge very quickly, which we could also confirm in our experiments. Since the overall objective function is convex, the minimum obtained by L-BFGS is an optimal solution. As initial guess for minimization, we choose an "average image"of the registered LR images, computed as $\widetilde{\boldsymbol{W}}^T \boldsymbol{y}$ where $\widetilde{\boldsymbol{W}}$ is $\boldsymbol{W}$ with normalized columns [4].

2.3   Experiments

The proposed framework was implemented based on Nvidia's CUDA platform and is available on our website[1]. All vectorial computations are performed on the GPU, obviating the need to frequently transfer large amounts of data between host and device memory. The cuBLAS library is used for standard operations like dot products, vector scaling and scaled multiply-add. The system matrix W is stored in both compressed row storage (CRS) and compressed column storage (CCS) formats as it is necessary to compute matrix-vector products for both W and its transpose efficiently. Sparse matrix multiplication and the CRS/CCS management are handled by the cuSPARSE library.

In our ex-vivo experiments, we measured a porcine liver with a PMD Cam-Cube 3.0 and a high-precision light-section sensor [8] simultaneously. The data acquired by the latter served as ground truth.

For quantitative evaluation, absolute distance statistics and the root-mean-square error (RMSE) between the super-resolution output and the ground truth data were calculated. For this purpose, we registered both using optical markers. To obtain robust results, 240 ToF frames were split into 15 even sets. For each set, super-resolution was performed with different upsampling factors and sequence lengths. Both runtimes and error measurements were then averaged over all sets. All calculations were performed on an Nvidia GTX 580. The required image registration was performed offline using a 2D affine registration framework [9].

3   Results

In Fig. 2, we compare nearest-neighbor upsampling of an LR frame to a pre-processed [2] and our super-resolved image. Note that our framework has the desirable property of preserving edges as compared to the state-of-the-art pre-processing system, which becomes even more evident with larger motion. Fig. 3 shows a 3D mesh reconstruction of both the raw data and our result.

---
[1] http://www5.cs.fau.de/research/software/

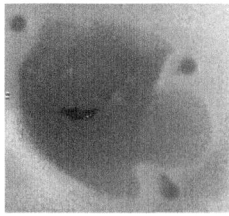 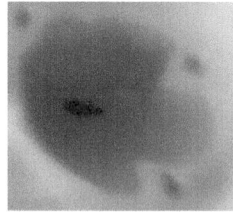 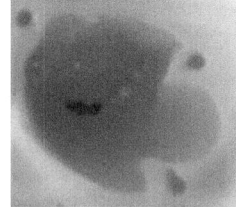

Fig. 2. Nearest neighbor (left) and preprocessed (middle) upsampling of one low-resolution range image, the range image obtained by super-resolution using 10 frames and upsampling factor of 2 (right).

	Raw	SR
RMSE	8.11 mm	6.29 mm
Median	4.92 mm	3.16 mm
Std.dev.	±0.34 mm	±0.16 mm

Table 1. Root-mean-square error (RMSE) and median as well as standard deviation of absolute distances to the ground truth mesh, averaged over 15 sets. Parameters for SR: 10 input frames and 2× upsampling factor.

Quantitative results regarding the errors are given in Tab. 1. All measured statistical properties were improved by our super-resolution framework. Further evaluation is performed on runtimes for different sequence lengths and upsampling factors (Fig. 5).

4 Discussion

In this paper, we presented a framework for super-resolution of preregistered ToF range images at interactive frame rates, running on off-the-shelf GPUs. Experiments on porcine liver data acquired with a PMD CamCube showed promising results regarding both accuracy and performance. We were able to decrease the RMSE by more than 20% on average from a single raw frame by upsampling 10

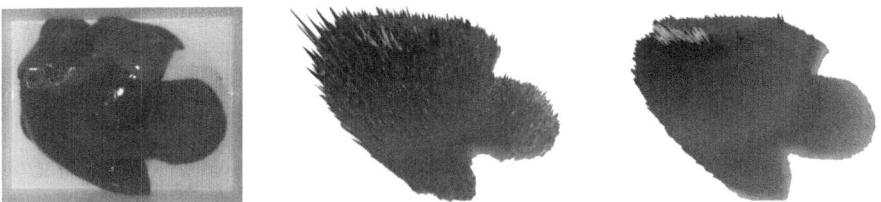

Fig. 3. The porcine liver measured for all experiments (left) and reconstructed meshes from raw data (middle) and after super-resolution of 10 frames with 2× zoom factor (right).

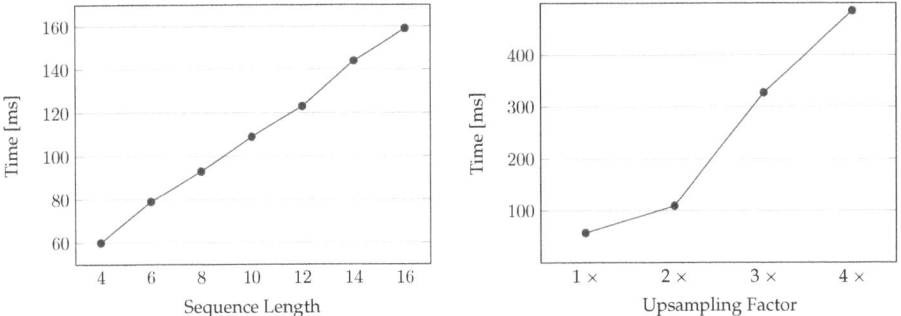

Fig. 4. Runtime analysis of our framework dependent on the number of input frames for an upsampling factor of 2 (left) and on the upsampling factor with 10 frames (right).

frames of 200×200 px. We computed the super-resolved image with an upsampling factor of 2 in 109 ms. Interactive frame rates were achieved for all evaluated sequence lengths given an upsampling factor of 2.

Future work will have to focus on integrating robust affine registration for a complete GPU accelerated system. Prior work by Ansorge et al. [10], using affine registration as an initialization for B-Spline registration in CUDA, strongly suggests that this is attainable. More sophisticated models that combine the registration step with the super-resolution optimization process have been proposed and may also be considered for use within our system.

Acknowledgement. The authors gratefully acknowledge funding of the Erlangen Graduate School in Advanced Optical Technologies (SAOT) by the German National Science Foundation (DFG) in the framework of the excellence initiative, as well as the support by the DFG under Grant No. HO 1791/7-1. This research was funded/supported by the Graduate School of Information Science in Health (GSISH) and the TUM Graduate School.

References

1. Cash D, Miga M, Glasgow S, et al. Concepts and preliminary data toward the realization of image-guided liver surgery. J Gastrointest Surg. 2007;11(7):844–59.
2. Wasza J, Bauer S, Hornegger J. Real-time preprocessing for dense 3-D range imaging on the GPU: defect interpolation, bilateral temporal averaging and guided filtering. Proc IEEE Int Conf Comput Vis. 2011; p. 1221–7.
3. Fuchs S, Hirzinger G. Extrinsic and depth calibration of ToF-cameras. Proc IEEE CVPR. 2008; p. 1–6.
4. Pickup LC. Machine learning in multi-frame image super-resolution; 2008. PhD Thesis, University of Oxford.
5. Schuon S, Theobalt C, Davis J, et al. High-quality scanning using time-of-flight depth superresolution. Proc IEEE Comput Soc Conf Comput Vis Pattern Recognit. 2008; p. 1–7.
6. Patil VH, Bormane DS, Patil HK. Real time super resolution image reconstruction. Proc ICIAS. 2007; p. 651–4.
7. Liu DC, Nocedal J. On the limited memory BFGS method for large scale optimization. Math Program. 1989;45(3):503–28.
8. Ettl S, Arold O, Yang Z, et al. Flying triangulation-an optical 3D sensor for the motion-robust acquisition of complex objects. Appl Opt. 2012;51(2):281–9.
9. Evangelidis GD, Psarakis EZ. Parametric image alignment using enhanced correlation coefficient maximization. IEEE Trans Pattern Anal Mach Intell. 2008;30:1858–65.
10. Ansorge RE, Sawiak SJ, Williams GB. Exceptionally fast non-linear 3D image registration using GPUs. IEEE Nucl Sci Symp Conf Rec. 2009; p. 4088–94.

Calibration of a Camera-Based Guidance Solution for Orthopedic and Trauma Surgery

Jessica Magaraggia[1], Adrian Egli[2], Gerhard Kleinszig[2], Rainer Graumann[2],
Elli Angelopoulou[1], Joachim Hornegger[1]

[1]Pattern Recognition Lab, University of Erlangen-Nuremberg, Erlangen, Germany
[2]Siemens AG, Healthcare Sector, Erlangen, Germany
jessica.magaraggia@informatik.uni-erlangen.de

Abstract. In orthopedic and trauma surgery, fracture reduction usually requires the use of metallic plates and their fixation by means of screws. The employment of guidance solutions during surgical procedures has become of great importance during the last decades. Our guidance solution exploits a small video camera placed directly on the instrument, for example a drill, and a set of small markers placed around the location where the drilling needs to be performed. A calibration step is required in order to determine the relative position of the instrument tip and axis w.r.t the coordinate system of the video camera. In this paper we describe a calibration method for our guidance solution. This calibration method exploits optical markers and a calibration plate whose geometry is known. Moreover, we show how we can exploit directly the image acquired by the video camera during the calibration in order to define an error measure to estimate the accuracy of the calibration. With this method, we achieved respectively an accuracy of 0.23 mm and 3.40 ° in the estimation of the instrument tip position and of the orientation of the instrument axis.

1 Introduction

In orthopedic and trauma surgery, guidance solutions are often exploited in order to help the surgeon fixing screws during a fracture reduction procedure. Typically, optical navigation solutions (e.g. VectorVision® from BRAINLAB AG. and Navigation System II from Stryker Inc.) use a stereo camera placed outside the operative field [1, 2]. Solutions based on video cameras have also been proposed. Diotte et al. [3], for example, exploited an augmented reality C-arm and a modified Schanz screw to determine the tip position of the drilling guide during the procedure by means of video images. Real-time display of its position is then possible on both video and X-ray images since they are coregistered after calibration of the device.

Our proposed solution does not require an augmented C-arm. We exploit a small video camera placed on the surgical instrument, e.g. a surgical drill. To our purpose, a calibration step is required in order to relate the position

H.-P. Meinzer et al. (Hrsg.), *Bildverarbeitung für die Medizin 2013*, Informatik aktuell,
DOI: 10.1007/978-3-642-36480-8_7, © Springer-Verlag Berlin Heidelberg 2013

of the axis and of the tip of the instrument to the camera. After the calibration, provided that optical markers are positioned where the instrument has to be inserted, it will be possible to exploit the images acquired from the video camera to determine the position of the attached instrument in real-time. Position feedback could be therefore provided to the surgeon during the procedure. A similar video camera based approach has been proposed by the medical company ActiViews, Inc. for percutaneous lung and liver interventions under CT-guidance. Their approach exploits the standard design of percutaneous instrumentation, such as biopsy needles and ablation probes that allows a camera-instrument calibration just relative to the individual instrument length. In comparison, we need to provide a full instrument calibration since we need to calibrate both tip position and axis direction of the instrument. In the following sections, we describe our calibration setup and the steps of the calibration procedure. Moreover, we propose a method for the estimation of the calibration error based directly on the images acquired from the video camera attached to the instrument.

2   Materials and methods

Our calibration setup is illustrated in Fig. 1. The calibration tool is made of a holder plate with an insertion guide that hosts the instrument axis and that is orthogonal to the plate's surface. Around its entry location, on the surface of the calibration plate, square optical markers are placed. The markers are similar to the ones proposed by Forman et al. [4]. The center of the entry location of the insertion guide is chosen to be the origin of our reference coordinate system M. The z-axis of M is also orthogonal to the plate surface (Fig. 2). The user has to position the instrument so that its axis is inserted into the guide and the tip reaches its bottom. The tip position is then defined by $\mathbf{P_M} = (0, 0, -d)^T$, where d is the depth of the guide, and the axis direction by $\mathbf{v_M} = (0, 0, 1)^T$, w.r.t M. The geometry of the markers is also known w.r.t M. As a consequence, the transformation matrix $\mathbf{T_C^M}$ from M to the camera coordinate system C can be determined exploiting a set of known point correspondences. The latter are defined between the corners of the markers in M and their corresponding points location in the images acquired by the camera. For the estimation of $\mathbf{T_C^M}$ we exploit the Perspective-n Points algorithm from Schweighofer et al. [5].

Once $\mathbf{T_C^M}$ is known, we can easily describe our tool position in the camera coordinate system as $D_C = (\mathbf{P_C}, \mathbf{v_C})$ where $\mathbf{P_C}$ and $\mathbf{v_C}$ are respectively the position of the instrument tip and axis orientation expressed in C

$$\begin{bmatrix} \mathbf{P_C} \\ 1 \end{bmatrix} = \mathbf{T_C^M} \begin{bmatrix} \mathbf{P_M} \\ 1 \end{bmatrix} \begin{bmatrix} \mathbf{v_C} \\ 1 \end{bmatrix} = \mathbf{T_C^M} \begin{bmatrix} \mathbf{v_M} \\ 1 \end{bmatrix} \tag{1}$$

One camera acquisition could suffice for the estimation of D_C. However, the accuracy of our estimation depends on the validity of our hypothesis that the instrument axis remains orthogonal to the calibration plate and that the instrument tip does not move. If small deviations of the instrument position occur, $\mathbf{v_M}$

and $\mathbf{P_M}$ no longer represent the correct axis orientation and tip position w.r.t M. Such deviations could occur naturally as a consequence of the instrument weight or could be induced by the user while holding the instrument. In order to reduce the influence of small deviations of the instrument position, we perform a set of measurements rotating the upper part of the instrument of approximately $360°$ about its axis $\mathbf{v_M}$. While rotating, the camera is continuously acquiring and for each frame, the relation described in 1 can be established. In the end, all measurements are combined together as described in the following in order to achieve a more robust estimation of D_C.

First of all, we observe that the instrument axis and tip are inside the field of view of the camera. Since the relative position between the camera and the instrument axis is fixed by construction, its position in the camera image does not change. Before starting the calibration procedure, we acquire an image I from our camera on a white background. From this image, we determine the tip position $\mathbf{I_P} = (x_P, y_P)^T$ and the axis orientation $\mathbf{v_P} = (v_X, v_Y)^T$ in the image coordinate system as shown in Fig. 3. $\mathbf{I_P}$ and $\mathbf{v_P}$ can be used as ground truth in order to obtain a measurement of the accuracy of our estimation.

For each image frame i, we get an estimation of $\mathbf{P_C^i}$ and $\mathbf{v_C^i}$. Since we calibrated our camera, we can exploit the intrinsic matrix and the distortion coefficients estimated during the camera calibration to project $\mathbf{P_C^i}$ and $\mathbf{A_C^i} = \mathbf{P_C^i} + \mathbf{v}$ onto the image plane [6]. After, $\mathbf{I_C^i}$ is calculated as the corresponding image tip of $\mathbf{P_C^i}$. Since $\mathbf{A_C^i}$ represents a point on the instrument axis, we calculate its correspondent image point $\mathbf{I_{A_C}^i}$. The vector $\mathbf{v_I^i} = \mathbf{I_{A_C}^i} - \mathbf{I_C^i}$ represents the orientation of the instrument axis in the image. We then define e_P^i and e_α^i respectively the tip position error and the angular error of the axis in the image by

$$e_P^i = ||\mathbf{I_C^i} - \mathbf{I_P}||_2 \qquad e_\alpha^i = \arccos \frac{\mathbf{v_I^i} \cdot \mathbf{v_P}}{||\mathbf{v_I^i}||_2 ||\mathbf{v_P}||_2} \qquad (2)$$

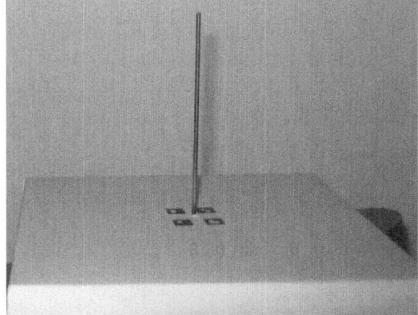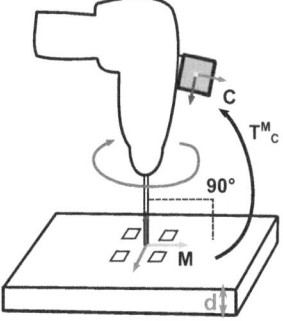

Fig. 1. Calibration plate and complete setup.

An overlay of the tracked tool tip and tracked axis onto 2-D or 3-D X-ray data sets or on video frames acquired from a video camera can be usually performed in order to have a feedback of the accuracy of the instrument position [2, 3]. However, this overlay requires a registration step between the tracker and the images on which the overlay is performed. In our case, no registration is required since 2 directly gives a feedback about the calibration accuracy.

We also define the weights w_P^i and w_α^i, that are respectively associated to the estimation of the tip position and angular orientation at the frame i

$$w_P^i = 1 - \frac{e_P^i}{\sum_{j=1}^N e_P^j} \qquad w_\alpha^i = 1 - \frac{e_\alpha^i}{\sum_{j=1}^N e_\alpha^j} \qquad (3)$$

According to 3, a smaller error in the estimation of $\mathbf{P}_C^i$ and $\mathbf{v}_C^i$ is associated respectively with a bigger w_P^i and w_α^i. Both weights are used to obtain a final estimation of the tip position $\overline{\mathbf{P}}_C$ and of the axis orientation $\overline{\mathbf{v}}_C$ according to 4. A position estimation $\mathbf{P}_C^i$ and an angular orientation $\mathbf{v}_C^i$ which returned a small estimation error contribute therefore more to the final estimation of the tip position and of the angular orientation $\overline{\mathbf{P}}_C$ and $\overline{\mathbf{v}}_C$

$$\overline{\mathbf{P}}_C = \frac{\sum_{i=1}^N w_\alpha^i \mathbf{P}_C^i}{\sum_{i=1}^N w_\alpha^i} \qquad \overline{\mathbf{v}}_C = \frac{\sum_{i=1}^N w_P^i \mathbf{v}_C^i}{\|\sum_{i=1}^N w_P^i \mathbf{v}_C^i\|_2} \qquad (4)$$

The instrument in camera coordinate system is then described by

$$\overline{D}_C := (\overline{\mathbf{P}}_C, \overline{\mathbf{v}}_C) \qquad (5)$$

For the evaluation of our calibration method, we positioned our instrument as depicted in Fig. 2 and rotated it of $360\,^\circ$ about its axis $\mathbf{v}_M$. Before starting the rotation, we turned our firewire camera on and continued acquiring while rotating. Our images were acquired uniformly over the whole span range of approximately $360\,^\circ$ with a resolution of 768×1024 obtaining 422 image-frames. For each frame i, we calculated e_P^i. The tip position that returned the minimum error for the whole sequence, $\mathbf{P}_C^{Min}$ and the current $\mathbf{v}_C^i$ were used for calculating $\mathbf{A}_C^i$ in each frame. Using $\mathbf{P}_C^{Min}$ instead of the corresponding $\mathbf{P}_C^i$ for each frame allows to investigate the error in the angular orientation independently from the error in the estimation of the tip position. For each frame also the angular error e_α^i was calculated. After, the whole set of measurements was used to get the final estimation of $\overline{D}_C$ as described in 4 and 5.

3   Results

The results of our instrument calibration are shown in Fig. 2. The reported errors are calculated according to 2. As concerning the tip position error, we used an empirically determined conversion factor $1\,\text{px} = 0.05\,\text{mm}$ in order to express our results in mm. This factor is proportional to the camera-markers distance. In Fig. 2(a) and Fig. 2(c) we show respectively the results of the tip position and of the axis orientation estimation evaluated for each frame separately. The position of the instrument tip and the axis orientation could be estimated with an accuracy of 1.39 ± 0.41 mm and $3.36 \pm 0.72\,°$. In Fig. 2(b) and Fig. 2(d) we report the errors obtained estimating $\mathbf{P_C^i}$ and $\mathbf{v_C^i}$ for the frame i considering also the previous $i-1$ frames according to 4. At the last frame, for which all the 422 frames available are considered, we obtained $e_P^N = 0.23$ mm and $e_\alpha^N = 3.36\,°$ where $N = 422$. The resulting $\mathbf{P_C^N}$ and $\mathbf{v_C^N}$ represent our final estimation $\overline{D}_C$, which reprojected onto the image lead to an angular error of $3.40\,°$. The final result of the calibration is depicted in Fig. 3.

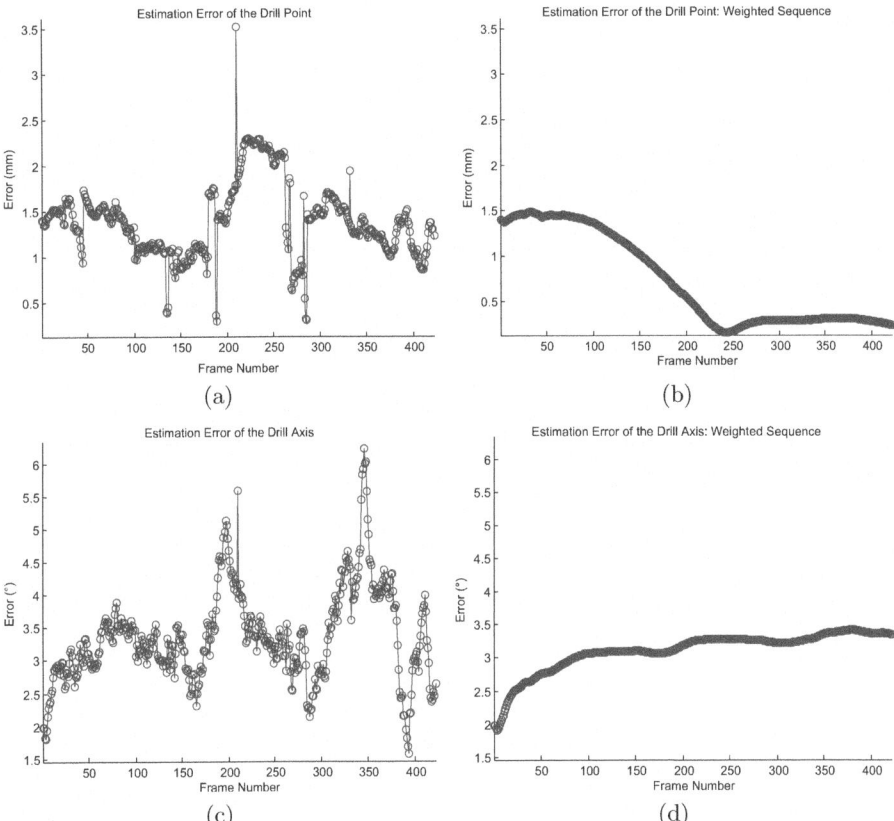

Fig. 2. Position error of the drill tip, (a) and (b), and angular error of the direction of the instrument axis, (c) and (d). In (a) and (c) each frame is considered individually. In (b) and (d), the error for the frame number i is calculated using the weighted average over the frame sequence from 1 to i.

Fig. 3. The result of the estimation of the position of the instrument tip and of the direction of the instrument axis are depicted in green. The reference position and orientation are depicted in red.

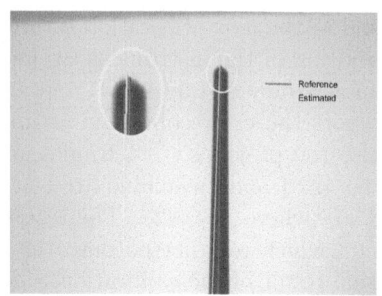

4   Discussion

In this paper we presented a calibration method for a camera-based guidance solution. The method allows to determine the instrument position and the instrument axis direction with an accuracy of 0.23 mm and 3.40 ° respectively. Optical tracking systems usually require about 2 minutes for instrument calibration. In our setup, the calibration required about 20 seconds. Our experiments showed that using the whole sequence of acquired camera images contributes to obtain a more stable result that is less dependent from small axis oscillations which could occur when the instrument is in place in the calibration plate. Moreover, we showed that we can exploit the fact that the instrument axis position in the camera image does not change in order to obtain an error measure for the accuracy of our calibration. We expect to obtain a better accuracy in the direction estimation modifying our calibration plate in order to improve the stability of the instrument when placed on the plate, since this would allow a further reduction of the oscillation of the instrument axis. In future work, we aim to reduce the angular error of the instrument axis estimation to a value below 1 °.

References

1. Nagel M, Schmidt G, Petzold R, et al. A navigation system for minimally invasive CT-guided interventions. Med Image Comput Comput Assist Interv. 2005; p. 33–40.
2. Reaungamornrat S, Otake Y, Uneri A, et al. Tracker-on-C for cone-beam CT-guided surgery: evaluation of geometric accuracy and clinical applications. Proc SPIE. 2012;8316.
3. Diotte B, Fallavollita P, Wang L, et al. Radiation-free drill guidance in interlocking of intramedullary nails. Med Image Comput Comput Assist Interv. 2012; p. 18–25.
4. Forman C, Aksoy M, Hornegger J, et al. Self-encoded marker for optical prospective head motion correction in MRI. Med Image Comput Comput Assist Interv. 2010; p. 259–66.
5. Schweighofer G, Pinz A. Robust pose estimation from a planar target. IEEE Trans Pattern Anal Mach Intell. 2006;28(12):2024–30.
6. Ma Y, Soatto S, Kosecka J, et al. An Invitation to 3-D Vision: From Images to Geometric Models. Springer; 2004.

Optimized Cortical Subdivision for Classification of Alzheimer's Disease With Cortical Thickness

Mirco Richter, Dorit Merhof

Visual Computing, University of Konstanz
mirco.richter@uni-konstanz.de

Abstract. In several studies, brain atrophy measured by cortical thickness has shown to be a meaningful biomarker for Alzheimer's disease. In this research field, the level of granularity at which values are compared is an important aspect. Vertex- and voxel-based approaches can detect atrophy at a very fine scale, but are susceptible to noise from misregistrations and inter-subject differences in the population. Regional approaches are more robust to these kinds of noise, but cannot detect variances at a local scale. In this work, an optimized classifier is presented for a parcellation scheme that provides a trade-off between both paradigms by increasing the granularity of a regional approach. For this purpose, atlas regions are subdivided into gyral and sulcal parts at different height levels. Using two-stage feature selection, optimal gyral and sulcal subregions are determined for the final classification with sparse logistic regression. The robustness was assessed on clinical data by 10-fold cross-validation and by testing the prediction accuracy for unseen individuals. In every aspect, superior classification performance was observed as compared to the original parcellation scheme which can be explained by the increased locality of cortical thickness measures and the customized classification approach that reveals interacting regions.

1 Introduction

Various image processing and classification methods to diagnose Alzheimer's disease (AD) and mild cognitive impairment (MCI) have been developed and gradually improved over the past decades. With dedicated segmentation, registration and feature extraction methods, biomarkers based on structural and functional imaging can detect subtle neurodegenerative changes [1]. As a result, the amount of observed variance between health groups is increasing for the sake of improved discrimination. All these developments are important for an early classification and treatment of MCI and AD [2]. Amongst others, the structural biomarker cortical thickness (CoT) that is based on segmented data from magnetic resonance imaging (MRI) has shown to be a significant biomarker for dementia. Regarding MCI and AD, gray matter structures that are affected by atrophy include the hippocampus, the parahippocampal gyrus, the cingulate, parts of the temporal, parietal and frontal lobe, and the occipital pole [3].

For the estimation of CoT, there exist two competing paradigms, the voxel- and the surface-based approach [4, 5]. In both cases, measures can be compared

H.-P. Meinzer et al. (Hrsg.), *Bildverarbeitung für die Medizin 2013*, Informatik aktuell,
DOI: 10.1007/978-3-642-36480-8_8, © Springer-Verlag Berlin Heidelberg 2013

at different levels of granularity: fine-grained methods using voxel and vertex values or coarse-grained methods using mean values of anatomically distinct regions of interest (ROIs). Fine-grained methods provide high dimensional feature sets for the detection of local changes. However, they are susceptible to noise introduced e.g. by registration to normal space or inter-subject differences. Also, the relatively small set of observations compared to the large number of variables renders dimensionality reduction a crucial problem. In contrast, region-based approaches create low dimensional spaces that are easier to handle and averaging of measurements compensates for noise such as subtle misregistrations. However, as a consequence changes at a local scale cannot be revealed.

To close the gap between both extremes of the scale of granularity, an anatomical parcellation method was presented previously that subdivides the cortex into gyral and sulcal subregions at different levels of height for which mean CoT values are computed [6]. In this work, this parcellation scheme is employed by a customized feature selection and classification approach that determines the optimal set from the original ROIs and the gyral and sulcal subregions. Section 2 describes the subject population and the imaging data, presents our approach including a summary of preprocessing steps and CoT measurement, and describes the classification approach and the evaluation of robustness. In Sections 3 and 4, we present and discuss the improvements achieved on clinical data.

2   Materials and methods

2.1   Image data and preprocessing

For this study, MRI images of 84 subjects were collected from the database of the Alzheimer's Disease Neuroimaging Initiative (ADNI) for the following four groups (diagnoses assigned according to the ADNI protocol available at http://adni.loni.ucla.edu): healthy elderly controls N (11 females / 10 males; age: 76.4 ± 6.6; education: 16.4 ± 2.8), patients with early MCI (eMCI) (10/11; age: 74.2 ± 8.0; edu.: 16.6 ± 2.8), late MCI (lMCI) (8/13; age: 72.3 ± 5.5; edu.: 16.7 ± 2.7), and AD (8/13; age: 75.4 ± 10.2; edu,: 15.0 ± 3.2). One-way ANOVA ensured that sex, age and education were not significantly different between the groups. For all subjects, MRI data was acquired on 3T GE Signa HDxt scanning devices in the same format, but from different sites. The distribution of sites was random across subjects. An IR-SPGR sequence was applied with TR = 6.98 ms, TE = 2.85 ms, and TI = 400 ms, resulting in 196 T1-weighted sagittal slices with 1.0 × 1.0 mm in plane spatial resolution of dimension 256×256 voxels and 1.2 mm slice thickness.

The images were preprocessed in the same fashion as described in [6] with tools from the FMRIB Software Library (FSL, www.fmrib.ox.ac.uk/fsl). In short, manual neck cropping was followed by automatic skull stripping using the Brain Extraction Tool. The extracted brain was segmented into white matter (WM), gray matter (GM) and cerebrospinal fluid using FAST that provides probabilistic voxel-wise membership values for each of the tissue classes. ROIs were defined according to the labels of the Harvard-Oxford probabilistic atlas (distributed with FSL) which comprises 48 cortical ROIs for each hemisphere. To transform the ROI labels from the atlas to each subject space, FLIRT and FNIRT performed spatial normalization of the original images to the MNI152 space by affine multi-resolution registration with normalized correlation as similarity function followed by non-linear free-form deformations. The labels of the Harvard-Oxford atlas were spatially transformed to the subject space by inverting these registrations. Using the GM segmentation, voxelwise CoT was estimated using minimum line integrals measured along an approximation of the medial GM layer [4, 6].

2.2   Feature selection and classification

The anatomical subdivision of the cortex into gyral and sulcal subregions was achieved by an adaption of a robust skeletonization approach for discrete volumetric objects with genus 0 [7]. Basically, the skeleton of the WM segmentation is computed that associates each skeleton point with at least two closest points on the WM surface. By measuring geodesic distances τ between those surface points, a pruning function is defined that can be thresholded to separate gyri and sulci at different height levels. An extension of this pruning function prevents the false detection of noisy features as gyral regions. Using thresholds $\tau \in [8, 20]$ mm in steps of 2 mm, seven gyral and seven sulcal subregions are created per ROI in addition to the ROI itself. These are denoted as $\mathcal{G}_\tau$, $\mathcal{S}_\tau$ and $\mathcal{W}$, respectively. For the whole brain, this results in 15 regions per ROI times the 96 ROIs of the Harvard-Oxford atlas, each represented by a mean CoT value. For a collection of n subjects, T_{ij} denotes the feature vector containing the mean CoT values for all subjects for the cortex label $i \in [1, 96]$ and the subregion $j \in [1, 15]$. Each T_{ij} was corrected for the covariates sex, age, and education by a linear regression model estimated for the normal group and normalized to z-scores.

As rather subtle differences in mean CoT are expected between the groups, and as the subregions of each ROI may contain redundant information, direct application of sparse logistic regression or a support vector machine might not be sufficient to maximize the gain of this rich feature set. Therefore, we propose a two-stage feature selection before the final classification, which comprises the following steps: The first stage eliminates redundancy in each ROI by determining for the gyral and sulcal subregions $\mathcal{G}_\tau$ and $\mathcal{S}_\tau$ those that maximize the Pearson's correlation of their mean CoT values T_{ij} with the group membership variable Y. The resulting set T'_{ij} with $i \in [1, 96]$ and $j \in [1, 3]$ contains the mean CoT values of the whole ROI, the best gyral and the best sulcal subregion.

Within the second stage, interactions between pairs of variables of the set T'_{ij} were considered as the selection criterion since enforcing interactions might result in higher stability and better performance of the final classification. Similar to the linear discrimination for pairs of mean CoT values in [3], linear regression was applied to optimize the linear model $Y = [T'_{ij} \; T'_{lm}] \, \beta + \epsilon$ for each pair of variables T'_{ij} and T'_{lm} with $(i, j) \neq (l, m)$. Here, β and ϵ denote the regression weights and error variables. Ranking each variable pair according to the coefficients of determination R^2, the best variables are filtered to form the set $\mathcal{D}_{LR}$. For

Table 1. AUC values of 10-fold cross-validation and prediction for the whole ROI set $\mathcal{D}_W$, the best gyral and best sulcal set $\mathcal{D}_{G_\tau}$, $\mathcal{D}_{S_\tau}$, and the sets $\mathcal{D}_{\mathrm{Corr}}$ and $\mathcal{D}_{LR}$ optimized by correlation and linear regression. First and second best values in bold.

| Group Pair | 10-fold Cross Validation | | | | | Prediction | | | | |
	$\mathcal{D}_W$	$\mathcal{D}_G$	$\mathcal{D}_S$	$\mathcal{D}_{\mathrm{Corr}}$	$\mathcal{D}_{LR}$	$\mathcal{D}_W$	$\mathcal{D}_G$	$\mathcal{D}_S$	$\mathcal{D}_{\mathrm{Corr}}$	$\mathcal{D}_{LR}$
N-eMCI	.74	.58	.59	**.80**	**.87**	.64	.58	.50	**.70**	**.81**
N-lMCI	**.69**	.52	.44	.65	**.83**	.58	.47	.54	**.67**	**.75**
N-AD	.93	.93	.86	**.97**	**.99**	.87	.89	.88	**.94**	**.96**
eMCI-lMCI	.53	.48	**.70**	.62	**.93**	.50	.51	**.67**	.65	**.82**
eMCI-AD	.84	**.93**	.89	.81	**.99**	.70	.78	**.79**	.75	**.90**
lMCI-AD	.60	**.81**	.71	.72	**.86**	.64	**.76**	.72	.72	**.82**

comparison, $\mathcal{D}_{\mathrm{Corr}}$ was created by selecting the best variables according to the correlation between T'_{ij} and Y, similar to the approach in [8]. For both sets, their size was fixed to 96, equal to the size of the original partitions.

For the six group pairs created from the four groups, the following feature sets were compared: $\mathcal{D}_j = \{T_{ij}\}$ with $j \in [1, 15]$ which denotes the 15 sets (i.e. whole ROI, seven gyral and seven sulcal sets), $\mathcal{D}_{\mathrm{Corr}}$ and $\mathcal{D}_{LR}$. For this purpose, sparse logistic regression with the elastic net (ENLR) was applied to each set [9]. The regression factor α that combines features of lasso and ridge regression was set to 0.5 for a trade-off between low and high number of features. Two tests of robustness were applied: At first, stratified 10-fold cross-validation with 20 repetitions for bias-free estimates, and second, evaluation of predictive accuracy by splitting the population into two equally sized training and test tests by random stratification and assessing mean values from 20 repetitions.

3   Results

For the first comparison using 10-fold cross-validation, curves of the receiver operator characteristic (ROC) are presented in Figure 1 (top) for the group pairs N-eMCI, N-lMCI and N-AD. The corresponding discriminative regions are highlighted on the surface of one healthy subject in Figure 1 (bottom). The mean values of the area under the ROC (AUC) are listed for both validations and for all groups in Table 1. In all cases, $\mathcal{D}_{LR}$ shows superior performance, while $\mathcal{D}_{\mathrm{Corr}}$ is better than all sets $\mathcal{D}_j$ in only two cases for 10-fold cross-validation, and in three cases for prediction. The three top regions identified using $\mathcal{D}_{LR}$ for N-eMCI are $\mathcal{G}_8$ in the right frontal pole, $\mathcal{S}_{14}$ in the left central opercular cortex, and $\mathcal{W}$ of the right planum temporale. For N-lMCI, the regions are $\mathcal{S}_{20}$ in the right middle temporal gyrus, $\mathcal{G}_8$ in the left parietal operculum cortex, and $\mathcal{S}_{20}$ in the right superior temporal gyrus. For N-AD, the regions are $\mathcal{G}_{18}$ in the right inferior temporal gyrus, $\mathcal{S}_{20}$ in the right inferior temporal gyrus, and $\mathcal{W}$ of the right cingulate gyrus.

4   Discussion

In this work, a classification method for Alzheimer's disease and mild cognitive impairment is presented that optimizes the selection of mean cortical thickness variables from a set provided by a cortical parcellation scheme. For this purpose, features are selected from this set by assessing the power to predict the group membership variable Y from each pair of mean CoT variables. In this way, the contribution of interacting variables could be enforced which was observed by a strong improvement in classification power validated for robustness by two different resampling techniques.

Traditional feature selection methods consider the correlation between a single predictor and Y [8]. This is beneficial for large feature spaces that require efficient methods. However, classification performance might get impaired as interactions between multiple variables are completely ignored. In this work, this problem was solved properly with linear regression using pairs of predictors. Due to the quadratic complexity, this approach is not directly applicable to high dimensional data, but a divide-and-conquer approach could achieve at least a good approximation of the complete ranking for the sake of quality.

Acknowledgement. The data used was obtained from the Alzheimer's Disease Neuroimaging Initiative (ADNI) database (http://adni.loni.ucla.edu), NIH grants U01 AG024904, P30 AG010129, K01 AG030514. As such, the investiga-

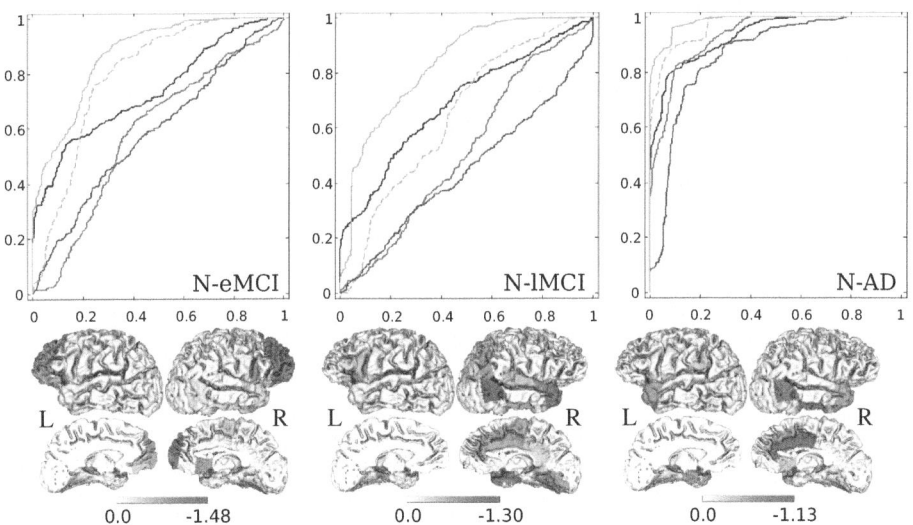

Fig. 1. *Top:* ROC curves assessed by 20-times repeated stratified 10-fold cross-validation of ENLR. $\mathcal{D}_W$ (black), best $\mathcal{D}_{G_\tau}$ (red), best $\mathcal{D}_{S_\tau}$ (blue), $\mathcal{D}_{\mathrm{Corr}}$ (green dashed line), and $\mathcal{D}_{LR}$ (green solid line). False positive rate on abscissa, true positive rate on ordinate. *Bottom:* Discriminative regions projected on the surface of one healthy subject for the group pairs N-eMCI (left), N-lMCI (middle) and N-AD (right). Colors from white to red are proportional to the negative regression weight (decreasing CoT).

tors within the ADNI contributed to the design and implementation of ADNI and/or provided data but did not participate in analysis or writing of this report. A complete listing of ADNI investigators is given in the Internet[1]. Furthermore, the work was supported by the DFG Research Training Group GK-1042 "Explorative Analysis and Visualization of Large Information Spaces".

References

1. Hampel H, Bürger K, Teipel SJ, et al. Core candidate neurochemical and imaging biomarkers of Alzheimer's disease. Alzheimer's & Dementia. 2008;4(1):38–48.
2. Small G, Bullock R. Defining optimal treatment with cholinesterase inhibitors in Alzheimer's disease. Alzheimer's & Dementia. 2011;7(2):177–84.
3. Lerch JP, Pruessner J, Zijdenbos AP, et al. Automated cortical thickness measurements from MRI can accurately separate Alzheimer's patients from normal elderly controls. Neurobiology of Aging. 2008;29(1):23–30.
4. Aganj I, Sapiro G, Parikshak N, et al. Measurement of cortical thickness from MRI by minimum mine integrals on soft-classified tissue. Hum Brain Mapp. 2009;30(11):3188–99.
5. Fischl B, Dale A. Measuring the thickness of the human cerebral cortex from magnetic resonance images. Proc Natl Acad Sci USA. 2000;97(20):11050–5.
6. Richter M, Bishop CA, Dukart J, et al. Skeleton-based gyri sulci separation for improved assessment of cortical thickness. In: IEEE 9th International Symposium on Biomedical Imaging; 2012. p. FR–PO.PA.37.
7. Reniers D, Jalba A, Telea A. Robust classification and analysis of anatomical surfaces using 3D skeletons. Eurographics Workshop on Visual Computing for Biomedicine. 2008; p. 61–8.
8. Zhou L, Wang Y, Li Y, et al. Hierarchical anatomical brain networks for MCI prediction: revisiting volumetric measures. PLoS One. 2011;6(7):e21935.
9. Zou H, Hastie T. Regularization and variable selection via the elastic net. Journal of the Royal Statistical Society, Series B. 2005;67(2):301–20.

---

[1] http://adni.loni.ucla.edu/wp-content/uploads/how_to_apply/ /ADNI_Acknowledgement_List.pdf

Quantifying Differences Between Primary Cortical Areas in Humans Based on Laminar Profiles in In-Vivo MRI Data

Juliane Dinse[1,2], Pablo Martin[1], Andreas Schäfer[1], Stefan Geyer[1],
Robert Turner[1], Pierre-Louis Bazin[1]

[1]Max Planck Institute of Cognitive and Brain Science, Stephanstr. 1a, 04103 Leipzig
[2]Simulation and Graphics Department, Faculty of Computer Science,
Otto-von-Guericke University Magdeburg
dinse@cbs.mpg.de

Abstract. This paper presents an approach for mapping the human cortical architecture in vivo based on quantitative MRI indices of myelin. We automatically construct laminar profiles in several primary cortical areas and investigate different sampling strategies. The results demonstrate that our method is able to distinguish these areas at specific cortical depths.

1 Introduction

The human brain is a complex organ, including a highly convoluted cortex. Functional activity occur in a $2-5$ mm thin sheet of neurons along the cortical surface, organized in six layers. The relative thickness of these layers changes in different areas of the brain which corresponds to different functional roles. In the early 20th century, neuroanatomists started to investigate areal differences [1], deriving comprehensive measures of the cortical laminar pattern. The myeloarchitecture mappings of the Vogts' described the anatomical features associated with the myelin sheaths of neuronal axons and included over 200 cortical areas. However, their findings were defined on subjective and qualitative measures on two-dimensional stained tissue sections of post-mortem brains.

Magnetic resonance imaging (MRI) enables scientists to measure structural and functional features in vivo. With an increased resolution and sensitivity, methods have evolved which are able to map the organization of the cortex by imaging the myelin content. Geyer et al. demonstrated that 7 Tesla MRI reveals local cortical differences in quantitative T1 images and can precisely depict the cortical boundaries [2]. Glasser and van Essen published a new method based on myelin content, as revealed by T1-weighted and T2-weighted MRI [3]. Clare and Bridge have investigated how reliably cortical areas and boundaries can be detected using MRI [4]. But to what extend are myelin-related laminar profiles in MR data specifiable between primary cortical areas?

To our knowledge, the approach presented here is the first ever published comparison of quantitative myelin-related laminar profiles between primary areas (motor, somatosensory and visual), based on in vivo MRI. We investigate

H.-P. Meinzer et al. (Hrsg.), *Bildverarbeitung für die Medizin 2013*, Informatik aktuell,
DOI: 10.1007/978-3-642-36480-8_9, © Springer-Verlag Berlin Heidelberg 2013

and compare two different methods of obtaining samples in regions-of-interest (ROIs): probabilistic atlases based on cytoarchitectonic data of post-mortem brains and manually sampling voxels in regions defined by macro-anatomical landmarks. Our results allow for a first quantitative comparison to the myeloarchitecture of the cortex and outline new possibilities of incorporating such information into new parcellation approaches. A proper mapping of the cortical organization will provide enhanced models of the human cortex for neuroimaging, especially if myelination patterns can be reproduced robustly in individual brains.

2   Materials and methods

Six MRI data sets with 0.7 mm^3 resolution have been acquired according to the MP2RAGE imaging sequence [5, 6]. The data is registered to the Montreal's Neurological Institute (MNI) brain space to preserve cortical geometry and resampled to 0.4 mm^3 resolution. The rigid registration includes six degrees of freedom and is optimized using a cost function of normalized mutual information. The cortex is extracted using in-house software [7] integrated in the MIPAV framework (http://mipav.cit.nih.gov/). The boundaries φ_{GW} between gray matter (GM) and white matter (WM) and φ_{GC} between GM and cerebrospinal fluid (CSF) estimated during the segmentation are represented as level set surfaces [8] and used to estimate l equi-distant laminae in-between ($l = 20$) with the following differential equation

$$\frac{\partial \varphi_d}{\partial t} + (\varphi_d - ((1 - \rho)\varphi_{GW} - \rho\varphi_{GC}))|\nabla\varphi_d| = \epsilon\kappa|\nabla\varphi_d| \qquad (1)$$

where $(1 - \rho)\varphi_{GW} - \rho\varphi_{GC}$ is the target laminae as a weighted average function of $\rho \in [0, 1]$ The cortical depth is computed at each point depending on the desired lamina and local curvatures. $\epsilon\kappa|\nabla\varphi_d|$ is a level set regularization term which avoids shocks and smooths the laminae. The real cortical layers are different from our estimated laminae. The relative thickness of the six cortical layers varies due to curvature, thus compensating for the folding. Our method only provides a coordinate system for measuring cortical depth. Based on the set of the equi-distant laminae $\{\varphi_d\}$, orthogonal profile curves can be generated as follows: from any starting location x, the projection onto the closest lamina φ_d is obtained as

$$x_d = x - \varphi_d(x)\frac{\nabla\varphi_d(x)}{|\nabla\varphi_d(x)|} \qquad (2)$$

and x_d is projected onto the next closest lamina, until a curved 3D profile is generated that intersects all the layered laminae.

The constructed profiles are the basis of this work. We select four ROIs of primary cortical areas: Brodmann Area BA 1 and BA 3b (somatosensory cortex), BA 4 (motor cortex) and BA 17 (visual cortex) within the left hemisphere. For the atlas-based sampling we use the probabilities given in the Jülich atlas [9].

We threshold the individual ROIs at the probability $p = 25\%$ in order to ensure a large enough sample size. The manually sampling on individual brains is guided by macro-anatomical landmarks which in primary areas show good correlation with microstructural borders. The profile analysis is done in MATLAB (MathWorks, Inc).

For each subject and each ROI, we calculate an average profile consisting of mean and standard deviation per lamina. To do so, the intensity histogram per lamina in individual subjects and ROIs is computed and a Gaussian curve is fitted to it based on a Maximum-Likelihood approach. The mean and standard deviation are derived from the distribution curve. For comparison among the overall intensities in the cortex, we compute histograms, their means and standard deviations for the entire hemisphere. We calculate the correlation coefficients of the profile for each ROI between all subjects, for each of the two different sampling methods, to ensure that the shapes follow the same pattern. Furthermore, we calculate the difference between the cortex and each ROI for each subject. Based on these difference measures, the mean and standard deviation are computed again. In order to verify the significance of the results, and to demonstrate that profiles can be distinguished at specific cortical depths, a z-test was carried out per lamina between 0.25 to 0.9 cortical depth. The range of the cortical depth has been limited due to partial volume effects at the WM/GM and GM/CSF interfaces. Based on the test outcome, a rejection rate R is calculated as number of rejected cases devided by all tested cases. Finally, the mean and standard deviations of the differences of manual sampled voxels are graphed in order to visually emphasize their areal distinction.

3   Results

The focus in the following sections is on BA 1, 3b and 4. However, BA 17 has been processed in the same way. The results are similar, but have been omitted due to space limitations. Fig. 1 depicts the different sampling methods in an individual brain. BA 1, 3b and 4 are anatomically in close vicinity, but related to different function, and should have different myelin-related profiles. In contrast to the manually sampled elements guided by macro-anatomical landmarks, Fig. 1 shows that samples of the probabilistic atlas overlap to a high degree. They also sample in neighboring regions. Fig. 2 (rows 1-3) shows the average profiles of all subjects in BA 1, 3b and 4 for both sampling strategies. All subjects have fairly consistent profiles, especially for the manually sampled ROIs. The profile shape in manually sampled ROIs are descriptive, in particular in BA 1. The correlation calculation for each ROI in both samplings always resulted in $r=1$ and $p=0$, meaning the profiles correlate well between subjects. When averages are grouped over the six subjects in each ROI and the cortex (Fig. 2, bottom row), it becomes obvious that the mean profiles in the individual ROIs of the manual sampling are much more distinct than those derived from the probabilistic profiles. After calculating the mean and standard deviation of the differences between the cortex and each ROI, both methods show some strong dissimilarities between primary areas and the cortex as a whole. In the manual sampling, all ROIs are also distinct from each other (Fig. 3) whereas the probabilistically sampled ROIs were very similar. The mean differences from the manual sampling are larger, standard deviations are smaller, or at least comparable. BA 4 and BA 3b follow the same profile pattern (location of increase and decrease of slope) with BA 4 always having larger differences between 0.3 to 0.8 of cortical depth. Using manual sampling this difference is more than doubled. BA 1 is also distinguishable from all other ROIs. The z-test for probabilistic sampling showed that on average in R=41.67 % of compared cases the profiles are distinguishable between each other (min: BA 4: 28.57 %, max: BA 1: 54.76 %). The z-test results for the manual samples were much higher with R=80.16 % on average (min: BA 1 and BA 3b: 78.57 %, max: BA 4: 83.33 %). In former studies, we saw that profile shapes changed with less than 1000 samples. In this study sample sizes for probabilistic atlases are on average: 20.848 (BA 1), 85.311 (BA 3b) and 79.305 (BA 4). The sizes for manual sampling are: 2.400, 1.810 and 2.660, respectively.

4   Discussion

We have shown that it is possible to compare quantitative areal differences in laminar profiles of T1 between primary areas in in vivo MRI data of the human cortex. The profiles of the subjects in each ROI show excellent consistency. The averaged profiles in each ROI show good agreement with architectonic differences published by Vogt & Vogt [1]. BA 4 is highly myelinated with their Bands of Baillarger mainly obscured, thus having shorter T1 values in a larger range of cortical depth (Fig. 2). However, BA 3b shows Bands of Baillarger and their corresponding profiles show higher T1 values in mid cortical depth. Also, the relative thickness of myelinated layers is reflected in the profiles. In summary, our proposed quantification method is able to model myelination relations in primary areas.

However, in this first analysis there are some limitations. The resolution of the data analyzed is not yet sufficient to reveal the full microstructure of the cortex. Some important features of the actual cortical layering are not repre-

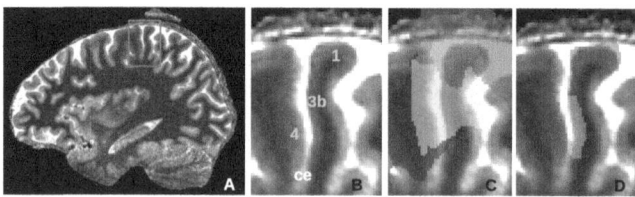

Fig. 1. A quantitative T1 map of the brain (A) with the areas in focus (B) in the central sulcus (ce). The probabilistic samples (C) overlap neighboring regions, whereas the manual samples (D) are within microstructural borders.

sented in the MRI data. Improved resolution will make it easier to deal with
partial voluming effects, especially in regions with highly folded structures (BA
1 and BA 17). Furthermore, the equi-distant laminae used do not confirm to
the actual cortical layering and thus will sometimes cross cortical layers. A more
accurate volume-preserving model which incorporates cortical curvature is under
investigation [10]. The problem of correct sampling is hard to resolve. Probabilistic ROIs from the Jülich atlas provide only an approximate localization due
to individual variations and include samples from neighboring areas. In large

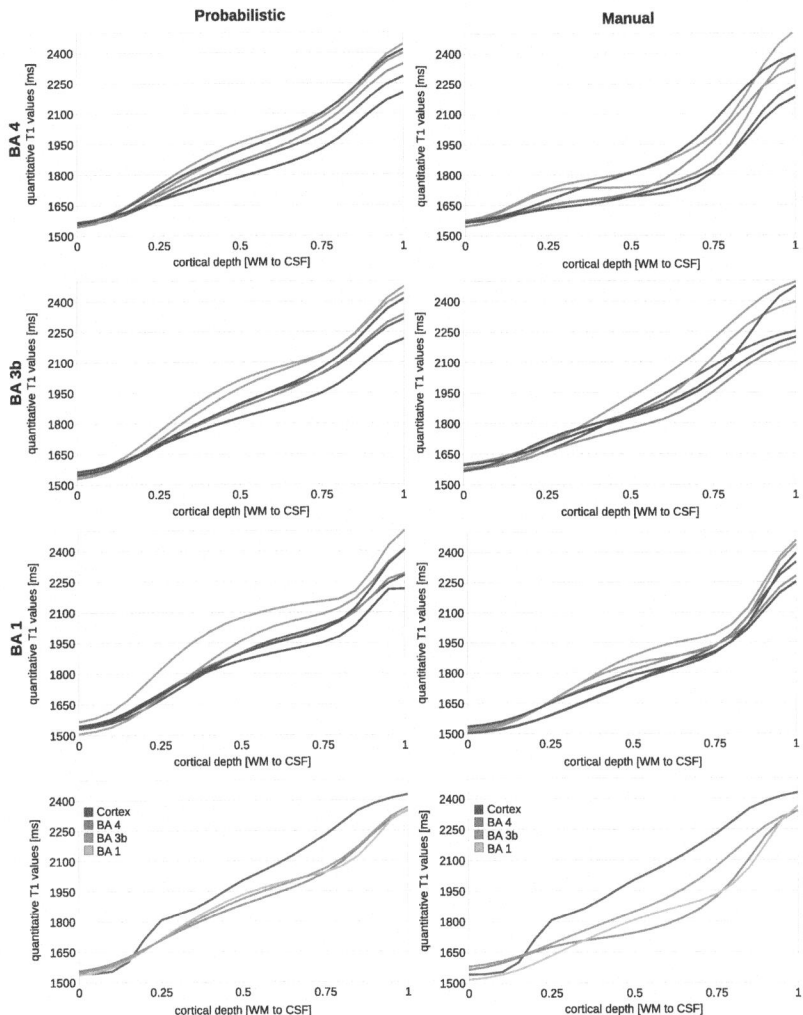

Fig. 2. Average profiles of primary cortical areas in focus (rows 1-3) each calculated in
six subjects. The bottom row plots the group average of the individual ROIs according
to the groups' average profile of the cortex.

Fig. 3. Mean and standard deviation of the differences between the cortex and each ROI in all cortical depths.

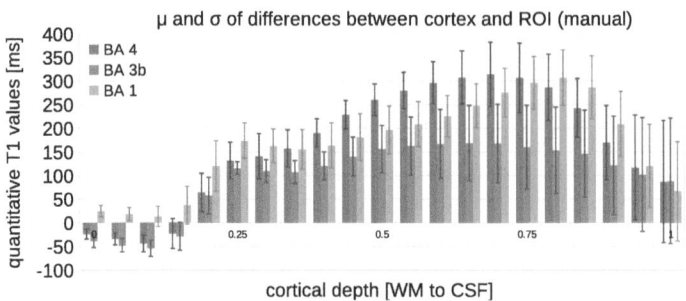

areas such as BA 17, the effect can be small, but in most places it will distort the profile. For these reasons, it is desirable to have subject-specific definitions of the areas. This study shows that it is possible to derive a quantitative model which can be obtained with high-resolution quantitative MRI and analysis of cortical profile differences. More work is needed to refine such a model, extend it to more areas and to finally segment and classify the areas in new subjects.

References

1. Vogt C, Vogt O. Allgem. Ergebnisse unserer Hirnforschung. 1. Mitteilung. Ziele und Wege unserer Hirnforschung. J Psychol Neurol. 1919;25.
2. Geyer S, Weiss M, Reimann K, et al. Microstructural parcellation of the human cerebral cortex–from Brodmann's post-mortem map to in vivo mapping with high-field magnetic resonance imaging. Front Hum Neurosci. 2011;5(19).
3. Glasser MF, Van Essen DC. Mapping human cortical areas in vivo based on myelin content as revealed by T1-and T2-weighted MRI. J Neurosci. 2011;31(32):11597–616.
4. Clare S, Bridge H. Methodological issues relating to in vivo cortical myelography using MRI. Hum Brain Map. 2005;26(4):240–50.
5. Marques J, Kober T, Krueger G, et al. MP2RAGE, a self bias-field corrected sequence for improved segmentation and T1-mapping at high field. NeuroImage. 2010;49(2):1271–81.
6. Hurley AC, Al-Radaideh A, Bai L, et al. Tailored RF pulse for magnetization inversion at ultrahigh field. MRM. 2010;63(1):51–8.
7. Bazin PL, Weiss M, Dinse J, et al. A computational pipeline for subject-specific, ultra-high resolution cortical analysis at 7 Tesla. Hum Brain Map. 2012;(abstract).
8. Sethian JA. Level set methods and fast marching methods: evolving interfaces in computational geometry, fluid mechanics, computer vision, and materials science. Cambridge University Press; 1999.
9. Eickhoff S, Stephan K, Mohlberg H, et al. A new SPM toolbox for combining probabilistic cytoarchitectonic maps and functional imaging data. NeuroImage. 2005;25(4):1325–35.
10. Waehnert M, Weiss M, Streicher M, et al. Do cortical layers conform to the Laplace equation? Hum Brain Map. 2012;(abstract).

Classification of Benign and Malignant DCE-MRI Breast Tumors by Analyzing the Most Suspect Region

Sylvia Glaßer[1], Uli Niemann[1], Uta Preim[2], Bernhard Preim[1], Myra Spiliopoulou[3]

[1]Department for Simulation and Graphics, OvG-University Magdeburg
[2]Department for Radiology, Municipal Hospital Magdeburg
[3]Knowledge Management and Discovery Lab (KMD), OvG-University Magdeburg
glasser@isg.cs.uni-magdeburg.de

Abstract. Classification of breast tumors solely based on dynamic contrast enhanced magnetic resonance data is a challenge in clinical research. In this paper, we analyze how the most suspect region as group of similarly perfused and spatially connected voxels of a breast tumor contributes to distinguishing between benign and malignant tumors. We use three density-based clustering algorithms to partition a tumor in regions and depict the most suspect one, as delivered by the most stable clustering algorithm. We use the properties of this region for each tumor as input to a classifier. Our preliminary results show that the classifier separates between benign and malignant tumors, and returns predictive attributes that are intuitive to the expert.

1 Introduction

Dynamic contrast enhanced magnetic resonance imaging (DCE-MRI) allows for perfusion characterization of breast tumors. DCE-MRI has high sensitivity but moderate specificity. So, it remains supplemental to conventional X-ray mammography and is frequently used to confirm the malignancy or benignity of lesions [1]. Malignant breast tumors often lead to neo-angiogenesis with increased tissue permeability and increased number of supporting vessels; this is usually reflected in a rapid contrast agent washing and/or washout. Hence, it is typical to define a region of interest (ROI) and to compute the ROI's average relative enhancement (RE) over time – the RE curve – for it. From the early RE and the curve's shape, the radiologist assesses the contrast agent washing and washout. Since a breast tumor is as malignant as its most malignant part, the RE curve of this ROI is used to determine the tumor's malignancy. In this study, we partition a ROI into regions that are homogeneous with respect to the RE curves of their voxels, and identify region features that contribute to predict malignancy.

The RE curves of the individual voxels are noisy by nature, so a major challenge lays in grouping them to homogeneous and spatially contiguous regions. Glaßer et al. propose a region merging method to this purpose [2], which is

H.-P. Meinzer et al. (Hrsg.), *Bildverarbeitung für die Medizin 2013*, Informatik aktuell,
DOI: 10.1007/978-3-642-36480-8_10, © Springer-Verlag Berlin Heidelberg 2013

used in [3] to study the role of tumor heterogeneity in predicting malignancy. Similar to our work is the study of Chen et al. [4], who perform clustering with fuzzy c-means and extract the most characteristic RE curve for the separation between benign and malignant tumors. However, our approach combines the identification of the most suspect region per tumor with the identification of predictive tumor characteristics that hold for multiple tumors.

2   Material and methods

In this paper, we study a set of 68 breast tumors. For each tumor, we apply multiple density-based clustering algorithms and identify the most suspect region. We extract the properties of this region and show that these properties contribute to distinguishing between benign and malignant tumors.

2.1   Tumor data

Our data set comprises 50 patients with 68 breast tumors. 31 tumors proved to be benign and 37 malignant (confirmation was carried out via histopathologic evaluation or by follow up studies after six to nine months). We included only lesions that have been detected in MRI. The data sets were acquired with a 1.0 T open MR scanner and exhibit the parameters: in-plane resolution $\approx 0.67 \times 0.67\,\mathrm{mm}^2$, matrix $\approx 528 \times 528$, number of slices ≈ 100, slice gap $= 1.5\,\mathrm{mm}$, number of acquisitions $= 5 - 6$ and total acquisition time $\approx 400\,\mathrm{sec}$. During and immediately after the bolus injection of contrast agent one pre-contrast and four to five post-contrast images were acquired per series. Since DCE-MRI data exhibit motion artifacts mainly due to thorax expansion through breathing and patient's movement, motion correction was carried out with MeVisLab (www.mevislab.de), employing the elastic registration developed by Rueckert et al. [5]. Next, the relative enhancement (RE) of a tumor, i.e. the percent aged signal intensity increase, is calculated [1] with $RE = (SI_c - SI)/SI \times 100$. Here, SI is the pre-contrast and SI_c is the post-contrast signal intensity. Each breast tumor was segmented by an experienced radiologist. The segmentation comprises only voxels exhibiting at least 50% RE at the first time step after the early post contrast phase.

2.2   Methods

Our approach consists of two steps: the extraction of the most suspect region for each tumor and the classification process over all tumors (Fig. 1).

Step 1: Extraction of the most suspect region of each tumor. We extract the most suspect region by determining descriptive perfusion parameters, three-time-point classes and applying density-based clustering.

The RE plotted over time yields RE curves that allow for the extraction of the descriptive perfusion parameters (Fig. 2(a)): washing (the steepness of

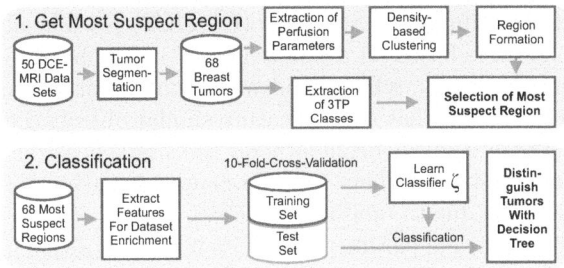

Fig. 1. Schematic overview of the presented approach. First, we determine each tumor's most suspect region. Second, we learn a classifier to predict malignancy.

the ascending curve), washout (the steepness of the descending curve), peak enhancement (the maximum RE value), integral (the area under the curve) and time to peak (the time when peak enhancement occurs), which are substitutes for physiological parameters like tumor perfusion and vessel permeability. Since peak enhancement and integral strongly correlate, we exclude peak enhancement from the subsequent analysis.

The three-time-point (3TP) method presented by Degani et al. [6] allows for an automatic RE curve classification based on three well chosen time points: t_1', the first point in time before the contrast agent injection, t_2', 2 min after t_1' and t_3', 4 min after t_2'. With the 3TP method, a RE change in the interval $\pm 10\%$ in the time between t_2' and t_3' will be interpreted as plateau, whereas RE changes higher than 10% and lower than -10% [6] are classified as increasing curve and washout curve, respectively. Since our study contains 5-6 time steps due to different scanning parameters, we assign the third time step to t_2' and the last time step to t_3'. The analysis of the initial contrast agent accumulation, i.e. the RE value at t_2', which is classified into slow, normal and fast in combination with the three curve shapes yields nine curve types (Fig. 2(b)). We compare the results of our clustering algorithms with the 3TP classes.

To evaluate the tumor enhancement, voxels with similar RE values are grouped into regions. We adapted and applied the following density-based clustering algorithms to our study: Density-based Spatial Clustering of Applications with Noise (DBSCAN) [7], Density-Connected Subspace Clustering (SUBCLU) [8],

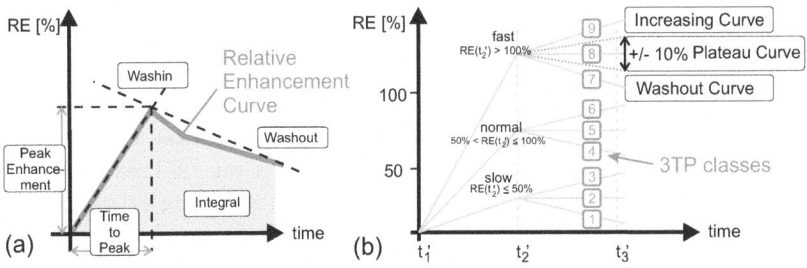

Fig. 2. In (a) a RE curve and its descriptive perfusion parameters are depicted. In (b), the 3TP classes based on RE at t_1', t_2', and t_3' are presented.

and Ordering Points to Identify the Clustering Structure (OPTICS) [9]. The algorithms separate objects into clusters based on estimated density distributions. They yield clusters with arbitrary shapes, which is advantageous for irregular and heterogeneous tumor parts. Objects that do not feature similar objects (i.e. objects with similar parameters) in a given neighborhood are marked as outliers. That's a further advantage, since outliers may be caused by a missing inter-voxel-correspondence over time due to motion artifacts.

Next, we employ each voxel's perfusion parameters and its relative position in the data set as observations. We apply DBSCAN, SUBCLU and OPTICS with the following parameters: the number of minimum points P_{min} for a cluster is set to 4, 6, and 8. The ϵ-value that determines the size of the neighborhood depends on the clustering. For DBSCAN and each P_{min} value, ϵ was automatically determined as suggested in [7]. For SUBCLU, we automatically estimate ϵ from the k-distances graph [7], as depicted in Fig. 3. We apply this approach to all four perfusion parameter sets and assign ϵ to the mean of the four estimated values. For OPTICS, we empirically set ϵ to 0.5 and 0.75. With $P_{min} \in \{4, 6, 8\}$, we get three configurations for DBSCAN and SUBCLU and six configurations for OPTICS yielding 12 clustering results per data set. Spatially connected clusters are maintained by a connected component analysis.

Fig. 3. Determination of ϵ based on the k-distances graph for a given P_{min} value. The graph maps the distance of an object to its k next neighbors (with $k = P_{min}$). A well suited ϵ can be detected at a position with increased slope. It is automatically determined by choosing the point with the biggest distance perpendicular to a line g connecting the first and the last point of the graph.

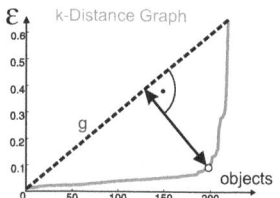

To select the most suspect region, we choose the clustering with the least outliers. Next, we reject all regions that contain less than three voxels. From the remaining regions, we choose the biggest region with an average RE curve of 3TP class 7. If no such region exists, we search for the 3TP class 9, 8, 4, 6, 5, 1, 3, 2 in that order. Although this is a user-defined ranking, we establish this empirical ranking based on definitions of the most malignant tumor enhancement kinetics: a present washout in combination with a strong washing (Fig. 2(b)).

Step 2: Data enrichment and classifier learning. In the second part, we combine the extracted data to learn a classifier ζ over our 68 breast lesions.

Data enrichment is carried out by including the following attributes of the tumor and its most suspect region: tumor size (in mm^3), number of tumor voxels, percent aged region size, number of region voxels, the similarity measures Purity (P), Jaccard index (J) and the F1 score (F_1) based on the comparison of our clustering and the 3TP-based division (we extracted and include values per tumor, per region and per outlier cluster), the region's mean perfusion parameters, the number of region voxels of each of the 3TP classes, the most prominent 3TP class (the 3TP class to which the majority of region voxels belong), the region's mean RE curve, the RE curve's 3TP class and the patient's age.

For our approach, we use the J4.8 classification algorithm of the Waikato Environment for Knowledge Analysis (Weka) library – a Java software library that encompasses algorithms for data analysis and predictive modeling [10]. J4.8 is based on the C4. 5 decision tree classification [11]. It performs 10-fold cross validation and requires at least two instances (two tumors) for each tree leaf. We worked iteratively, reducing the features under consideration and aiming to avoid features that are obviously predictive (such as tumor size), so that the predictive power of other features is highlighted. As a result, we came up with the classifier ζ (Fig. 4) that was learned on 18 of the original ca. 40 features.

3   Results

We learned a decision tree (Fig. 4) that employs eight of the 18 features and classifies 46 of the 68 lesions correctly. Features closer to the root of the tree are more important than those at lower levels, because the former help in splitting a larger set of tumors. We can see that the most important attributes are the heterogeneity of the tumor, as identified by the clustering algorithm (represented by J_{Tumor} and J_{Outlier}) and the age of the patient. The most prominent 3TP class, the number of voxels in the 3TP class 9 ($\#(3TP_9)$) and 6 ($\#(3TP_6)$), the contrast agent washing ($RE(t_3)$), and washout are also important.

4   Discussion

We presented a new method that combines within-tumor clustering and tumor classification to predict tumor malignancy, and we reported on our preliminary results on a data set with 68 breast tumors. Our first results indicate that the identification of the most suspect region with clustering and the exploitation of

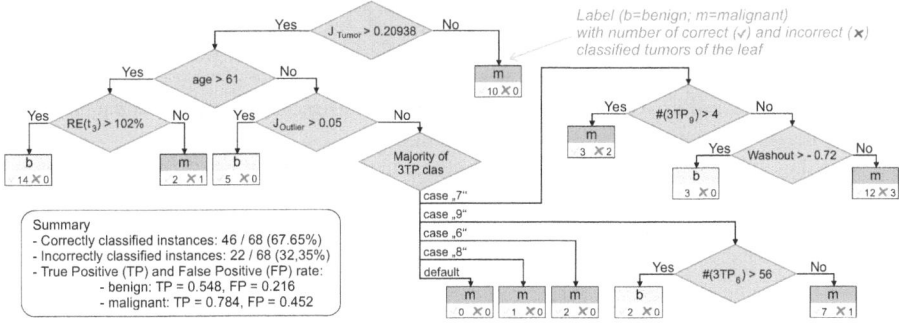

Fig. 4. Learned decision tree: the attributes at the upper part of the tree are the most important ones.

this region's features in classification are promising steps in tumor separation. The low sensitivity of our results must be attributed to the specific tumor type, for which it is difficult to distinguish between benignity and malignancy. In the future, we want to deepen and expand our findings in several directions. We intend to use 5-fold cross-validation and more rigid statistics on the 68-tumor data set, since it is very small for training. A further challenge arises from correlated tumors; which come from the same patient. We intend to apply dedicated methods for such instances within a bigger study in the future.

Acknowledgement. This work was partially supported by the DFG projects SPP 1335 "Scalable Visual Analytics" and SP 572/11-1 "IMPRINT: Incremental Mining for Perennial Objects".

References

1. Kuhl CK. The current status of breast MR imaging, part I. Radiology. 2007;244(2):356–78.
2. Glaßer S, Preim U, Tönnies K, et al. A visual analytics approach to diagnosis of breast DCE-MRI data. Comput Graph. 2010;34(5):602–11.
3. Preim U, Glaßer S, Preim B, et al. Computer-aided diagnosis in breast DCE-MRI: quantification of the heterogeneity of breast lesions. Eur J Radiol. 2012;81(7):1532–8.
4. Chen W, Giger ML, Bick U, et al. Automatic identification and classification of characteristic kinetic curves of breast lesions on DCE-MRI. Med Phys. 2006;33(8):2878–87.
5. Rueckert D, Sonoda L, Hayes C, et al. Nonrigid registration using free-form deformations: application to breast MR images. IEEE Trans Med Imaging. 1999;18(8):712–21.
6. Degani H, Gusis V, Weinstein D, et al. Mapping pathophysiological features of breast tumors by MRI at high spatial resolution. Nat Med. 1997;3:780–2.
7. Ester M, Kriegel HP, Sander J, et al. A density-based algorithm for discovering clusters in large spatial databases with noise. Proc KDD. 1996; p. 226–31.
8. Kailing K, Kriegel HP, Kröger P. Density-connected subspace clustering for high-dimensional data. Proc SIAM Data Mining. 2004; p. 246–57.
9. Ankerst M, Breunig MM, Kriegel HP, et al. OPTICS: Ordering points to identify the clustering structure. Proc ACM SIGMOD Conf Management Data. 1999; p. 49–60.
10. Holmes G, Donkin A, Witten IH. WEKA: a machine learning workbench. Proc Intelligent Information Systems. 1994; p. 357–61.
11. Quinlan JR. C4.5: Programs for Machine Learning. Morgan Kaufmann Publishers; 1993.

Quantification of Changes in Language-Related Brain Areas in Autism Spectrum Disorders Using Large-Scale Network Analysis

Caspar J. Goch[1], Bram Stieltjes[2], Romy Henze[2,3], Jan Hering[1],
Hans-Peter Meinzer[1], Klaus H. Fritzsche[1,2]

[1]Medical and Biological Informatics, DKFZ Heidelberg
[2]Quantitative Imaging-based Disease Characterization, DKFZ Heidelberg
[3]Child and Adolescent Psychiatry, Heidelberg University Hospital
c.goch@dkfz.de

Abstract. Diagnosis of autism spectrum disorders (ASD) is difficult, as symptoms vary greatly and are difficult to quantify objectively. Recent work has focused on the assessment of non-invasive diffusion tensor imaging based biomarkers of the disease that reflect the microstructural characteristics of neuronal pathways in the brain. While tractography-based approaches typically analyse specific structures of interest, a graph-based large-scale network analysis of the connectome can yield comprehensive measures of the global architecture of the brain. Aim of this work was to assess the concept of network centrality as a tool to perform structure specific analysis within the global network architecture. Our approach was evaluated on 18 children suffering from ASD and 18 typically developed controls using magnetic resonance imaging based cortical parcellations in combination with diffusion tensor imaging tractography. We show that the reduced capacity for comprehension of language in ASD is reflected in the significantly ($p < 0.001$) reduced network centrality of Wernicke's area while the motor cortex, that was used as a control region, did not show any significant alterations. Our results demonstrate the applicability of large-scale network analysis tools in the domain of region-specific analysis and may be an important contribution to future diagnostic tools in the clinical context of ASD diagnosis.

1 Introduction

Diffusion tensor imaging (DTI) has been increasingly used in the investigation of white matter alterations in autism spectrum disorder (ASD) patients [1]. Especially the study of the human connectome via large-scale network analysis and its application to the assessment of ASD and other mental illnesses has gathered a lot of interest in the recent years [2]. A large part of this interest has been focused on the study of differences of the global network for different diseases. Recent findings in an analysis of high-functioning autism patients demonstrate differences between high-functioning autism patients and healthy controls in the

H.-P. Meinzer et al. (Hrsg.), *Bildverarbeitung für die Medizin 2013*, Informatik aktuell,
DOI: 10.1007/978-3-642-36480-8_11, © Springer-Verlag Berlin Heidelberg 2013

clustering coefficient and the characteristic path length for the whole brain connectivity network [3].

While such an analysis of global network characteristics provides a good indicator for existing deviations of patients' from a healthy brain architecture, the applied measures may not necessarily be specific to the changes caused by one disease. In ASD for example, patients typically suffer significant reduction in communication capabilities while showing little to no reduction in motor control. The integrity of the language pathways has been suggested as a marker of ASD [4]. These specific changes however, are not reflected by global measures such as efficiency, small worldness, or clustering coefficient.

Based on the concept of centrality assessment [5], we present an approach that can complement a global characterization by analysing how a disease affects the global relationship of a specific set of nodes to the rest of the connectome. According to the symptomatology in ASD mentioned above, we focus our analysis on network hubs in the brain that are known to be involved in language processing and comprehension, namely Wernicke's area, which focuses on comprehension of speech, and Broca's area, which focuses on the motor control of speech. Recent research regarding the comprehension of speech suggests a different extent of the associated Wernicke's area [6]. The algorithms for network creation and network statistics were made available online as part of the diffusion component of the toolkit MITK[1] [7].

2   Materials and methods

2.1   Data acquisition

Evaluation was performed on a group of 18 right-handed children (16 m/2 f) with a mean (SD) chronological age of 9.7 (2.1) with a diagnosis of Asperger Syndrome or High Functioning Autism. The control group of 18 typically developed children of age 9.7 (1.9) was matched for age, sex and IQ. Data acquisition was done using a 1.5 T scanner (Siemens Avanto). T1 images for parcellation were taken with the following settings: MPRAGE TR/TE/TI/α = 1.9 s/4 ms/1.1 s/8°, FOV = 256 × 256 mm^2, matrix = 256 × 256, scan time 6 min). Diffusion weighted imaging was performed using single shot EPI with a dual bipolar diffusion gradient and a double spin echo for reduction of eddy currents with the following parameters: TR/TE 4700/78, FOV 192 mm, data matrix of 96 × 96 yielding an in-plane resolution of 2.0 mm, 50 axial slices with a thickness of 2.0 mm and no gap, with 6 gradient directions (b=1000 s/mm^2) and a b=0 image. This scheme was repeated 15 times.

2.2   Preprocessing and network construction

The entire image processing pipeline is depicted in Fig. 1. The T1 image was used to create a parcellation of the brain using freesurfer [8] as well as a binary mask

---

[1] http://www.mitk.org/

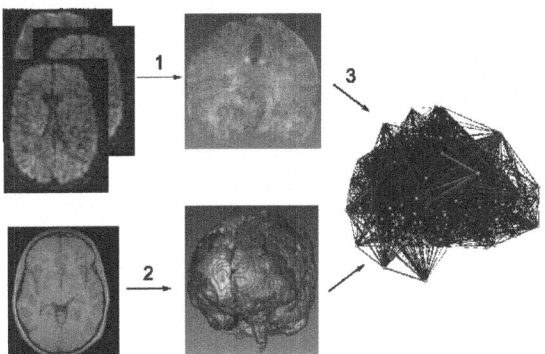

Fig. 1. Preprocessing pipeline.
1. Diffusion images are used to create a fiber image.
2. Anatomical MR image is used to create a parcellation of the brain.
3. Parcellation and fiber image are used to create a network.

of the brain. DWI images were motion and eddy-current corrected using FSL [9]. Q-ball images were then generated using solid angle reconstruction as provided by MITK [7]. Fiber tractography was performed on the q-ball images using the global tractography approach as presented by Neher et al. [10] using the brain mask to restrict the search space for possible fibers. The same settings were used to track each subject: 10^7 iterations, particle length of 3.4 mm, particle width of 1.2 mm, particle weight of 0.0018, start temperature of 0.1, end temperature of 0.001, energy balance of 0, minimal fiber length of 19 mm and curvature threshold of 45°. 5 patients and 3 controls were excluded due to heavy image artifacts and a resulting failure of the processing pipeline.

Connectivity matrices were created from the tractography result and the parcellation. DWI data and T1 images were registered using ANTs[2] for affine registration. Each label of the freesurfer segmentation was represented by one node if at least one fiber originated or ended within it. Two nodes were linked by an edge if at least one fiber connected the corresponding volumes. If a fiber ended either before encountering grey matter or outside of the brain mask it was assigned to a projected label. In the first case this was done by either extending it linearly until meeting either grey matter or background. In the second by retracting step by step until encountering either white matter or grey matter. If a fiber could not be assigned two different labels it was disregarded.

2.3 Assessment of subject specific nodal centralities

The betweenness centrality c is a measure for how central a given node is for the efficiency of the network. It describes how many shortest paths between any two nodes a and b pass through a given node n [5]

$$c(n) = \sum_{a \neq n \neq b} \frac{\sigma_{ab}(n)}{\sigma_{ab}} \tag{1}$$

where σ_{ab} is the number of shortest paths from node a to node b and $\sigma_{ab}(n)$ the number of those that pass through node n. As an area of interest might

---

[2] http://www.picsl.upenn.edu/ANTS/

consist of more than one node as defined by the freesurfer parcellation we propose to calculate a betweenness centrality for each area of interest by averaging the betweenness centrality of all composing nodes. We averaged the unweighted betweenness centrality for (always left and right hemisphere) Broca's area, Wernicke's area and the primary motor cortex. The primary motor cortex was used as a control region as no significant change was expected.

3   Results

The results of the network analysis can be seen in Fig. 2. A statistically relevant difference for the betweenness centrality of the Wernicke's area ($p < 0.001$) was found, for the primary motor cortex ($p = 0.707$) and Broca's area ($p = 0.269$) no such difference is visible.

4   Discussion

We presented an approach using large-scale structural network analysis and graph theoretical measures to analyse the impact of ASD on the betweenness centrality of brain areas responsible for the comprehension of speech.

For children suffering from autism spectrum disorders these areas show a significant reduction of importance in their relation to the rest of the brains connectome. On the other hand areas responsible for the motor control, for speech and in general, show no such reduction in importance. These observations correspond to known symptoms of ASD where patients show communication deficits but usually no significant impact on motor control [3].

While these results are promising, the low number of subjects coupled with a high failure rate during pre-processing need to be addressed. Our results suggest, that the betweenness centrality in the examined areas is a good measure to differentiate between ASD and controls. However we have not examined whether it may be used to distinguish between ASD and other neurological diseases, which might have a similar impact on the hubs of language comprehension. We also did not study the stability of our results with regard to the choice of other parcellation or tracking methods on the results, although our chosen method showed remarkable stability against the difference in the number of fibers found using global tractography. Tractography results for the ASD group as described by the number of fibers (SD) are with 6100 (1700) lower and more variable than for the control group 7970 (770). The control average does not include a single outlier at 56089 fibers, which was included in the evaluation and produced centrality measures similar to the rest of the group. This suggests the betweenness centrality to be a robust measure for quantifying the changes in the involvement of different brain areas in ASD.

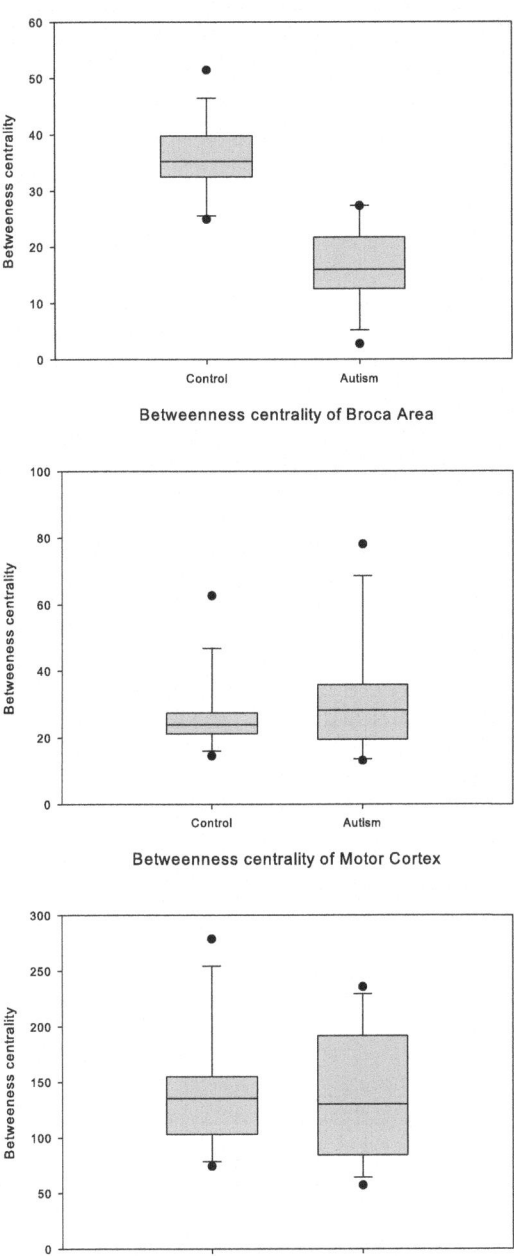

Fig. 2. Betweenness centrality of Wernicke's area, Broca's area and the primary motor cortex comparing control subjects and patients suffering from ASD. The betweenness centrality represents how integrated the corresponding area is in the connectome.

Further research is necessary to compare our method to other structure-specific analysis methods that are based on the quantification of diffusivity measures within the desired region of interest, as demonstrated in the literature [1]. Our approach, although focusing on specific areas, inherently takes the global changes of the entire network into consideration. With its combination of high sensitivity and robustness, we are confident, that it will be a valuable tool in the diagnosis of ASD.

References

1. Travers BG, Adluru N, Ennis C, et al. Diffusion tensor imaging in autism spectrum disorder: a review. Autism Res. 2012;5(5):289–313.
2. Bullmore E, Sporns O. Complex brain networks: graph theoretical analysis of structural and functional systems. Nat Rev Neurosci. 2009;10:186–98.
3. Li H, Xue Z, Ellmore TM, et al. Network-based analysis reveals stronger local diffusion-based connectivity and different correlations with oral language skills in brains of children with high functioning autism spectrum disorders. Hum Brain Mapp. 2012.
4. Lewis WW, Sahin M, Scherrer B, et al. Impaired language pathways in tuberous sclerosis complex patients with autism spectrum disorders. Cereb Cortex. 2012.
5. Freeman LC. A set of measures of centrality based on betweenness. Sociometry. 1977;40(1):35–41.
6. DeWitt I, Rauschecker JP. Phoneme and word recognition in the auditory ventral stream. Proc Natl Acad Sci U S A. 2012;109:E505–E514.
7. Fritzsche KH, Neher PF, Reicht I, et al. MITK diffusion imaging. Methods Inf Med. 2012; p. 441–8.
8. Fischl B, van der Kouwe A, Destrieux C, et al. Automatically parcellating the human cerebral cortex. Cereb Cortex. 2004;14(1):11–22.
9. Jenkinson M, Beckmann CF, Behrens TEJ, et al. FSL. Neuroimage. 2012;62(2):782–90.
10. Neher PF, Stieltjes B, Reisert M, et al. MITK global tractography. Proc SPIE. 2012;8314:83144D–83144D–6.

Personalisierte Modellierung der Progression primärer Hirntumoren als Optimierungsproblem mit Differentialgleichungsnebenbedingung

Andreas Mang[1], Jenny Stritzel[1], Alina Toma[1,2], Stefan Becker[1,2],
Tina A. Schuetz[1,3], Thorsten M. Buzug[1]

[1]Institut für Medizintechnik, Universität zu Lübeck (UL)
[2]Centre of Excellence for Technology and Engineering in Medicine (TANDEM)
[3]Graduiertenschule für Informatik in Medizin und Lebenswissenschaften, UL
mang@imt.uni-luebeck.de

Kurzfassung. Die vorliegende Arbeit liefert einen neuartigen Ansatz für die Individualisierung bildbasierter, biophysikalischer Modelle der Progression primärer Hirntumoren. Das verwendete mathematische Modell ist etabliert. Es basiert auf einer parabolischen, partiellen Differentialgleichung (PDG). Die Modellierung der Migration von Tumorzellen entlang der Nervenbahnen der weißen Substanz wird durch eine Integration von Diffusionstensordaten realisiert. Die Modellindividualisierung basiert auf der Lösung eines Parameteridentifikationsproblems. Der verwendete Ansatz führt auf ein Optimierungsproblem mit Differentialgleichungsnebenbedingung. Eine qualitative und quantitative Analyse für patientenindividuelle Bildgebungsdaten demonstriert die phänomenologische Validität des verwendeten Modells. Die gute Übereinstimmung zwischen der geschätzten Zustandsfunktion (Lösung des direkten Problems) und der Observable (gewonnen aus den Bildgebungsdaten) bestätigt die Methodik.

1 Einleitung

Die Prognose für Patienten mit der Diagnose einer aggressiven Manifestation primärer Hirntumoren ist fatal [1]. Eine zentrale Schwierigkeit für eine erfolgreiche Therapie ist das Vermögen einzelner tumoröser Zellen, in gesundes Gewebe vorzudringen. Infiltrierte Areale sind in klinischen in-vivo Bildgebungsdaten nicht detektierbar. Als Präventivmaßnahme wird typischerweise das proximal zum Tumorkern gelegene, gesund erscheinende Gewebe ebenfalls behandelt. Die Vorgehensweise ist in der Regel konservativ und empirisch. Dies macht es notwendig Verfahren zu entwickeln, die (i) eine systematische Analyse der Bilddaten erlauben, (ii) in einem besseren Verständnis der Pathophysiologie münden und (iii) es erlauben, prädiktive Faktoren aus patientenindividuellen Daten abzuleiten.

Ein vielversprechendes Werkzeug für eine systematische Bewertung einer Pathologie ist die mathematische Modellierung. Ein zentrales Problem liegt in der Modellindividualisierung. Diese ist nicht nur zwingend notwendig, um prädiktive Verfahren entwickeln zu können, sondern auch, um auf systematische Art

H.-P. Meinzer et al. (Hrsg.), *Bildverarbeitung für die Medizin 2013*, Informatik aktuell,
DOI: 10.1007/978-3-642-36480-8_12, © Springer-Verlag Berlin Heidelberg 2013

und Weise die phänomenologische Validität des Modells zu bestätigen. In der Literatur existieren zwei Verfahrensklassen zur Individualisierung bildbasierter Modelle des Wachstums primärer Hirntumoren [2, 3, 4]. Eine Möglichkeit ist die Verwendung einer Wandernde-Wellen-Lösung (WWL) [2]. Dieser Ansatz wurde in [3] in der Gestalt erweitert, dass die Heterogenität des Gewebes und der Verlauf der Nervenbahnen in die WWL einfließen. Allerdings sind starke Vereinfachungen vorzunehmen.

Betrachtet man die Problemstellung der Individualisierung einer PDG bezüglich vorliegender Daten existiert hierfür ein natürlicher, theoretischer Rahmen – die Theorie der optimalen Steuerung. Dieser Ansatz führt auf ein Optimierungsproblem mit Differentialgleichungsnebenbedingungen. In [4] wurde erstmals ein derartiges Verfahren für die Individualisierung eines bildbasierten, mathematischen Modells der Progression primärer Hirntumoren vorgestellt. Primäre Zielsetzung dieser Arbeit ist die Entwicklung hybrider Verfahren für die nicht-rigide Bildregistrierung [5]. Die vorliegende Arbeit ist durch [4] motiviert. Der zentrale Beitrag ist die Individualisierung eines diffusionstensorgestützten Modells und dessen phänomenologische Validierung basierend auf Bildgebungsdaten von 12 Patienten. Nach unserem besten Wissen ist dies die erste Arbeit, in der eine Individualsierung eines diffusionstensorgestützten Modells basierend auf der Theorie der optimalen Steuerung vorgestellt wird. Darüber hinaus wird eine Quantifizierung der Modelgüte für Bildgebungsdaten von 12 Patienten vorgenommen.

2 Material und Methoden

Im Folgenden wird zunächst das direkte Problem (Bestimmung der Zustandsfunktion unter Kenntnis der Systemparameter) und dann das zugehörige inverse Problem (Bestimmung der Systemparameter aus einer Observablen (im einfachsten Fall eine verrauschte Messung der Zustandsfunktion)) besprochen.

2.1 Direktes Problem

Das verwendete Modell ist etabliert ([6, 7] und Referenzen darin). Es basiert auf einer parabolischen PDG. Die Zustandsfunktion u modelliert die Dichte tumoröser Zellen in zerebralem Gewebe und ist von der Gestalt $u : \bar{\Omega}_B \times [t^0, \tau] \to \mathbf{R}_0^+$. Hierbei repräsentiert $\Omega_B \subset \Omega := (\omega_1^1, \omega_2^1) \times \cdots \times (\omega_1^d, \omega_2^d) \subset \mathbf{R}^d$, $d \in \{1, 2, 3\}$, mit Rand $\partial\Omega_B$ und Abschluss $\bar{\Omega}_B$, das durch das Gehirn eingenommene Gebiet; Ω_B setzt sich aus $\Omega_G \subset \Omega_B$ (graue Substanz) und $\Omega_W \subset \Omega_B$ (weiße Substanz) mit $\Omega_W \cap \Omega_G = \emptyset$ zusammen. Das Intervall $[t_0, \tau] \subset \mathbf{R}_0^+$ markiert den betrachteten Zeitraum. Das zugehörige Anfangsrandwertproblem ist durch

$$\partial_t u = \mathcal{L}(w, u) + \phi_\gamma(u) = \nabla \cdot (w \nabla u) + \gamma u(u - u_L), \quad \text{auf } \Omega_B \times (t_0, \tau] \quad (1)$$

$$\partial_n u = 0, \qquad\qquad\qquad\qquad\qquad \text{auf } \partial\Omega_B \times (t_0, \tau] \quad (2)$$

$$u(x, t_0) = u_I \exp\left(\|x_I - x\|_2^2 / 2\sigma_I^2\right), \qquad\qquad x \in \Omega_B \quad (3)$$

erklärt. Der Differentialoperator $\mathcal{L}$ beschreibt das Migrationsverhalten der Krebszellen und ϕ_γ die Zellvermehrung. Weiter ist $w : \Omega \to \mathbf{R}^{d \times d}$ ein Tensorfeld, $\gamma > 0$

die Wachstumsrate und $u_L > 0$ eine obere Schranke für die Zellpopulation. Gl. (2) schreibt homogene NEUMANN-Randbedingungen und (3) mit $x_I \in \Omega_B$, $\sigma_I > 0$ und $u_I > 0$ die Anfangsbedingungen vor. Das Modell für das Tensorfeld ist durch $w = \alpha \psi$, $\alpha : \Omega \to \mathbf{R}_0^+$, $\alpha = \kappa_W \alpha_W + \kappa_G \alpha_G$, $\kappa_l > 0$, $\alpha_l : \Omega \to [0,1]$, $l \in \{G, W\}$, $\psi = \Psi$, $\Psi : \Omega \to \mathbf{R}^{d \times d}$, für $x \in \Omega_W$ und $\psi = \mathrm{diag}(1, \ldots, 1) \in \mathbf{R}^{d \times d}$ sonst, erklärt. Die Koeffizienten κ_l parametrisieren die Ausbreitungsgeschwindigkeit in dem zugehörigen Gebiet Ω_l. Die Funktionen α_l repräsentieren unscharfe Gewebekarten; $\Psi : \Omega \to \mathbf{R}^{d \times d}$ ist ein durch Bildgebung gewonnenes Diffusionstensorfeld. über eine Skalierungsvorschrift ist es möglich, die Anisotropie des Tensorfeldes, kontrolliert über den Parameter $\beta > 0$ zu steuern. Im Folgenden wird für das direkte Problem (1)–(3) die kompakte Darstellung $\mathcal{C}(m, u) = 0$ mit der Inversionsvariablen m verwendet. Details zum Vorwärtsmodell, der Implementierung und den verwendeten Daten für die Simulation können [7] entnommen werden.

2.2 Inverses Problem

Ein natürlicher Formalismus für die Individualisierung eines auf einer PDG basierenden Modells ist durch die restringierte Optimierungsaufgabe

$$\min_{m,u} \mathcal{J}(m, u) \quad \text{u. d. N.} \quad \mathcal{C}(m, u) = 0, \quad m_L \le m \le m_U \tag{4}$$

erklärt. Die Differentialgleichungsnebenbedingung $\mathcal{C}(m, u) = 0$ in (4) wird als Zustandsgleichung bezeichnet, u ist die Zustandsfunktion, m repräsentiert die Inversionsvariablen und $m_L \in \mathbf{R}^{n_P}$ bzw. $m_U \in \mathbf{R}^{n_P}$, $n_P \in \mathbf{N}$, schreiben eine untere bzw. obere Schranke für die Inversionsvariable m vor. Typischerweise wird $\mathcal{J}$ als ein TIKHONOV-Funktional, das aus einem Defektfunktional $\mathcal{D}$ und einem Regularisierungsfunktional $\mathcal{R}$ besteht, modelliert [8]. Das Defektfunktional wird i. A. als L^2-Norm der Differenz zwischen Zustandsfunktion u und der Observablen y modelliert [4, 8]. In [4, 5] wird für die Bestimmung einer zu u äquivalenten Observablen y die Verwendung eines Klassifikators vorgeschlagen. Es bestehen allerdings Unsicherheiten inwiefern die berechnete Wahrscheinlichkeitskarte für die Gewebetypen tatsächlich mit der durch die Zustandsfunktion u getragenen Information Übereinstimmt [5]. Aus diesem Grund werden in der vorliegenden Arbeit zunächst manuelle Expertensegmentierungen des Tumors in kontrastmittelangereicherten T1 gewichteten (T1w+K) und T2 gewichteten (T2w) MRT Daten als Observable verwendet. Um eine äquivalente Information aus der Zustandsfunktion u abzuleiten, wird die in [2] vorgeschlagene Hypothese für die Detektionsschwelle in T1w+K (Schwellwert: 16% der maximalen Zelldichte) und T2w Daten (Schwellwert: 80% der maximalen Zelldichte) verwendet. Die manuelle Segmentierung liefert die binären Kennsätze $\mathcal{Y}^{h,1,k}$ und $\mathcal{Y}^{h,2,k}$ für den T1w+K bzw. den T2w Datensatz. Die Schwellwertbildung resultiert in den zugehörigen Kennsätzen $\mathcal{U}^{h,1}$ und $\mathcal{U}^{h,2}$. Um die Übereinstimmung der binären Kennsätze zu quantifizieren, schlagen wir das (semi-diskrete) Zielfunktional

$$\mathcal{J}^h(u, m) = -\frac{1}{2} \sum_{k=1}^{n_S} \int_0^\tau \delta(t - t_{\mathrm{aq}}^k) \sum_{l=1}^{n_B} \left(\frac{2 \#(\mathcal{U}^{h,l}(u, t) \cap \mathcal{Y}^{h,l,k})}{\#\mathcal{U}^{h,l}(u, t) + \#\mathcal{Y}^{h,l,k}} \right) \mathrm{d}t \tag{5}$$

vor. In (5) repräsentiert $n_S \in \mathbf{N}$ die Anzahl der Akquisitionszeitpunkte t^k_{aq} (im vorliegenden Fall ist n_s wegen der typischen, klinischen Datenlage auf einen Zeitpunkt beschränkt), $n_B \in \mathbf{N}$ die Anzahl der binären Kennsätze pro Patient (d. h. $n_B = 2$) und $\#\mathcal{X}$ die Kardinalität einer Menge $\mathcal{X}$. Wegen der Gestalt von (5) wird für die Optimierung ein robustes, ableitungsfreies Suchverfahren verwendet [9]. Ein Regularisierungsfunktional ist in der vorliegenden Implementierung nicht vorgesehen. Die Wahl der Schranken m_L und m_U wird zusammen mit der Wahl der zu optimierenden Parameter im folgenden Abschnitt präzisiert.

2.3 Modellparameter

Zum derzeitigen Entwicklungsstadium muss eine Vielzahl an empirischen Annahmen einfließen, um eine solide Lösung des inversen Problems zu garantieren. Schwierigkeiten liegen in den Unsicherheiten in der (manuellen) Segmentierung und den Parameterbereichen, in den Partialvolumenartefakten und in der Spärlichkeit der Daten (ein Zeitpunkt mit präoperativen Daten; Darstellung des Tumors als Niveaumenge). Um die assoziierten Unsicherheiten für die Inversionsvariablen zu reduzieren, werden folgende Annahmen getroffen: Die Initialbedingungen werden festgehalten ($u_I = u_L$, $\sigma = 0.2$; x_I wird aus dem Tumorkennsatz (T1w+K) als Massenmittelpunkt bestimmt). Das Zeitfenster zwischen Auftreten der Pathologie bis zum Zeitpunkt der Bildakquisition wird basierend auf Erfahrungen aus Vorwärtsexperimenten abgeschätzt. Die Inversion wird für unterschiedliche Zeitfenster durchgeführt. Das quantitativ beste Resultat wird verwendet. Die verbleibenden Parameter werden optimiert. Es gilt $m := (\kappa_W, s, \beta, \gamma) \in \mathbf{R}^4$, mit $\kappa_G = s\kappa_W$. Um den Suchraum auf einen biophysiologisch sinnvollen Bereich zu beschränken, werden folgende Parameterschranken (basierend auf Erfahrungen aus Vorwärtsexperimenten und plausiblen Werten aus der Literatur (siehe bspw. [2, 4, 6])) verwendet: $m_L = (1.00\,\mathrm{E}\text{-}07\,\mathrm{m}^2/\mathrm{d}, 1, 1, 0.05/\mathrm{d})$, $m_U = (5.00\,\mathrm{E}\text{-}07\,\mathrm{m}^2/\mathrm{d}, 10, 4, 0.15/\mathrm{d})$ und $m_I = (3.00\,\mathrm{E}\text{-}07\,\mathrm{m}^2/\mathrm{d}, 5, 1, 0.1/\mathrm{d})$.

3 Ergebnisse

Ein exemplarisches Resultat für die Modellkalibrierung ist in Abb. 1 (oben,links) dargestellt. Die obere Reihe zeigt die reinen Simulationsergebnisse. In der mittleren Reihe ist das Simulationsergebnis nach Schwellwertbildung den (affin mit dem Atlas registrierten) T1w+K Daten überlagert. In der unteren Reihe sind die Simulationsergebnisse den T2w Daten gegenübergestellt. Eine Quantifizierung der Güte der Kalibrierung erfolgt über den DICE-Koeffizient (mittlere überdeckung) $\mathcal{D}^h_M$ und den mittleren HAUSDORFF-Abstand $\mathcal{D}^h_H$. Die Ergebnisse sind ebenfalls in Abb. 1 zusammengetragen. Basierend auf dem DICE-Koeffizient wurde für drei der zwölf Patienten (P_i, $i = 1, \ldots, 12$) eine unzureichende Übereinstimmung zwischen Zustandsfunktion und Bilddaten festgestellt (Schwellwert für $\mathcal{D}^h_D$: 66% Übereinstimmung, (gestrichelte, horizontale Linie in Abb. 1 (oben rechts; unten links))). Die Auswertung in Abb. 1 stellt sowohl die Ergebnisse für das gesamte Patientenkollektiv ($K_G := \{P_1, \ldots, P_{12}\}$)

als auch für die Patienten, für welche die Simulation als erfolgreich gewertet wurde, dar ($K_E := K_G \setminus \{P_2, P_3, P_6\}$). Zur Einordnung des mittleren HAUSDORFF-Abstandes ist die Voxeldiagonale der T1w+K (grün) und der T2w (blau) Daten als vertikale Linie in Abb. 1 (rechts, unten) eingezeichnet.

4   Diskussion

In der vorliegenden Arbeit wurde ein neuartiger Ansatz zur Individualisierung eines tensorgestützten, mathematischen Modells der Progression primärer Hirntumoren basierend auf einem Problem der optimalen Steuerung vorgestellt. Hierauf aufbauend wurde eine phänomenlogische Validierung der Methodik für präoperative Daten von 12 Patienten vorgenommen. Eine quantitative und qualitative Analyse der Resultate zeigt eine gute Übereinstimmung der Simulation und den Expertensegmentierung des Tumors. Im Detail liefert die Auswertung eine gute Übereinstimmung in 9 der 12 Patientendaten. Diskrepanzen treten vornehmlich dann auf, wenn große anatomische Unterschiede zwischen Atlas (Simulationsraum) und den patientenindividuellen Daten vorliegen. Ein weiteres zentrales Problem sind durch den Tumor induzierte, morphologische Veränderungen, die von dem derzeitigen Modell nicht abgebildet werden (Gewebedeformation). Eine

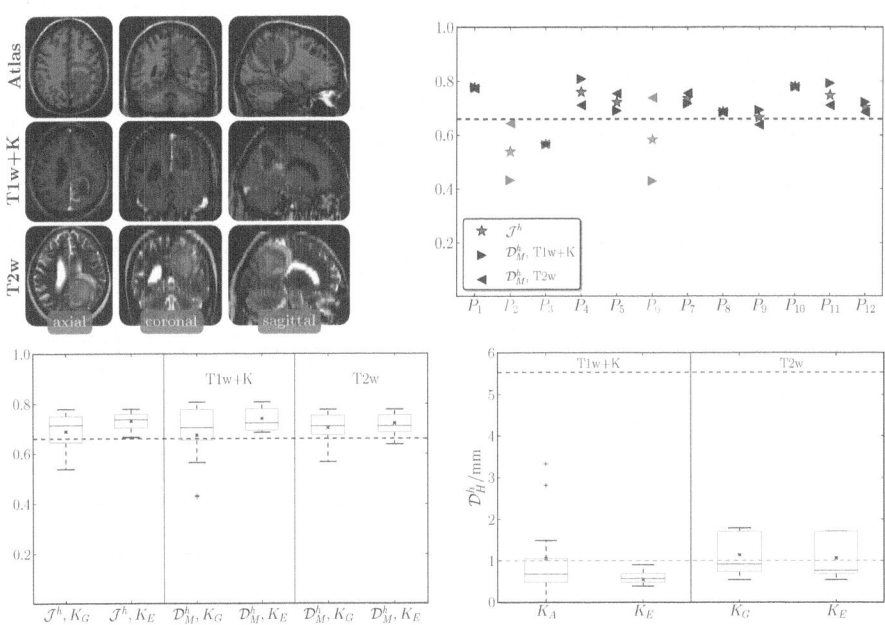

Abb. 1. Qualitative und quantitative Analyse der Resultate. Obere Reihe: Exemplarisches Resultat für die Modellkalibrierung (links) und DICE-Koeffizient für die patientenindividuellen Datensätze (rechts). Untere Reihe: Box-Whisker-Plots zur Auswertung des DICE-Koeffizienten (links) und des HAUSSDORF-Abstandes (rechts).

Simulation in den Patientendaten ist nicht möglich, da jeweils nur ein präoperativer Datensatz vorliegt (d. h. die Initialbedingungen können nicht direkt in den Bilddaten etabliert werden). Die Ziele für weiterführende Arbeiten sind vielseitig. Von der Berücksichtigung der Gewebedeformation [4] wird eine Verbesserung der Resultate erwartet. Weiter gilt es zu untersuchen inwiefern funktionelle Bildgebung für eine Kalibrierung des Modells gewinnbringend eingesetzt werden kann. Zudem soll für das Zielfunktional eine L^2-Distanz zwischen Zustandsvariable und Observable verwendet werden mit dem Ziel, den direkten Zugang zu etablierten numerischen Verfahren zu ermöglichen [8]. Hierfür ist es notwendig, einen Zusammenhang zwischen der Zustandsvariablen und den Intensitätsmustern in den Bilddaten zu etablieren. Neben der in [4, 5] vorgeschlagenen Verwendung von Klassifikatoren, ist eine übertragung der berechneten Zelldichte in Intensitätsmuster denkbar. Ein weiteres unserer zukünftigen Ziele ist es, derartige Verfahren für hybride Ansätze in der nichtrigiden Bildregistrierung einzusetzen [5, 10].

Danksagung. Diese Arbeit wird gefördert durch die Europäische Union und das Land Schleswig-Holstein (AT,SB) [Fördernummer 122-09-024] und die Exzellenzinitiative des Bundes (TAS) [Fördernummer DFG GSC 235/1]. Wir danken Christian Mohr, Thomas Eckey und Dirk Petersen vom Institut für Neuroradiologie der Universität zu Lübeck für die Unterstützung.

Literaturverzeichnis

1. Maher EA, Furnari FB, Bachoo RM, et al. Malignant glioma: Genetics and biology of a grave matter. Genes Dev. 2001;15(11):1311—33.
2. Swanson KR, Rostomily RC, Alvord EC. A mathematical modelling tool for predicting survival of individual patients following resection of glioblastoma: A proof of principle. Brit J Cancer. 2008;98(1):113–9.
3. Konukoglu E, Clatz O, Menze BH, et al. Image guided personalization of reaction-diffusion type tumor growth models using modified anisotropic eikonal equations. IEEE T Med Imaging. 2010;29(1):77–95.
4. Hogea C, Davatzikos C, Biros G. An image-driven parameter estimation problem for a reaction-diffusion glioma growth model with mass effects. J Math Biol. 2008;56(6):793–825.
5. Gooya A, Pohl KM, Bilello M, et al. GLISTR: Glioma image segmentation and registration. IEEE T Med Imaging. 2012;31(10):1941–54.
6. Murray JD. Mathematical biology. 3rd ed. New York: Springer; 2008.
7. Mang A, Toma A, Schuetz TA, et al. Eine effiziente Parallel-Implementierung eines stabilen Euler-Cauchy-Verfahrens fuer die Modellierung von Tumorwachstum. Proc BVM. 2012; p. 63–8.
8. Adavani SS, Biros G. Multigrid algorithms for inverse problems with linear parabolic PDE constraints. SIAM J Sci Comput. 2008;31(1):369–97.
9. Plantenga TD. HOPSPACK 2.0 user manual. Albuquerque, NM and Livermore, CA: Sandia National Laboratories; 2009. SAND2009-6265.
10. Mang A, Toma A, Schuetz TA, et al. A generic framework for modeling brain deformation as a constrained parametric optimization problem to aid non-diffeomorphic image registration in brain tumor imaging. Meth Inf Med. 2012;51:429–40.

Segmentierung der lumbalen Bandscheiben in MRT-Bilddaten

Regina Pohle-Fröhlich[1], Christian Brandt[1], Timmo Koy[2]

[1]iPattern – Institut für Mustererkennung, Hochschule Niederrhein, Krefeld
[2]Klinik für Orthopädie und Unfallchirurgie, Universität Köln
regina.pohle@hsnr.de

Kurzfassung. In dem Beitrag wird eine dreistufige vollautomatische Methode für die Segmentierung der lumbalen Bandscheiben in MRT-Daten vorgeschlagen. Diese besteht aus der Detektion der Wirbelsäule mittels horizontaler Symmetrietransformation, Lokalisierung der Bandscheiben durch ein lokales Schwellwertverfahren und Konturverfolgung kombiniert mit einer Graphsuche zur endgültigen Segmentierung. Die Leistungsfähigkeit des entwickelten Verfahrens wird anhand des Vergleichs mit einer manuellen Segmentierung eingeschätzt.

1 Einleitung

Mit zunehmendem Alter treten abhängig von der mechanischen Belastung, von Verletzungen, von der Ernährung und von genetischen Faktoren bei vielen Menschen chronische Veränderungen der Bandscheiben auf. Die Diagnose derartiger Veränderungen erfolgt in der klinischen Praxis bevorzugt anhand von MRT-Bildern. T_2-Relaxationszeiten geben dabei Auskunft über den Wassergehalt, den Kollagengehalt sowie die Kollagenstruktur des Bandscheibengewebes. Zur objektiven Quantifizierung der Bandscheibenveränderung anhand der mittleren T_2-Zeiten ist zuvor eine zuverlässige Segmentierung der Bandscheiben in den Bildern erforderlich. Diese Segmentierung erfolgt zumeist in geometrisch identisch aufgenommenen T_1-Bildern, da sich hier die Bandscheiben besser von der Umgebung abgrenzen lassen.

In der Literatur werden verschiedene Ansätze zur automatischen und semiautomatischen Segmentierung von Bandscheiben in MRT-Aufnahmen beschrieben. So nutzen Seifert u.a. einen modellbasierten Ansatz, bei dem die generalisierte Hough-Transformation in Verbindung mit einem Active Shape Modell verwendet wird [1]. In [2] wird eine Atlas-basierte Segmentierung eingesetzt. Die Nutzung von modellbasierten Methoden mit nur einem Formmodell für alle Bandscheiben lieferte bei Tests für die Bilddaten in unserer Studie viele fehlerhafte Segmentierungsergebnisse, da das Aussehen der Bandscheiben teilweise stark variierte. Für die Ableitung eines zuverlässigeren Formmodells hätte pro Bandscheibenposition eine große Anzahl von Bandscheiben manuell segmentiert werden müssen. Diese Daten standen für die Studie nicht zur Verfügung. Eine andere Arbeit beruht auf einem Ansatz zur Textursegmentierung [3]. Dieser wurde jedoch aufgrund

H.-P. Meinzer et al. (Hrsg.), *Bildverarbeitung für die Medizin 2013*, Informatik aktuell,
DOI: 10.1007/978-3-642-36480-8_13, © Springer-Verlag Berlin Heidelberg 2013

der geringen Größe der Bandscheibenregionen in unserer Studie verworfen. Das in [4] diskutierte Graphschnitt-Verfahren wurde in einer Voruntersuchung ebenfalls getestet. Aufgrund der ungleichmäßigen Helligkeitsverteilung innerhalb der Bandscheibenregion wurde bei diesem Ansatz die Region des Anulus fibrosus, die meist etwas dunkler als die des Nucleus pulposus war, häufig nicht erfasst. Schließlich ist in der Literatur noch der Einsatz der Wasserscheidentransformation beschrieben [5]. Aufgrund des hohen Rauschanteils in den Daten lieferten Tests jedoch kein zufrieden stellendes Ergebnis. Auch die Segmentierung mit einer markerbasierten Wasserscheidentransformation war nicht geeignet, da hier die gleichen Probleme wie bei der Segmentierung mit den Graphschnitten auftraten.

2   Gewählte Segmentierungsmethode

Die Segmentierung der lumbalen Bandscheiben erfolgt bei dem hier vorgestellten Verfahren, welches für die Auswertung von T_1-Bilddaten entwickelt wurde, in drei Stufen. Nach einer anisotropen Diffusion zur kantenerhaltenden Bildglättung wird zuerst mittels winkelabhängiger horizontaler Symmetrietransformation die Mittelachse der Wirbelsäule in den Aufnahmen bestimmt. Danach werden in einem zweiten Schritt durch den Einsatz eines Schwellwertverfahrens die Bandscheiben entlang der Mittelachse lokalisiert. Zur endgültigen Segmentierung der Bandscheiben wird abschließend ein Konturverfolgungsalgorithmus in Kombination mit einer Graphsuche eingesetzt. Auf die einzelnen Schritte wird im Folgenden näher eingegangen.

2.1   Horizontale Symmetrietransformation zur Positionsbestimmung der Wirbelsäule

Betrachtet man die Bilddaten (Abb. 1a), so fällt auf, dass sowohl die Wirbelsäule als auch die Bandscheiben selbst im Gegensatz zu den restlichen sichtbaren Strukturen im Bild einen hohen Grad an Symmetrie aufweisen. Zur Charakterisierung der an einem Bildpunkt vorliegenden Symmetrie eignet sich die Symmetrietransformation von Reisfeld [6]. Die Symmetrie für jeden Punkt p und jede Richtung ψ wird danach definiert als

$$S_{\sigma(p,\psi)} = \sum_{(i,j)\in\Gamma(p,\psi)} D_\sigma(i,j)P(i,j)r_i r_j \qquad (1)$$

Die Menge $\Gamma(p,\psi)$ bezeichnet hierbei alle Punktepaare p_i und p_j mit dem Symmetriezentrum p und einer Symmetrierichtung ψ, die sich als Mittelwert aus den Gradientenrichtungen θ_i und θ_j der beiden betrachteten Punkte bezogen auf die horizontale Achse ergibt. $D_\sigma(i,j)$ ist eine Gewichtung in Form einer zweidimensionalen Gauß-Funktion, die regelt, in wie weit entfernter liegende Bildpunkte zur Symmetrie beitragen sollen. Der Wert für σ wird in unserem Fall abhängig von der Bildgröße so gewählt, dass direkt benachbart liegende Pixel p_i und

p_j dreimal mehr zur Symmetrie beitragen als wenn sie sich am weitesten voneinander entfernt befinden würden. $P(i,j)$ bezeichnet ein Phasengewicht und berechnet sich nach Reisfeld wie folgt

$$P(i,j) = (1 - \cos(\theta_i + \theta_j - 2\alpha_{ij}))(1 - \cos(\theta_i - \theta_j)) \qquad (2)$$

mit α_{ij} als dem Winkel zwischen der Geraden durch die beiden Punkte p_i und p_j und der horizontalen Achse. Es liefert einen maximalen Symmetriewert, wenn die Gradientenrichtungen der beiden betrachteten Punkte in genau entgegengesetzte Richtung verlaufen. Für r_i und r_j wird die Gradientenstärke an den beiden betrachteten Punkten verwendet, da diese im Gegensatz zu der bei Reisfeld verwendeten logarithmischen Skalierung der Gradientenstärke die besseren Ergebnisse lieferte.

In Tests hat sich herausgestellt, dass die vertikale Symmetrie innerhalb der Wirbelsäule weniger stark ausgeprägt ist als die von anderen Strukturen. Deshalb werden bei der Auswertung der Bilddaten nur die horizontalen Symmetrien betrachtet. Eine horizontale Symmetrie liegt in unserem Fall vor, wenn die für zwei betrachtete Punkte p_i und p_j ermittelte mittlere Symmetrierichtung ψ nur $\pm 15^o$ von der horizontalen Achse abweicht. Das Ergebnis der Symmetrietransformation für jeden Pixel ergibt sich durch Aufsummieren der Symmetriewerte über den zulässigen horizontalen Winkelbereich. Da die lumbale Wirbelsäule in der Sagitalebene eine starke S-förmige Krümmung aufweist, muss die Lage der horizontale Achse für die einzelnen Bildzeilen angepasst werden. Eine grobe Abschätzung der Krümmung reicht jedoch aus, weil bei der zulässigen Symmetrierichtung eine Abweichung von $\pm 15^o$ zugelassen wird. Zur Bestimmung der mitt-

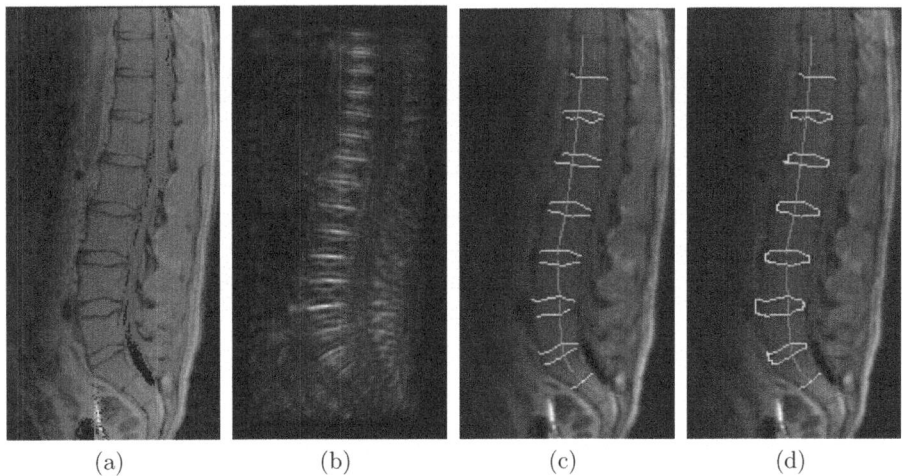

(a)   (b)   (c)   (d)

Abb. 1. a) T_1-Aufnahme der Wirbelsäule, b) Ergebnis der Symmetrietransformation, c) approximierte Bezier-Kurve (rot) und Ergebnis nach der Konturverfolgung ausgehend von den detektierten Startpixeln, d) Endergebnis der Bandscheibensegmentierung.

leren Krümmung wurde eine manuelle Segmentierung der vorderen Längsbänder der Wirbelsäule in 10 Beispielbildern unterschiedlicher Probanden durchgeführt. Anschließend wurde aus den berechneten Winkeln für jede Zeile ein mittlerer Krümmungswinkel bestimmt, um den die horizontale Achse in allen Bilddaten korrigiert wird. Das Ergebnis der Symmetrietransformation ist für das Beispielbild in Abb. 1b zu sehen.

Zur Identifikation der ungefähren Lage der Wirbelsäule im Bild wird über die obersten 50 Zeilen jedes Bildes das integrierte Zeilenprofil erstellt, da die Krümmung der Wirbelsäule in diesem Bereich nur gering ist. In diesem Zeilenprofil wird der Maximalwert bestimmt, der sich mittig innerhalb der Wirbelsäule befindet. Ausgehend von diesem Startpixel wird in einem rechteckigen Bereich von 20x10 Pixeln, der in Abhängigkeit von der jeweiligen Krümmung der Wirbelsäule positioniert wird, nach weiteren Pixeln mit maximaler Symmetrie gesucht. Dieser Suchbereich wird solange auf die zuletzt gefundene Position verschoben, bis die letzte Zeile erreicht ist. Die sich ergebenden Punkte liefern in etwa die Mittellinie der Wirbelsäule. An diese detektierten Mittellinienpunkte wird eine Bezier-Kurve angepasst (Abb. 1c).

2.2 Lokalisierung der Bandscheiben

Im nächsten Schritt wird entlang der berechneten Bezier-Kurve das Grauwertprofil ermittelt (Abb. 2). Es ist deutlich zu erkennen, dass aufgrund der dunkleren Grauwerte die Begrenzung der Bandscheiben gut zu finden ist. Eine reine Suche nach lokalen Minima ist jedoch nicht anwendbar, da die Daten trotz Bildglättung immer noch stark verrauscht sind. Weiterhin enthalten die Bilddaten Shading, so dass ein lokales Schwellwertverfahren zur Identifikation der Bandscheibenposition eingesetzt wird. In einigen Fällen werden bei dieser Vorgehensweise jedoch zu viele Startpixel gefunden. In einem Korrekturschritt wird, wenn mehrere ausgewählte Startpixel einen geringeren euklidischen Abstand als 3 Pixel besitzen, nur derjenige Pixel mit dem niedrigsten Grauwert weiter betrachtet.

2.3 Ermittlung der Bandscheibenkontur

Ausgehend von den Startpixeln wird jeweils eine Konturverfolgung nach links in Richtung der abnehmenden x-Koordinaten und nach rechts in Richtung der aufsteigenden x-Koordinaten vorgenommen. Als Start- und Stoppkriterium für die

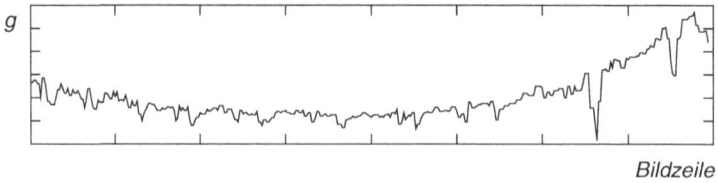

Abb. 2. Grauwert g entlang der approximierten Bezier-Kurve als Funktion der Bildzeile.

Konturverfolgung wird die Streuung von fünf Pixeln, die vertikal übereinander liegen und je nach Richtung einen um eins größeren oder kleineren Spaltenindex als der aktuelle Pixel aufweisen, ausgewertet. Liegt diese Streuung für einen betrachteten Pixel oberhalb des Schwellenwerts von $t = 3$, so startet die Konturverfolgung. Die Verfolgung wird dann solange fortgesetzt, bis die Streuung unter den Schwellenwert fällt, da dann entweder die Kontur nicht mehr sicher detektierbar oder das vordere bzw. hintere Längsband der Wirbelsäule erreicht ist. Das Ergebnis dieser Verfolgung ist für das Beispiel in Abb. 1c zu sehen. Das Schließen der Lücken zwischen zwei gefundenen linken bzw. rechten Konturendpunkten erfolgt mittels Graphsuche, wobei der Grauwert eines Pixels seine Knotenkosten festlegt. Da mit diesem Verfahren Wege mit minimalen Kosten zwischen zwei Punkten gefunden werden, ist sichergestellt, dass die Verbindungen auf den Grenzen der Bandscheiben verlaufen, weil diese geringere Grauwerte als ihre Umgebung aufweisen. Das Ergebnis der Segmentierung nach der Verbindung der Endpunkte ist in Abb. 1d dargestellt.

3   Ergebnisse

Die Bewertung der erzielten Segmentierungsergebnisse erfolgte unter zwei verschiedenen Gesichtspunkten. Zuerst wurde untersucht, ob die Methode zur Detektion der Mittelachse der Wirbelsäule korrekte Ergebnisse liefert. Zur Evaluation standen in diesem Fall 84 Bilder zur Verfügung. Die visuelle Auswertung ergab, dass in 82 Bildern die ermittelten Spline-Kurven korrekt innerhalb der Wirbelsäule positioniert waren. In zwei Bildern gingen durch die anisotrope Diffusion die Begrenzungen der Bandscheiben der Brustwirbelsäule Th10 bis Th12 teilweise verloren, so dass in diesem Bereich kaum horizontale Symmetrie vorlag und dadurch die Kurven falsch positioniert wurden.

Anschließend wurde die korrekte Detektion der Bandscheiben untersucht. Hierfür lagen manuelle Segmentierungen von 212 Bandscheiben in 33 Bildern, die auf einem Tablet-PC erstellt wurden, vor. Von diesen Bandscheiben konnten mit dem vorgeschlagenen Verfahren 187 vollautomatisch segmentiert werden, was einer Erkennungsrate von 88,2% entspricht. Die restlichen 25 Bandscheiben wiesen teilweise einen so geringen Kontrast zur Umgebung auf, so dass sie bei der Konturverfolgung nur in Teilen segmentiert wurden.

Da bei der späteren objektiven Charakterisierung von Bandscheibenveränderungen Kenngrößen berechnet werden, die von einer Unterteilung der segmentierten Fläche in drei Teilsegmente (Nucleus pulposus, vorderer und hinterer Anulus fibrosus) ausgehen, wurde zur Bewertung der Güte der Segmentierung zunächst der Anteil der korrekt segmentierten Fläche sowie das Auftreten von Unter- bzw. Übersegmentierung betrachtet. Im Vergleich zur manuellen Segmentierung wurden durchschnittlich 91% $\pm$ 5,4% der Fläche korrekt erkannt. Pro Bandscheibe wurden im Durchschnitt 16,2 $\pm$ 10,8 Pixel zu wenig detektiert. Bezogen auf die mittlere Fläche der Bandscheibenregion entspricht das einem Wert von 9% zuwenig detektierter Objektfläche. Die Übersegmentierung betrug 18,7 $\pm$ 12,3 Pixel, was 10% zuviel detektierter Objektfläche gleichkommt. Um die Qualität der Ergebnisse besser einschätzen zu können, wurde in einem nächsten Schritt untersucht, wie weit die Konturpunkte des Segmentierungsergebnisses von der Objektgrenze in der manuellen Segmentierung entfernt sind. Für die detektierten Bandscheiben ergab sich im Durchschnitt eine mittlere Abweichung zwischen beiden Konturen von 0,6 ± 0,3 Pixeln. Der maximal auftretende mittlere Fehler zwischen den Konturpunkten betrug 1,9 Pixel. Um festzustellen, wie weit die detektierten Punkte maximal von der manuell segmentierten Kontur entfernt sind, wurde der Hausdorff-Abstand bestimmt. Dieser betrug im Durchschnitt 2,7 ± 1,5 Pixel.

Zum Vergleich wurden fünf manuelle Segmentierungen eines Bildes, die zu unterschiedlichen Zeitpunkten erstellt wurden, miteinander verglichen. Hier ergab sich eine durchschnittliche mittlere Konturabweichung von 0,5 ± 0,2 Pixeln und ein durchschnittlicher Hausdorff-Abstand von 1,6 ± 0,5 Pixeln. Die durchschnittliche Flächenüberdeckung lag bei 90,9% ± 4,5% und die durchschnittliche Unter- und Übersegmentierung betrugen 8,9% bzw. 7,2% bezogen auf die mittlere Objektgröße.

4   Diskussion und Resümee

Die vorgeschlagene vollautomatische Segmentierungsmethode lieferte Ergebnisse, die im Bereich der Genauigkeit der manuellen Segmentierung liegen. Eine Verbesserung des vorgeschlagenen Verfahrens könnte erreicht werden, indem die lokale Schwellwertsegmentierung zur Lokalisierung der Bandscheibenposition auf die gesamte Region der Wirbelsäule angewandt wird. Dazu müssten jedoch zunächst noch das vordere und hintere Längsband detektiert werden.

Literaturverzeichnis

1. Seifert S, Wächter I, Schmelzle G, et al. A knowledge-based approach to soft tissue reconstruction of the cervical spine. IEEE Trans Med Imaging. 2009;28(4):494–507.
2. Michopoulo S, Costaridou L, Panagiotopoulos E, et al. Atlas-based segmentation of degenerated lumbar intervertebral disk from MR images of the spine. IEEE Trans Biomed Eng. 2009;56(9):2225–31.
3. Chevrifils C, Cheriet F, Aubin C, et al. Texture analysis for automatic segmentation of intervertebral disks of scoliotic spines from MR images. IEEE Trans Inf Technol Biomed. 2009;13(4):608–20.
4. Carballido-Gamio J, Belongie S, Majumdar S. Normalized cuts in 3-D for spinal MRI segmentation. IEEE Trans Med Imaging. 2004;23(1):36–44.
5. Chevrifils C, Cheriet F, Grimard G. Watershed segmentation of intervertebral disk and spinal canal from MRI images. LNCS. 2007;4633:1017–27.
6. Reisfeld D, Wolfson H, Yeshurun Y. Context-free attentional operators: The generalized symmetry transform. Int J Computer Vis. 1995;14(2):119–30.

Ein kubusbasierter Ansatz zur Segmentierung von Wirbeln in MRT-Aufnahmen

Robert Schwarzenberg[1,2], Bernd Freisleben[2], Ron Kikinis[1],
Christopher Nimsky[3], Jan Egger[1,2,3]

[1]Surgical Planning Laboratory, Brigham and Women's Hospital,
Harvard Medical School
[2]Dept. of Mathematics and Computer Science, University of Marburg
[3]Dept. of Neurosurgery, University of Marburg
rs@bwh.harvard.edu

Kurzfassung. In diesem Beitrag präsentieren wir ein graphbasiertes Verfahren zur volumetrischen Wirbelsegmentierung in MRT-Aufnahmen, das zur Segmentierung eine würfelförmige Vorlage nutzt. Dabei kann der Nutzer den Grad Δ (Smoothness-Term) der Abweichung von einem regulären Kubus bestimmen. Der Algorithmus generiert einen gerichteten zwei-terminalen Graphen (s-t-Netzwerk), wobei die Knoten des Graphen einer würfelförmigen Untermenge der Voxel entsprechen. Die Gewichtung der terminalen Kanten, die jeden Knoten mit einer virtuellen Quelle s und einer virtuellen Senke t verbinden, repräsentieren die Affinität eines Voxel zum Wirbel (Quelle) und zum Hintergrund (Senke); eine Menge unendlich gewichteter, nicht-terminaler Kanten realisiert den Smoothness-Term. Nach der Konstruktion wird in polynomialer Laufzeit ein minimaler s-t-Schnitt berechnet, der die Knoten in zwei disjunkte Mengen teilt, aus denen anschließend das Segmentierungsergebnis ermittelt wird. Die quantitative Auswertung einer C++ Implementierung des Algorithmus ergab einen durchschnittlichen Dice Similarity Coefficient von 81,33% bei einer maximalen Laufzeit von einer Minute.

1 Einleitung

Die demographische Entwicklung hat zu einem höheren Anteil älterer Patienten geführt, die einen operativen Eingriff an der Wirbelsäule benötigen [1, 2]. Dabei sind vor allem durch Veränderungen der ligamentären und ossären Strukturen degenerative Erkrankungen der Wirbelsäule weit verbreitet und die konsekutive Zunahme der Spinalkanalstenosen haben vermehrt Einschränkungen der Patienten im Alltag zur Folge. Zur präoperativen Evaluation der spinalen Knochenstruktur werden bevorzugt Computertomographie (CT)-Scans angefertigt, u.a. weil knöcherne Strukturen so besser erkennbar sind, als z.B. in Magnetresonanztomographie (MRT)-Aufnahmen [3].

In diesem Beitrag wird die Möglichkeit der MRT-Segmentierung im Hinblick auf die Rekonstruktion der Wirbelkörper vorgestellt. Potentiell wird so die Anzahl der CT-Scans zum Zweck der präoperativen Evaluierung von Wirbelkörpern

H.-P. Meinzer et al. (Hrsg.), *Bildverarbeitung für die Medizin 2013*, Informatik aktuell,
DOI: 10.1007/978-3-642-36480-8_14, © Springer-Verlag Berlin Heidelberg 2013

reduziert, da die Knochenstruktur durch die vorgestellte Methode auch in MRT-Aufnahmen gut erkennbar wird. Zudem wird der Zeitaufwand der präoperativen Maßnahmen durch eine automatische Segmentierung verringert.

In der Literatur finden sich mehrere Ansätze zur (semi-)automatischen Segmentierung von Wirbeln aus MRT-Aufnahmen. Bei dem Ansatz von Stern et al. [4] wird die Segmentierung durch eine Optimierung der Parameter eines dreidimensionalen deterministischen Modells der Wirbelsäule durchgeführt. Dabei wird nach der besten Übereinstimmung des deterministischen Modells mit der Wirbelsäule aus der Patientenaufnahme gesucht. Weese et al. [5] benutzen ein polygonales Modell der Wirbel und eine manuelle Initialisierung. Eine interne Energie entspricht der statistischen Form, eine externe Energie beruht auf den Bildgradienten. Der iterative Ansatz besteht aus zwei Schritten: Im ersten Schritt wird versucht, die Oberfläche zu erkennen, in einem zweiten Schritt wird das Modell angepasst. Das Verfahren von Ghebreab et al. [6] nutzt eine manuelle Initialisierung des ersten Wirbels und die Form der Wirbelsäule. Für die Repräsentation der Oberfläche wird eine B-Spline-Oberfläche mit 12x12 Kontrollpunkten genutzt, und zur Segmentierung benachbarter Wirbel wird ein statistisches Modell verwendet.

2   Material und Methoden

Der hier vorgestellte Algorithmus konstruiert in einem ersten Schritt ein zweiterminales Flussnetzwerk $F = ((V(G), E(G)), c, s, t)$, wobei $V(G) \backslash \{s, t\}$ eine Menge von Knoten bezeichnet, die wiederum einer Untermenge der Bildvoxel entspricht. $E(G)$ bezeichnet eine Menge von Kanten und c eine Funktion, die jeder Kante eine nicht-negative, reale Kapazität zuordnet. Außerdem besteht das Netzwerk aus einer Quelle $s \in V(G)$ und einer Senke $t \in V(G)$. Nach der Konstruktion des Netzwerks wird in polynomialer Zeit ein minimaler s-t-Schnitt (S, T) berechnet [7], aus dem anschließend das Segmentierungsergebnis wie folgt ermittelt wird:

– ein Knoten $v \in S$ wird dem Wirbelkörper zugeordnet und
– ein Knoten $v \in T$ wird dem Hintergrund zugeordnet.

Die betrachteten Voxel befinden sich entlang einer Menge von Strahlen, die ihren Ursprung alle in einem benutzerdefinierten Saatpunkt innerhalb des Wirbelkörpers haben. Hierbei besteht jeder Strahl aus der gleichen Menge von auf dem Strahl äquidistant verteilten Voxeln und alle Voxel der gleichen Ebene – z.B. die Menge der zweiten Voxel auf allen Strahlen – bilden eine Würfelform (Abb. 1, links).

Die terminalen Kanten des Netzwerks, die jeden Knoten mit s und t verbinden, repräsentieren die Grauwertunterschiede zwischen einem Voxel und seinem Vorgängervoxel auf demselben Strahl. Ist die Differenz klein (< 20), so wird davon ausgegangen, dass die beiden Voxel innerhalb einer homogenen Region des Bildes liegen (z.B. innerhalb des Wirbelkörpers), so dass die Kante, die den entsprechenden Knoten mit der Quelle verbindet, hoch gewichtet wird. Bei einer

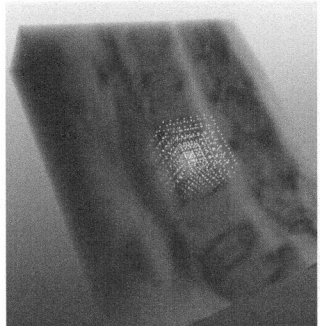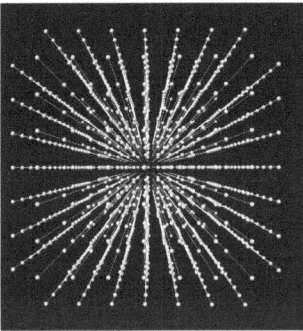

Abb. 1. Verteilung der Knoten eines Graphen (links) und Visualisierung der z-Kanten (rechts).

großen Differenz (> 20) kann von einem Objekt-Hintergrund-Übergang ausgegangen werden, so dass hier die entsprechende Kante zur Senke hoch gewichtet wird. Die terminalen Kantengewichtungen des ersten und des letzten Voxels auf jedem Strahl stellen außerdem sicher, dass der Saatpunkt dem Wirbelkörper und der letzte Voxel dem Hintergrund zugeordnet wird.

Um sicherzustellen, dass jeder Strahl nur genau einmal geschnitten wird, wird eine Menge von nicht-terminalen, ∞-gewichteten Kanten eingeführt, die jeden Knoten $v_{i_r} \in V(G) \backslash \{s, t, v_1\}$ mit seinem Vorgänger $v_{(i-1)_r} \in V(G) \backslash \{s, t\}$ auf einem Strahl r verbinden (Abb. 1, rechts) [8, 9]

$$A_z = \{(v_{i_r}, v_{(i-1)_r})\} \tag{1}$$

Einen Strahl r einmal zu schneiden verursacht, aufgrund von A_z, Kosten von mindestens ∞, da $(v_{i_r}, v_{(i+1)_r})$ geschnitten werden muss, gdw $v_{(j \leq i)_r} \in S$ und $v_{(j>i)_r} \in T$. Einen Strahl zweimal zu schneiden, würde Kosten von mindestens $2 \cdot \infty$ verursachen. Da jedoch der Saatpunkt v_1 in S liegt, während der letzte Knoten auf jedem Strahl T zugeordnet ist, muss ein Strahl von einem minimalen s-t-Schnitt genau einmal geschnitten werden. Im Fall eines scharfen Objekt/Hintergrund-Übergangs muss dieser Schnitt, aufgrund der hohen Gewichtung der terminalen Kante zur Senke, genau vor dem ersten Knoten im Hintergrund verlaufen.

Typische Herausforderungen im Kontext von graphbasierten Segmentierungen sind starke Abweichungen innerhalb der anatomischen Struktur, die einen zu frühen Schnitt zur Folge haben, sowie homogene Objekt/Hintergrund-Übergänge, die einen Überlauf des Segmentierungsergebnisses verursachen. Der Ansatz begegnet diesen Problemen, indem er dem Nutzer erlaubt, einen Smoothness-Term zu definieren, der die Objekt-Hintergrund Distanz $\Delta \in \mathbf{N_0}$ zweier benachbarter Strahlen beschränkt. Hierzu wird eine weitere Menge von nicht-terminalen, ∞-gewichteten Kanten eingeführt

$$A_{xy} = \{v_{i_r}, v_{\max\{i-\Delta, 1\}_{r'}}\} \tag{2}$$

wobei r und r' aus einer Vierernachbarschaft stammen (Abb. 2). Ein Δ-Wert von Null hat somit eine reguläre Würfelform zur Folge, bei einem Δ-Wert $>$ Null sind entsprechende Abweichungen, abhängig von der Voxeldistanz auf den einzelnen Strahlen, möglich (Abb. 3).

Abb. 2.   Topologie
der (x, y)-Kanten:
$\Delta = 0$ (links) und
$\Delta = 1$ (rechts).

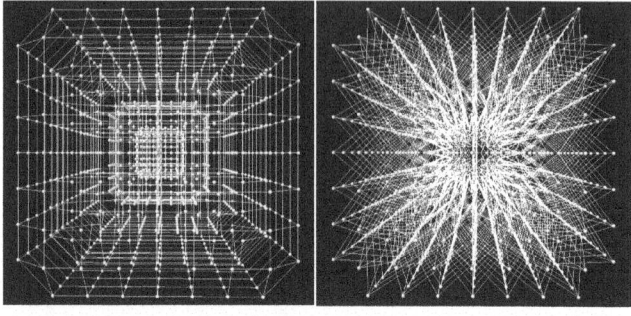

Abb. 3.
Segmentierungsergebnis
für $\Delta = 0$ (links) und
$\Delta = 2$ (rechts).

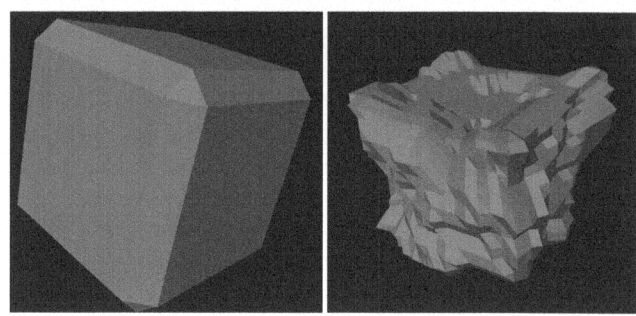

3   Ergebnisse

Zur Evaluation des vorgestellten Segmentierungsverfahrens wurde eine C++
Implementierung innerhalb der medizinischen Bildverarbeitungsplattform Me-
VisLab (www.mevislab.de, Version 2.2.1) realisiert und anhand von zehn Wirbeln in zwei sagittalen, T2-gewichteten MRT-Datensätzen ($160 \times 160 \times 35$ und
$160 \times 160 \times 23$) getestet. Die Tests lieferten bei einem direkten Vergleich mit
manuell vorgenommen Schicht-für-Schicht-Segmentierungen einen durchschnittlichen Dice Similarity Coefficient (DSC) [10] von 81,33% (Tab. 1). Abb. 4 zeigt
Segmentierungsergebnisse unseres Ansatzes (Cube-Cut).

Dabei hatten die rechenaufwendigsten Parametereinstellungen eine maximale Terminierungszeit von unter einer Minute (Netzwerkkonstruktion, s-t-Schnitt
und Triangulierung des Segmentierungsergebnisses)[1]. Manuell erstellte Segmentierungen, für die ein Mediziner Schicht-für-Schicht die Außengrenzen eines Wirbelkörpers in den Aufnahmen einzeichnete, dauerten dagegen 6,65 bis 10 Minuten, so dass die automatische Segmentierung die präoperativen Evaluierungs-
maßnahmen um 2,35 (min.) bis 15,65 Minuten (max.) verkürzte.

4   Diskussion

In diesem Beitrag wurde ein graphbasierter Ansatz zur Wirbelsegmentierung in
MRT-Aufnahmen vorgestellt, wobei der Graph anhand einer würfelförmigen Vor-

---

[1] 2,1 GHz, 4 GB RAM x64 PC,Windows 7 Home Premium (SP1)

Tabelle 1. Evaluierungsergebnisse für zehn Wirbel. Die Abkürzungen man., aut., Vol., Vox. und DSC stehen für manuell, automatisch, Volumen in cm^3, Voxel und Dice Similarity Coefficient in %.

	man. Vol.	aut. Vol.	man. Vox.	aut. Vox.	DSC
min.	15,42	16,64	1892	2041	71,64
max.	33,83	28,78	5240	4320	86,69
$\mu \pm \sigma$	24,97 ± 6,15	23,48 ± 5,12	3750	3152	81,33 ± 5,07

lage konstruiert wird und die Knoten des Graphen nicht gleichverteilt und nicht äquidistant innerhalb der MRT-Aufnahme gesampelt werden. Dadurch liefert ein anschließender minimaler s-t-Schnitt - in Abhängigkeit von einem benutzerdefinierten Smoothness-Term (Abweichung) - auch eine würfelförmige Segmentierung zurück.

Unseres Wissens nach ist dies das erste Mal, dass bei einem graphbasierten Ansatz die Knoten anhand einer würfelförmigen Vorlage verteilt wurden und der minimale s-t-Schnitt somit auch ein würfelförmiges Segmentierungsergebnis bevorzugt. Das vorgestellte Verfahren kann auch zur Segmentierung anderer, vergleichbarer, kubusförmiger Zielstrukturen genutzt werden und eignet sich besonders um homogenen Objekt/Hintergrund-Übergängen zu begegnen, die eine automatische Segmentierung des Objektes erschweren. Es ist geplant das Verfahren in der Zukunft zu verfeinern, so bietet sich z.B. eine komplexere Kantendetektion an (gradient magnitude). Außerdem sollen die Segmentierungsergebnisse noch auf Formgleichheit untersucht werden.

Bei den aktuellen Parametereinstellungen kam es vor, dass Ecken der Wirbel nicht genau segmentiert wurden. Abb. 5 zeigt ein Beispiel, bei dem die Konturen zweier Ecken eines Wirbels (Kreise) „abgeschnitten" wurden. Dieser Ungenauigkeit kann durch eine Verdichtung der Strahlen und dadurch auch einer Verdichtung der Knoten entgegengewirkt werden. Dies würde jedoch eine höhere Laufzeit zur Folge haben. Eine andere Möglichkeit wäre, anstatt eines Kubus

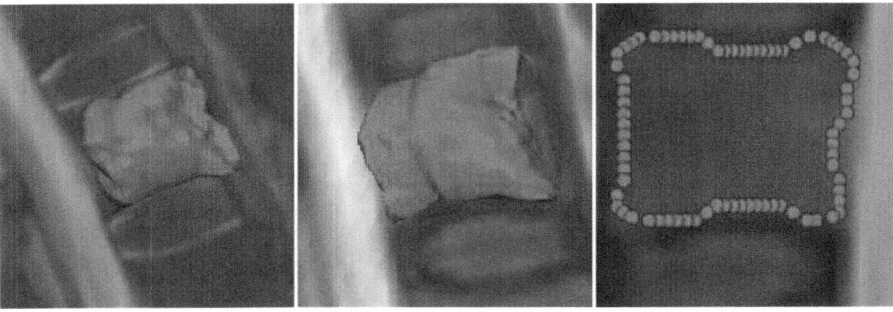

Abb. 4. 3D-Segmentierungsergebnisse (links und Mitte) und 2D-Perspektive auf ein Segmentierungsergebnis mit benutzerdefiniertem Saatpunkt in Blau (rechtes Bild).

eine dem Wirbel besser angepasste Vorlage für den Aufbau des Graphen zu verwenden, zum Beispiel mit Würfelseiten, die leicht nach innen gewölbt sind.

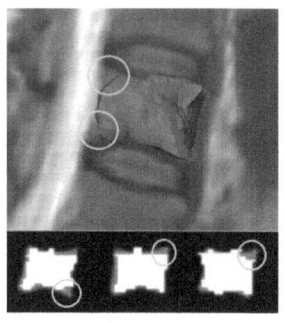

Abb. 5. Beispiel einer Segmentierung, bei der zwei Ecken des Wirbels (Kreise) nicht ausreichend segmentiert wurden. Im unteren Bildteil sind die manuellen Segmentierungen (rot) und die automatischen Segmentierungsergebnisse (weiß) in mehreren 2D-Schichten übereinandergelegt.

Danksagung. Wir danken Thomas Dukatz für sein Mitwirken an der Studie, Fraunhofer MeVis in Bremen für die Kollaboration und Horst-Karl Hahn für die Unterstützung und dem NIH (Grant 8P41EB015898-08).

Literaturverzeichnis

1. Joaquim AF, Sansur CA, Hamilton DK, et al. Degenerative lumbar stenosis: update. Arq Neuropsiquiatr. 2009;67(2B):553–8.
2. Hicks GE, Morone N, Weiner DK. Degenerative lumbar disc and facet disease in older adults: prevalence and clinical correlates. Spine (Phila Pa 1976). 2009;34(12):1301–6.
3. Richard PJ, George J, Metelko M, et al. Spine computed tomography doses and cancer induction. Spine (Phila Pa 1976). 2010;35(4):430–3.
4. Štern D, Vrtovec T, Pernuš F, et al. Segmentation of vertebral bodies in CT and MR images based on 3D deterministic models. Proc SPIE. 2011;7962.
5. Weese J, Kaus M, Lorenz C, et al. Shape constrained deformable models for 3D medical image segmentation. In: Insana M, Leahy R, editors. Information Processing in Medical Imaging. vol. 2082. Springer; 2001. p. 380–7.
6. Ghebreab S, Smeulders AW. Combining strings and necklaces for interactive three-dimensional segmentation of spinal images using an integral deformable spine model. IEEE Trans Biomed Eng. 2004;51(10):1821–9.
7. Boykov Y, Kolmogorov V. An experimental comparison of min-cut/max-flow algorithms for energy minimization in vision. IEEE Trans Pattern Anal Mach Intell. 2004;26(9):1124–37.
8. Li K, Wu X, Chen DZ, et al. Optimal surface segmentation in volumetric images: a graph-theoretic approach. IEEE Trans Pattern Anal Mach Intell. 2006;28(1):119–34.
9. Egger J, Kapur T, Dukatz T, et al. Square-cut: a segmentation algorithm on the basis of a rectangle shape. PLoS ONE. 2012;7(2):e31064.
10. Zou KH, Warfield SK, Bharatha A, et al. Statistical validation of image segmentation quality based on a spatial overlap index. Acad Radiol. 2004;2:178–89.

Computer-Assisted Analysis of Annuloplasty Rings

Bastian Graser[1], Mathias Seitel[1,2], Sameer Al-Maisary[3],
Manuel Grossgasteiger[4], Tobias Heye[5], Hans-Peter Meinzer[1], Diana Wald[1],
Raffaele de Simone[3], Ivo Wolf[1,6]

[1]Div. of Medical and Biological Informatics, German Cancer Research Center
(DKFZ), Germany
[2]Mint Medical GmbH, Germany
[3]Dept. of Heart Surgery, University of Heidelberg, Germany
[4]Dept. of Anesthesiology, University of Heidelberg, Germany
[5]Dept. of Radiology, University of Heidelberg, Germany
[6]Faculty of Computer Science, Mannheim University of Applied Science, Germany
b.graser@dkfz.de

Abstract. Over 40.000 annuloplasty rings are implanted each year in
the United States to treat mitral regurgitation. The rings come in different sizes and shapes. However it is unclear, which ring is most suitable
for the individual patient. Here we present a preoperative annuloplasty
planning software to determine an eligible ring. It provides fast interactive methods to create 4D mitral annulus models based on arbitrary
image data. Created models can be analyzed geometrically and compared to existing annuloplasty ring models. This way, forces caused by a
specific annuloplasty ring can visualized, which enables preoperative simulation and eventually improves operation results. Using our software,
we evaluated the size changes caused by five commercially available annuloplasty rings on the mitral annuli of 39 patients. The results suggest
that the annuloplasty ring should be selected for each patient specifically.

1 Introduction

Mitral regurgitation is a wide spread disease, which affects about 2% of the
population in the USA [1, 2]. The symptoms vary from reduced stamina and
shortness of breath to cardiac arrhythmia. Cause for these symptoms is a leakage of the mitral valve in the systolic phase. In severe cases, surgical treatment
is necessary. A mitral reconstruction can be performed, which includes implan-
tation of an annuloplasty ring. This way the patient's mitral annulus (MA) is
stabilized and the leaking can be stopped. However, the quality and durability
of the treatment are unpredictable. A major influencing factor for successful
treatment is the use of an annuloplasty ring with a suitable shape and size.

Annuloplasty rings are available in a large variety (Fig. 1). Shape and size
are important factors to the durability and quality of the treatment and should
be chosen carefully considering the appearance of the MA of the individual patients [3, 4]. Yet, most surgeons perform just coarse measurements during the

H.-P. Meinzer et al. (Hrsg.), *Bildverarbeitung für die Medizin 2013*, Informatik aktuell,
DOI: 10.1007/978-3-642-36480-8_15, © Springer-Verlag Berlin Heidelberg 2013

operation by placing a template of a ring onto the visible mitral valve of the opened, non-beating heart and decide visually, if it fits. For a more replicable result, the measurement should be done preoperatively with the heart in a natural condition using medical imaging techniques. Methods performing semi-automatic and automatic MA measurements on ultrasound or computer tomography images have been proposed [5, 6, 7]. However, precise results can only be received by manual measurement, especially when the given image is of low quality. With this study we present a software application to analyze the patients MA. To the best of our knowledge this is the first time software is proposed to simulate annuloplasty ring forces preoperatively.

2   Material and methods

The developed software is based on the free open-source Toolkit MITK[1] and can be divided into two modules: Mitral Annulus Modeling and Mitral Annulus Analyze.

2.1   Mitral annulus modeling

The Mitral Annulus Modeling module allows extracting the patient specific annulus shape from images of any modality (eg. ultrasound, computer tomography, magnetic resonance). The image data can be 3D or 4D recordings. All common file formats of medical images including some vendor-specific variants for 3D/4D ultrasound data are supported. The dataset is displayed in three 2D windows, representing the axial, coronal and the sagittal view directions. A fourth window depicts a 3D visualization of the data by showing all 2D views in their current position as intersecting planes. At first, the dataset is reoriented by the user. The axial plane is translated and rotated, so it resembles the mitral

---

[1] www.mitk.org

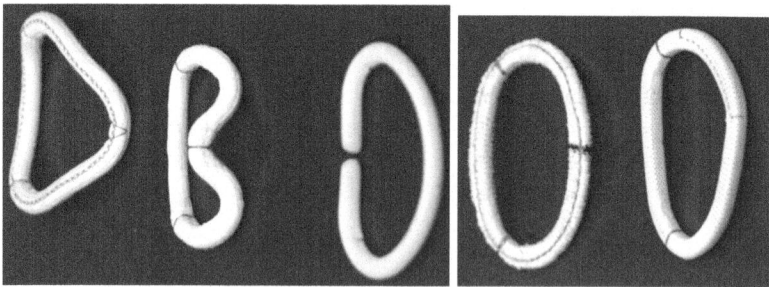

Fig. 1. Annuloplasty rings used for evaluation. Left: Edwards Lifescience Myxo ET-logix, Edwards Lifescience GeoForm and Edwards Lifescience Classic. Right: St. Jude Medical Rigid Saddle and Edwards Lifescience IMR ETlogix.

annulus plane and contains the anterior and posterior commissure points. Subsequently the sagittal plane is turned, so it contains both commissure points as well. Eventually the user marks the commissure points on the intersection line of both planes. If the dataset is time-resolved, this procedure is done for all time steps of the image data. If subsequent time steps are similar due to a high temporal solution, some time steps can be skipped. The plane orientation and the position of the commissure points of these time steps are interpolated linearly. Afterwards the mitral annulus shape is defined. A coarse mitral annulus model is placed in the image data. Its position and size is determined by the selected commissure points, while the orientation is defined by the planes. The model consists of 16 points, which are connected by subdivision curves [8] to resemble the round shape of the mitral annulus. For each point the user adjusts the distance to the center of the mitral annulus and the vertical position of the point to ensure it is located in the annulus tissue. The final result is a precise 4D model of the patients MA.

2.2   Mitral annulus analyze

Previously created MA models can be analyzed with the Mitral Annulus Analyze module. By comparing the points and orientation of the model, several parameters are measured: Perimeter, diameter, annulus height, surface size, cardiac displacement and cardiac velocity (Fig. 2).

Additionally the selected model can be compared to different annuloplasty rings. The application places the annuloplasty ring model according to the position and orientation of a patient's MA model. The size of the annuloplasty ring can be chosen freely. Subsequently, the deviation of both models is interpreted

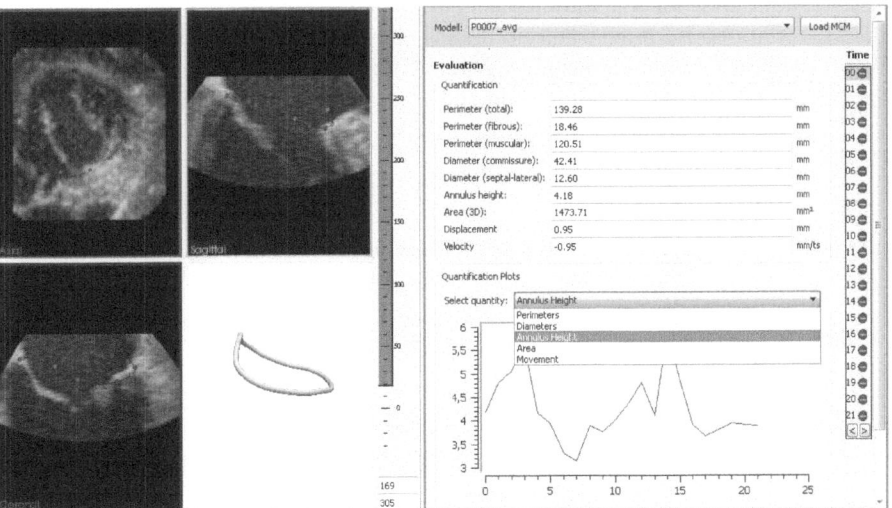

Fig. 2. Geometrical analysis of the obtained patient specific annulus model.

as tissue tension that would be caused by the ring. The results are presented by colorizing the model and displaying the tissue displacement as directed arrows (Fig. 3). So far, we provide five annuloplasty ring models for comparison. Additional rings can be added easily by using the method described in section 2.1 on 3D image data of a specific ring.

3   Results

We had access to time resolved transesophageal-echography image data of 39 patients. All patients underwent mitral surgery in which an annuloplasty ring was implanted. An expert created 4D mitral models of all patients using our proposed software. To minimize user errors, the expert created three models per patient on separate days, which were then averaged into one model. The average time needed for modeling one patient was about 15 minutes and decrease with growing expertise and practice. Using Mitral Annulus Analyze module, we compared the patients' mitral annuli to five different annuloplasty rings. These were Classic, Geoform, IMR ETlogix and Myxo ETlogix by Edwards Lifescience as well as Rigid Saddle Ring by St. Jude Medical (Fig. 4). In this comparison we used five different sizing methods. We scaled the rings with the commissure diameter of the patients MA (equal size) and then increased (oversized) and decrease (undersized) the annuloplasty ring diameter by two and four millimeters. Results are shown in Fig. 4.

4   Discussion

The comparison (Fig. 4) between the five annuloplasty rings and patients collective show, that all five annuloplasty rings cause a similar average resizing of the MA of about 1.1 mm, when no under- or oversizing of the ring is performed. When implanting an undersized ring, the Myxo ETlogix causes the least tension on the mitral annulus tissue, while the most tension is caused by Classic. In the case of an oversizing, the Myxo ETlogix causes the highest tension and the GeoForm pulls the least on the tissue.

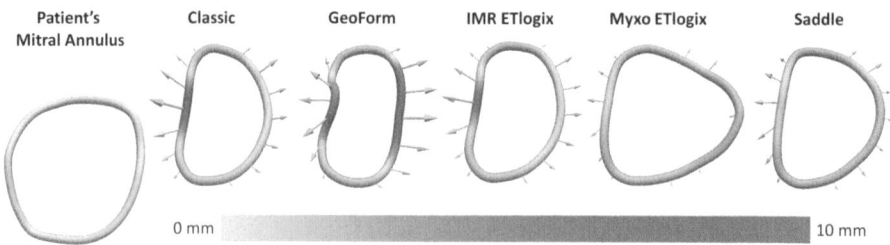

Fig. 3. Visualization of the mitral annulus tissue displacement caused by five different annuloplasty ring types on a specific patient.

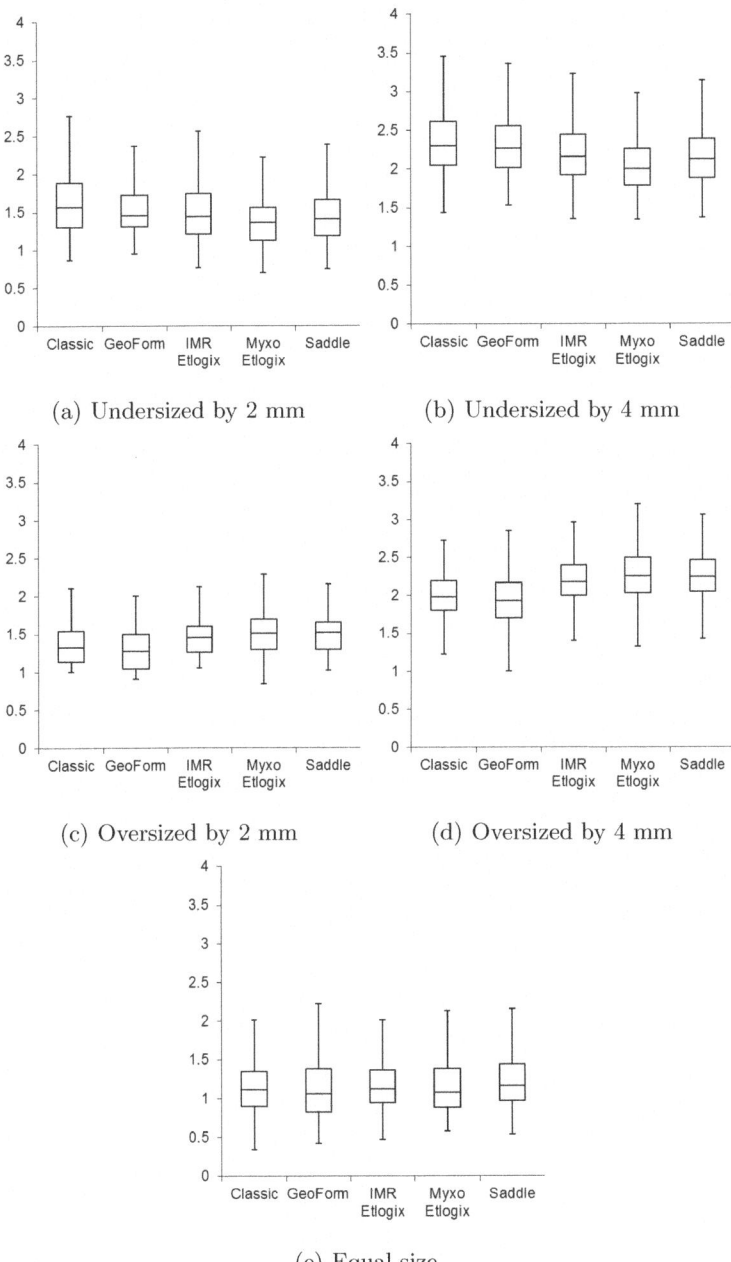

(a) Undersized by 2 mm

(b) Undersized by 4 mm

(c) Oversized by 2 mm

(d) Oversized by 4 mm

(e) Equal size

Fig. 4. Box-Whisker plots showing the average tissue displacement caused by five different annuloplasty rings on 39 patients. Whiskers are set to minimum and maximum values. The annuloplasty ring was sized using different strategies.

The higher the displacement, the higher the risk of a ring dehiscence. However, it is difficult to make a general statement about the amount of acceptable force. This depends on the mitral annulus tissue elasticity, which varies a lot between patients [9]. The decision, which ring is most eligibility, has to be made for each patient individually. In order to do so a specific analysis is necessary. This is possible with the proposed software. The depicted forces (Fig. 3) enable the physician to decide preoperatively for a suitable annuloplasty ring that causes a desired deformation of the individual patient's MA.

Acknowledgement. This study was supported by the Research Training Group Graduiertenkolleg 1126 funded by the German Research Foundation (DFG).

References

1. Singh JP, Evans JC, Levy D, et al. Prevalence and clinical determinants of mitral, tricuspid, and aortic regurgitation (the Framingham Heart Study). Am J Cardiol. 1999;83(6):897–902.
2. Nkomo, Gardin, Skelton, et al. Burden of valvular heart diseases: a population-based study. Lancet. 2006;368(9540):1005–11.
3. Adams DH, Anyanwu AC, Rahmanian PB, et al. Large Annuloplasty Rings Facilitate Mitral Valve Repair in Barlow's Disease. Ann Thorac Surg. 2006;82(6):2096–101.
4. Braun J, van de Veire NR, Klautz RJM, et al. Restrictive mitral annuloplasty cures ischemic mitral regurgitation and heart failure. Ann Thorac Surg. 2008;85(2):430–6.
5. Graser B, Wald D, Seitel M, et al. A robust model-based approach to detect the mitral annulus in 3D ultrasound. Proc SPIE. 2013;(in press).
6. Ionasec RI, Voigt I, Georgescu B, et al. Patient-specific modeling and quantification of the aortic and mitral valves from 4D cardiac CT and TEE. IEEE Trans Med Imaging. 2010;29(9):1636–51.
7. Voigt I, Mansi T, Ionasec R, et al. Robust physically-constrained modeling of the mitral valve and subvalvular apparatus. Proc MICCAI. 2011.
8. Dubuc S. Interpolation through an iterative scheme. J Math Anal Appl. 1986;114(1):185–204.
9. Edwards MB, Draper ERC, Hand JW, et al. Mechanical testing of human cardiac tissue: some implications for MRI safety. J Cardiov Magn Reson. 2005;7(5):835–40.

Texture-Based Detection of Myositis in Ultrasonographies

Tim König[1], Marko Rak[1], Johannes Steffen[1], Grit Neumann[2],
Ludwig von Rohden[2], Klaus D. Tönnies[1]

[1]Institut für Simulation & Graphik, Otto-von-Guericke-Universität Magdeburg
[2]Klinik für Radiologie & Nuklearmedizin, Otto-von-Guericke-Universität Magdeburg
tim.koenig@st.ovgu.de

Abstract. Muscle ultrasonography is a convenient technique to visualize healthy and pathological muscle tissue as it is non-invasive and image acquisition can be done in real-time. In this paper, a texture-based approach is presented to detect myositis in ultrasound images automatically. We compute different texture features like wavelet transform features and first-order grey-level intensity statistics of a relevant central image patch carrying structure and intensity information of muscle tissue. Using a combination of these information we reached an accuracy of classification of 92.20 % with our approach on a training data set of 63 clinically pre-classified data sets.

1 Introduction

An automatically computer-supported detection of myositis may serve different purposes and goals: it can save time for radiologists during the diagnosis and it gives a second, independent result, which can be taken into consideration. A well trained process may also be capable of early diagnosis and categorization. Moreover, it will help young professionals with only a small degree of experience identifying myositis in ultrasound images.

Neuromuscular disorders often cause structural muscle changes that can be seen in ultrasound images. Infiltration of fat and fibrous tissue increase muscle echo intensity, i.e. the reference image of the muscle will become brighter. Thus, myositis can be found by measuring muscle thickness. As healthy muscles contain only little fibrous tissue only a few reflections will occur during image acquisition resulting in a low echo intensity and thus a relatively dark image (Fig. 1). It is assumed that the replacement of muscle tissue with fat and fibrosis is the main cause of increased muscle echo intensity as they increase the number of reflections within the muscle and therefore the mean grey value of the muscle in the ultrasound image (Fig. 1)[1].

Under these assumptions a texture-based analysis should be adequate to detect myositis. Using texture as discriminating feature in ultrasound images has a long history in image analysis. Most methods use a combination of spectral and first-order statistical features as these reflect the nature of deterministic

H.-P. Meinzer et al. (Hrsg.), *Bildverarbeitung für die Medizin 2013*, Informatik aktuell,
DOI: 10.1007/978-3-642-36480-8_16, © Springer-Verlag Berlin Heidelberg 2013

tissue-related variation and non-deterministic influences from image generation (e.g. [2] for classification of liver tumors, [3] for classification of breast tumors, or [4] for the classification of arterioscleroric tissue). Both, differences in grey-level intensity and in the micro-structure between healthy and pathological muscle tissue can be used to compute representative and distinctive features. In contrast to [5], who required training to select texture features and a manually specified region-of-interest (ROI), we believe that - similar to [4] - selection of features reflecting micro-structural change will result in a robust method that requires little to no user input.

Fig. 1 shows that the texture of pathological muscle tissue images is more unstructured or diffuse, containing smaller contrast changes compared to the texture of healthy muscle tissue images, which seem to be more directed or structured containing higher contrast changes caused by the relatively dark regions of the healthy muscles. We propose a texture analysis method that applies a wavelet decomposition computing features carrying structure information as well as first-order grey-level intensity statistics.

Fig. 1. Ultrasound images including healthy (left) and pathological (right) muscle tissue.

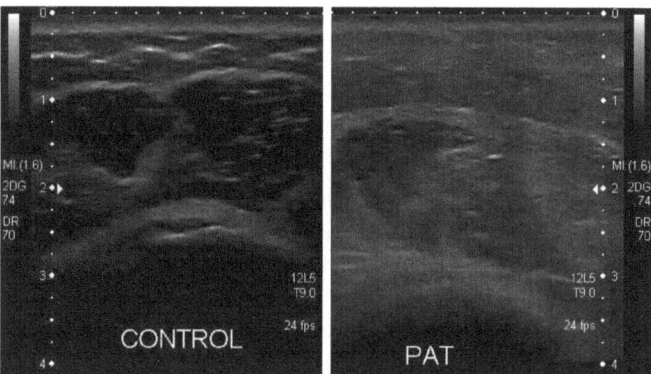

2   Materials and methods

Feature extraction and classification are performed on 63 clinical ultrasound images including 14 images of healthy muscles and 49 images of pathological muscle tissues. The images have a pixel resolution of 350 px × 500 px covering an area of 2.8 cm × 4.0 cm. The data contains scans of various muscles from upper and lower human limbs as well as scans acquired by different angulation of the 9 MHz linear transducer. All images were pre-classified by radiological experts allowing a comparison of our analysis results with these ground truth assumptions.

2.1 Feature extraction

In the feature extraction, we focus on two features of the wavelet decomposition and two features of the first-order grey-level intensity statistics: the reverse bi-orthogonal 1.1 and 1.3 wavelet transform features [6] carrying non-directional information of the muscle tissue micro-structure and also the grey-level entropy and variance as first-order statistic features. These features measure similar attributes compared to [2] and especially [4]. They were selected from a range of features by visual inspection of scatter plots of all possible pairs of features.

Since the data does not include a segmentation of the muscle tissue and a manual search of a window for which the features are computed would be inefficient we specified during image acquisition that the relevant muscle structures are located near the center of the ultrasound image. Hence, we place a ROI of size 60 px × 60 px in the center of the image and compute the four texture features for each pixel p in the ROI (Fig. 2). Texture computation requires the definition of a window with suitable size around p. We experimented with window sizes between 80 px × 80 px and 220 px × 220 px for determining the optimal size.

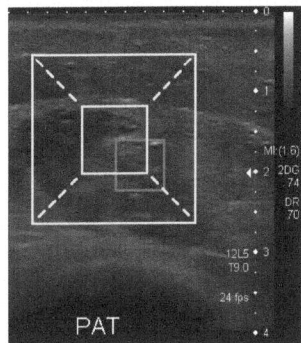

Fig. 2. Feature extraction for each pixel of a central ROI (red) of 60 px × 60 px with different window sizes (yellow) from 80 px × 80 px up to 220 px × 220 px. This results in 3600 feature vectors per image for a fixed window size. Each feature vector contains the four different features.

2.2 Classification

To classify the images we use the k-nearest neighbor algorithm (kNN) [7] based on closest training samples in feature space. The kNN classification is then cross-validated by the leave-one-out method. Thus, the kNN classifier was trained on the feature subset of $N-1$ images – each image contains 3600 feature vectors for a fixed windows size – to validate the class of the N-th image (with $N = 63$). This process is repeated such that each image is used once for validation. However, the choice of k is highly dependent on the problem and the data set. Hence, we experimented with k varying from 2 up to 128.

Finally, for each k and each window size a single misclassification error per image (SCE) as well as the mean misclassification error over all images (MCE) is computed to evaluate the results of our approach. The SCE is estimated by the ratio of the number of correctly classified pixels to the number of falsely classified pixels of the ROI. The mean misclassification error is then computed by averaging of the SCE's.

3   Results

Fig. 3 shows the MCE for all window sizes for $k = 64$ (MCE#k64) as well as the minimum (MCE#Min) and maximum mean misclassification error (MCE#Max) for each window size for all k-values. Our approach reaches its lowest error rate of 7.80% at a window size of 180 px × 180 px used for feature extraction and training of the classifier. The smallest window size of 80 px × 80 px produces the highest error rate with 25.16 %. The MCE differs with respect to the parameter k only between 0.38 % and 3.08 % depending on particular window sizes.

The results of the SCE for a fixed window size of 180 px × 180 px and a fixed $k = 64$ are shown in Fig. 4. The results can be used for classification into pathological and healthy tissue by assigning the class of the majority of pixels in the ROI. Most (60 of 63 cases) of the evaluated images reach a low misclassification error ≤ 30 %, thus, more than 70 % of the ROI pixels are classified correctly. In 29 of 63 cases more than 99 % of the pixels were classified correctly. Only 3 of 63 ultrasound images (4.76 %) show a misclassification rate ≥ 50 %.

4   Discussion

Using non-directional wavelet transform features and first-order grey-level intensity statistics combined with the presented approach of computing features for

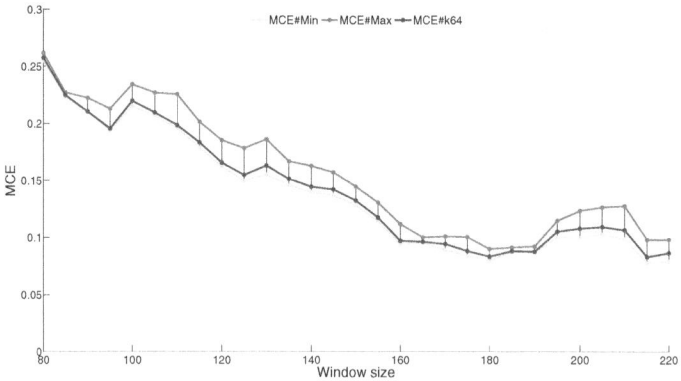

Fig. 3. Results of the MCE for all analyzed window sizes for $k = 64$ (MCE#k64). The upper red line displays the maximum mean misclassification error (MCE#Max) of all k-values, the lower green line shows the results of the minimum mean misclassification error (MCE#Min) of all k-values.

each pixel of the ROI with various window sizes provides a stable texture-based analysis for detecting myositis in ultrasonographies.

The choice of the window size impacts the classification results. Too small windows (range from 80 px × 80 px to 150 px × 150 px) result in worse classification rates (Fig. 3) since those windows do contain enough relevant information. Too large windows (range from 190 px × 190 px to 220 px × 220 px) carry the risk that too many other kinds of tissues and structures are observed within the selected window and thus the results can be falsified strongly. Determining the proper window position and size also depends on the location of the muscle tissue in the image, on the resolution of the image and on the kind of scanned muscles. There might be no optimal solution for all data sets. Hence, some imaging protocol should be used for image generation that fixes important parameters such as the anatomic region so that different windows sizes can be determined for different protocols. The selection of the k-values of kNN has little influence on the classification rate. However, smaller k-values result in slightly worse classification rates than higher k-values.

As mentioned, a window size of 180 px × 180 px resulted in best classification rates. Nevertheless, 3 of 63 images have been misclassified (Fig. 4) because those images include feature characteristics that are inconsistent with our initial assumptions that the texture of pathological muscle tissue images is more diffuse with smaller contrast changes compared to the texture of healthy muscle tissue images with structured tissue and higher contrast changes (Fig. 5). A reason for this could be the different procedures which were used during image acquisition or the fact that our data set contains images from different muscles.

Although our data set is insufficient for clinical reliable results, we have shown that texture analysis can be used as a robust, automatic method to anal-

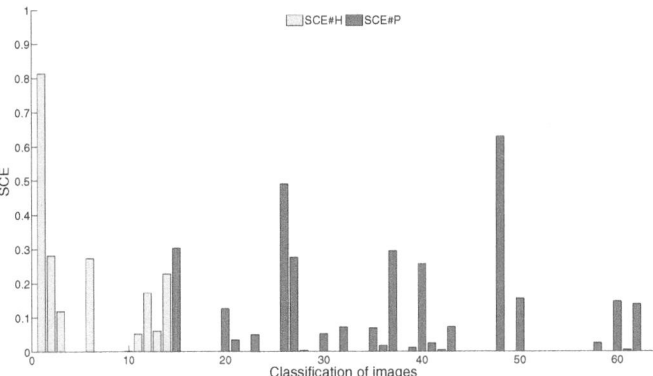

Fig. 4. Results of the SCE for a fixed window size of 180 px × 180 px and a fixed $k = 64$. The green bars represent the SCE of healthy muscle tissue images (SCE#H) and the red bars of the pathological muscle tissue images (SCE#P).

Fig. 5. Examples of misclassified images for healthy (left, SCE of 81.30%) and pathological (right, SCE of 62.88%) muscles.

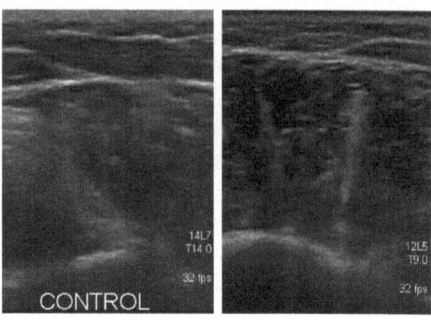

yse myositis from ultrasound images. Future work will focus on an evaluation of a larger number of images including more patients acquired with consistent imaging protocols to prevent variations caused by different acquisition parameters, positions, and orientations of the transducer or anatomical regions as well as maximization of unpreventable variations within the data like patient specific variation, i.e. age, gender and fat rate, to get a representative sample set. Furthermore, an application of the proposed method to other muscles could be possible, if one would select different window positions and sizes for each muscle group. An integration of staging of myositis is a topic which is worth of further research.

Different classification techniques will be evaluated, i.e. SVM, as we decided on the kNN classifier because of visual separability of our feature space. However, this assumption could be a misinterpretation of the visual observations caused by the dimensional down-projection of the feature space for visualization.

References

1. Pillen S, van Alfen N. Skeletal muscle ultrasound. Neurol Res. 2011;33(10):1016–24.
2. Wu CM, Chen YC, Hsieh KS. Texture features for classification of ultrasonic liver images. IEEE Trans Med Imaging. 1992;11(2):141–52.
3. Huang YL, Wang KL, Chen DR. Diagnosis of breast tumors with ultrasonic texture analysis using support vector machines. Neural Comput Appl. 2006;15(2):164–9.
4. Tsiaparas NN, Golemati S, Andreadis I, et al. Comparison of multiresolution features for texture classification of carotid atherosclerosis from B-mode ultrasound. IEEE Trans Inf Technol Biomed. 2011;15(1):130–7.
5. Pohle R, Fischer D, von Rohden L. Computergestützte Gewebedifferenzierung bei der Skelettmuskelsonographie. Ultraschall Med. 2000;21(6):245–52.
6. Mallat SG. A theory for multiresolution signal decomposition: the wavelet representation. IEEE Trans Pattern Anal Mach Intell. 1989;11(7):674–93.
7. Cover T, Hart P. Nearest neighbor pattern classification. IEEE Trans Inf Theory. 1967;13(1):21–7.

Segmentierung von Kolonpolypen in NBI-Bildmaterial mittels gaborfilterbasierten Multikanal-Level-Sets

Cosmin Adrian Morariu[1], Sebastian Gross[2,3], Josef Pauli[1], Til Aach[2]

[1]Lehrstuhl Intelligente Systeme, Universität Duisburg-Essen
[2]Lehrstuhl für Bildverarbeitung, RWTH Aachen
[3]Medizinische Klinik III, Universitätsklinikum Aachen
adrian.morariu@uni-due.de

Kurzfassung. Das Narrow Band Imaging (NBI) erleichtert die Differenzierung zwischen Adenomen und harmlosen Darmwandgebilden (Hyperplasten) durch eine kontrastreiche Blutgefäßdarstellung. Dadurch wird eine automatische Segmentierung der Blutgefäße und Klassifizierung der Kolonpolypen hinsichtlich ihrer Entartungsfähigkeit ermöglicht. Eine erste Voraussetzung besteht in der automatisierten Trennung der Polypenoberfläche von der umliegenden Darmwand. In dieser Arbeit wird ein Verfahren vorgestellt, welches die Nachahmung der Fähigkeiten des Menschen zur Mustererkennung umsetzt. Die kombinierte Einbeziehung von Farbe und Textur gelingt mit Hilfe eines Gaußschen Farbmodells und Gaborfilterbasierten Aktiven Konturen. Eine Lokalisierungsgenauigkeit von 81% und eine Spezifität von 94% gewährleisten eine akkurate Polypensegmentierung durch die vorgestellte Level-Set-Methode und verprechen eine erfolgreiche Erkennung auch anderer Gewebe im Rahmen optischer sowie radiologischer Untersuchungen.

1 Einleitung

In Deutschland nimmt Darmkrebs mit über 68.000 jährlichen, auf beide Geschlechter annähernd gleich verteilten Erkrankungsfällen eine führende Position unter den malignen Krankheiten ein [1]. Ein Kolonkarzinom entsteht in den meisten Fällen während eines zeitlich lang andauernden Prozesses aus Vorstufen (Adenomen). Deswegen verspricht die Früherkennung von Darmkrebs gute Heilungsaussichten. Die Polypenentfernung (Polypektomie) während der Koloskopie birgt jedoch auch gewisse Risiken wie schwere Blutungen und Darmwandperforationen. Folglich sollten nur Polypen mit Entartungspotential der Polypektomie unterzogen werden. Die Inspektion der Polypenoberflächenstruktur einschließlich vaskulärer Muster liefert ein gutes Entscheidungsmaß in dieser Hinsicht. Im Rahmen einer Studie [2] wurde die Bedeutung von Narrow Band Imaging (NBI) bei der Differenzierung zwischen Adenomen und harmlosen Darmwandgebilden (Hyperplasten) während der optischen Koloskopie ergründet. Die Verwendung zweier ausgewählter, enger Bandpassbereiche des Weißlichts führt aufgrund der

H.-P. Meinzer et al. (Hrsg.), *Bildverarbeitung für die Medizin 2013*, Informatik aktuell,
DOI: 10.1007/978-3-642-36480-8_17, © Springer-Verlag Berlin Heidelberg 2013

starken Absorption des Lichts dieser Wellenlängen – grün (530–550 nm) und blau (390–445 nm) – durch das im Blut enthaltene Hämoglobin zu einer Hervorhebung der Blutgefäße. Dabei zeichnen sich Adenome in der Regel durch eine ausgeprägtere Blutgefäßstruktur aus. Ausgehend von einer solchen, vom Arzt erzeugten NBI-Bildaufnahme soll die Polypenoberfläche automatisch detektiert werden. Diese wird anschließend untersucht, um die darauf befindlichen Blutgefäßstrukturen zu segmentieren und daraus geeignete Merkmale für eine erfolgreiche Klassifizierung zu extrahieren [3].

Für die Segmentierung der Kolonpolypen in NBI-Bildmaterial wurden bereits mehrere Verfahren vorgeschlagen. Die Generalisierte Hough Transformation für Ellipsen in [4], sowie das Template Matching elliptischer Vorlagen mit dem Kantenbild in [5] verwerten hauptsächlich die (meistens) elliptische Form der Polypen. Im Gegensatz zu geometrischen Level-Sets [6] gewährleisten die parametrischen Aktiven Konturen (Snakes, sowie Aktive Strahlen in [4]) eine explizite Repräsentation der Kurve.

2 Material und Methoden

Die besondere Herausforderung der Polypenlokalisierung in endoskopischem Bildmaterial leitet sich aus den unterschiedlichen Aufnahmebedingungen und der biologischen Vielfalt der Polypen ab. Die Hinzunahme von Farbe und Textur als Segmentierungsmerkmale soll eine Lösung dafür repräsentieren. Unter Verwendung des in [7] vorgestellten Gaußschen Farbmodells wird das menschliche Sehvermögen nachgebildet. Die RGB-Werte des Originalbildes werden durch dieses Modell in einen wiederum dreikanäligen, der Gegenfarbtheorie des menschlichen Sehens entsprechenden Farbraum transformiert. Die Werte jedes neu entstandenen Farbkanals werden zur Texturcharakterisierung mit einer Filterbank bestehend aus 20 Gaborfiltern gefaltet. Durch die Beträge der resultierenden Filterantworten wird jedem Bildpixel ein 60-dimensionaler Merkmalsvektor zugewiesen. Anschließend erfolgt mittels Hauptachsentransformation (Principal Component Analysis) eine Dimensionsreduktion des 60-dimensionalen Merkmalsraums auf die ersten 4 Hauptkomponenten. Diese enthalten einen über alle Polypenbilder gemittelten Varianzanteil von 80,17%. Die Bildpixel werden unter Verwendung der assoziierten 4-dimensionalen Merkmalsvektoren mithilfe des K-Means-Verfahrens geclustert. Mit $K = 2$ findet die Unterscheidung der beiden Klassen Polypoberfläche bzw. Hintergrund statt. Für das Polypendatenset diente dieses von weiteren Parametern unabhängige Segmentierungsverfahren lediglich zur adäquaten Dimensionierung der Gaborfilterbank. Die K-Means-Segmentierung wird anschließend durch Aktive Konturmodelle, die auf multidimensionalen Merkmalsräumen operieren [8], ersetzt. Die Evaluierung des Verfahrens erfolgt auf dem in [4] verwendeten Polypenbilderset (jeweils 586 x 502 Pixel), das am Universitätsklinikum Aachen an unterschiedlichen Patienten mit einem NBI-Zoom-Endoskop (Olympus Exera II CV-180) aufgenommen wurde. Das Dataset, bestehend aus 184 NBI-Bildern, enthält 104 Trainigsbilder zur Verfahrensentwicklung und Parameteroptimierung und 80 Testbilder für die Evaluierung.

Tabelle 1. Abklingen η der Amplitude der zweidimensionalen Gaußfunktion am Rand der Filtermaske der Breite W (bezogen auf die Maximalamplitude).

W	2σ	4σ	6σ	8σ
η	60,65%	13.53%	1,11%	0.03%

Die Segmentierung von Textur erfordert eine gleichzeitige Betrachtung im Ortsbereich wie im Frequenzbereich, wobei die Gabofilter einen hervorragenden Kompromiss zwischen Orts- und Frequenzauflösung bieten. Im zweidimensionalen Bereich repräsentiert ein Gaborfilter

$$h(x,y) = \frac{1}{2\pi\sigma^2} e^{-\frac{x^2+y^2}{2\sigma^2}} e^{2\pi j(Ux+Vy)} \tag{1}$$

eine orientierte, komplexe Sinusfunktion, die durch eine zweidimensionale Gaußsche Einhüllende moduliert wird. Gemäß einer nachrichtentechnischen Interpretation wird dem Gaußschen Signal eine Bandbreite im Bereich der Trägerfrequenz F der komplexen Sinusfunktion zugewiesen. F bezeichnet dabei die Frequenz der in horizontaler Richtung verlaufenden Sinusschwingung und somit gleichzeitig die Trägerfrequenz des Gaborfilters. Die Frequenzkoordinaten U und V werden aus der Trägerfrequenz und der Orientierung durch $U = F \cdot cos\phi$, $V = F \cdot sin\phi$ berechnet.

In der vorliegenden Arbeit wurden 20 unterschiedliche Gaborfilter, erstellt mithilfe von 5 Trägerfrequenzen und 4 Orientierungen, eingesetzt. Bei der Orientierungswahl wurde die Erfassung horizontaler, vertikaler, sowie diagonaler Strukturen beabsichtigt. Dieses Ziel wird durch $\phi = 0, \frac{\pi}{2}, \frac{\pi}{4}, -\frac{\pi}{4}$ erreicht.Wenn die Standardabweichung der Gaußschen Einhüllenden den Wert σ annimmt, wird die Größe der Filtermaske auf 6σ festgelegt. Bei diesem Wert ist die einhüllende Gaußfunktion bereits auf 1,11% der Maximalamplitude abgeklungen. Größere Fenstermaße würden somit die Ergebnisse nicht wesentlich beeinflussen, aber dafür den Berechnungsaufwand erhöhen. Tabelle 1 zeigt den Zusammenhang zwischen Filtermaskengröße W und dem Amplitudenabklingen η der zweidimensionalen Gaußfunktion. Mit $\sigma = 10$ resultiert eine Kernelgröße von 61x61 Pixel. Die Standardabweichung der komplexen Einhüllenden beeinflusst die Frequenzbandbreite des Filters.

Jeder der 20 Gaborfilter wird mit den drei Farbkanälen des Gaußschen Farbraummodells gefaltet und ergibt somit 60 Merkmalsbilder. Per Pixel werden die für verschiedene Parametersets (F, ϕ, σ) erzielten Beträge der Filterantworten als Merkmale gewählt. Die mithilfe des K-Means-Clusterings empirisch optimierten Parameter $F = \{0,043; 0,053; 0,063; 0,073; 0,083\}$ (Zyklen pro Pixel), sowie $\phi = \{0, \frac{\pi}{2}, \frac{\pi}{4}, -\frac{\pi}{4}\}$ und $\sigma = 10$ ergeben $N = 60$ Merkmalsbilder, welche als Eingangsgrößen des Multikanal-Level-Set-Algorithmus dienen.

I_i mit $i = 1, ..., N$ stellt den i-ten Kanal des ursprünglichen Bildes I dar. Für jeden Kanal bezeichnen m_i und n_i die Mittelwerte von I_i innerhalb beziehungsweise außerhalb der Kontur $\mathcal{C}$. Unter Verwendung der impliziten Darstellung der Kurve $\mathcal{C} = \{(x,y)|\Phi(x,y,t) = 0\}$ durch die Level-Set-Funktion Φ ergibt sich der

Zero-Level-Set, wobei $\Phi(x, y, t) < 0$ außerhalb und $\Phi(x, y, t) > 0$ innerhalb der Kurve $\mathcal{C}$ gilt. Mit $m = (m_1, ..., m_N)$ und $n = (n_1, ..., n_N)$ definiert

$$\frac{\partial \Phi}{\partial t} = \delta(\Phi)[\mu \operatorname{div}\left(\frac{\nabla \Phi}{|\nabla \Phi|}\right) - \frac{1}{N}\sum_{i=1}^{N}\lambda_i(I_i - m_i)^2 + \frac{1}{N}\sum_{i=1}^{N}\gamma_2(I_i - n_i)^2] \qquad (2)$$

die Update-Gleichung des Zero-Level-Sets, welche nach jeder neuen Iteration der Gaborfilterbasierten Aktiven Konturen den Zero-Level-Set aktualisiert. Für alle 60 Kanäle werden die Intensitätsmittelwerte inner- beziehungsweise außerhalb der Kontur während jeder Iteration neu ermittelt. Die linke Seite dieser Gleichung wird im diskreten Bereich durch einen Differenzenquotient mit dem Zeitschritt Δt=0,5 implementiert. Damit ist es möglich, zum Zeitpunkt t_{n+1} die neue Kontur $\Phi^{t_{n+1}}$ aus der alten Kontur Φ^{t_n} und den Intensitätsmittelwerten $m_i(t_n)$, respektive $n_i(t_n)$, abzuleiten. Der mit μ gewichtete Ausdruck $\operatorname{div}\left(\frac{\nabla \Phi}{|\nabla \Phi|}\right)$ repräsentiert die Krümmung der Kontur und wird mithilfe finiter Differenzen implementiert.

Der Algorithmus iteriert für jedes einzelne Bild solange, bis die quantitative Veränderung zwischen zwei Iterationen unter eine Abbruchschwelle S fällt. Die Prüfung der Konvergenz hat den Zero-Level-Set $\mathcal{C}_{n+1} = \{(x, y)|\Phi(x, y, n + 1) = 0\}$ zum Zeitpunkt $t = n + 1$ als Ausgangspunkt. In einer beschränkten, durch einen Betragswert kleiner als 0,5 charakterisierten Umgebung dieser Kontur werden die aktuellen Level-Set-Werte den vorherigen Werten Φ_n gegenübergestellt. Es wird anschließend innerhalb dieser Region die Summe der so bestimmten Betragsdifferenzen über die gesamte Konturlänge ermittelt und mit dem für die Trainingsbilder optimierten Schwellwert $S = \Delta t \cdot 0,0324$ verglichen. Die Konvergenz des Algorithmus wird somit bei Erfüllung der Ungleichung

$$\sum_{1}^{Laenge(\mathcal{C}_{n+1})} (|\Phi_{n+1} - \Phi n|) < \Delta t \cdot 0,0324 \quad \text{für } |\Phi_{n+1}| < 0,5 \qquad (3)$$

erreicht. Mit einem Zeitschritt $\Delta t = 0,5$ ergibt sich der Schwellwert 0,0162.

Um eine Reduktion des Rechenaufwandes zu erreichen, wird das 502x586 Pixel große Eingangsbild um den Faktor 0,4 herunterskaliert. Die Initialkontur $\Phi_0(x, y) = \Phi(x, y, 0)$ wird ausgehend von einer binären Maske über eine Distanztransformation festgelegt. Das Binärbild enthält Elemente ungleich Null innerhalb eines im Bild zentrierten Kreises mit einem Radius von 55 Pixeln.

Eine morphologische Nachbearbeitung der Ergebnisse zur Erhaltung einer einzigen zusammenhängender Region wird mithilfe einer Reihe von Erosionen und Dilatationen realisiert. Als strukturierende Elemente für diese Operationen wurden Kreise verschiedener Radien (zwischen 5 und 15 Pixel) eingesetzt.

3   Ergebnisse

Für jedes Polypenbild steht eine handsegmentierte Maske (Goldstandard) in Form eines Binärbildes zur Verfügung. Ein pixelweiser Vergleich der beiden Masken führt auf vier mögliche Kombinationen, die nach der Polypenlokalisierung auftreten können. Korrekt lokalisierte Polypenpixel werden als „richtig positiv"(RP) bezeichnet, während korrekt detektierte Hintergrundpixel als „richtig negativ"(RN) zählen. Die Menge „falsch negativ"(FN) besteht aus Polypenpixel, die fälschlicherweise als Hintergrundpixel eingestuft werden. Die Kenngröße „falsch positiv"(FP) quantifiziert die als Polypenpixel erkannten Hintergrundpixel. Die Sensitivität = RP/(RP+FN) beschreibt die Anzahl korrekt erfasster Polypenpixel bezogen auf die Gesamtheit aller Polypenpixel, während sich mit Hilfe der Spezifität = RN/(RN + FP) der Anteil der korrekt klassifizierten Hintergrundpixel an allen Hintergrundpixeln quantifizieren lässt. Die Genauigkeit = (RN + RP)/(RN + RP + FP + FN) definiert die Summe der insgesamt korrekt erkannten Pixeln in Relation zur Gesamtpixelanzahl.

Das beste Genauigkeitsergebnis (80,7%) der Gaborfilterbasierten Aktiven Konturen ergibt sich für $\mu = 1000$ nach 300 Iterationen (Tab. 2). Die korrespondierende mittlere Spezifität von 94,22% bleibt mit $\sigma = 6,34$ für alle Polypen auf einem relativ konstanten Niveau, während die Sensitivität von 61,04% größeren Schwankungen unterlegen ist ($\sigma = 22,34\%$). In Tab. 2 sind die Resultate des neuen Verfahrens sowie die Ergebnisse der in [4] und [5] vorgestellten Methoden eingetragen.

4 Diskussion

Durch das in der vorliegenden Veröffentlichung erläuterte Verfahren ist die Verbesserung der automatischen Lokalisierung von Dickdarmpolypen in koloskopischen Bilddaten um 19,16% (in Vergleich zu den bisherigen Methoden aus Tabelle 2) gelungen. Die Spezifität beträgt annähernd 95%, was für die anschließende Blutgefäßsegmentierung und Polypenklassifizierung von großer Bedeutung ist. Die inkorrekte Einstufung von Hintergrundpixeln als Polypenpixel würde bedeuten, dass sich der mittels Support-Vector-Machine durchgeführte Klassifikationsprozess auf falschen Daten beläuft. Die unvollständige Detektion eines

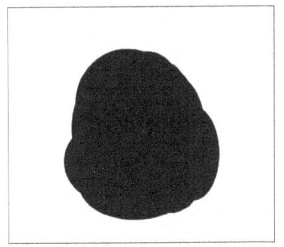 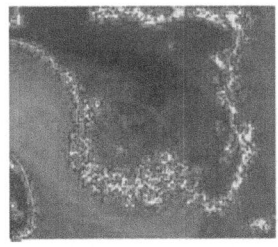 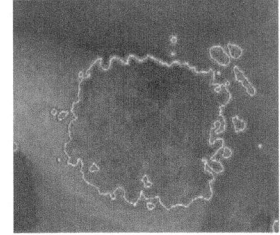

(a) Ground Truth   (b) Chan-Vese-Verfahren   (c)   Gaborfilterbasierte
                          (250 Iter.)   Aktive   Konturen   (250
                                                             Iter.)

Abb. 1. Ergebnisse. Im Vergleich zum Chan-Vese-Verfahren verbessern die Gaborfilterbasierten Aktiven Konturen (hier vor morphologischer Nachbearbeitung) die Texturerkennung.

Tabelle 2. Vergleich der Verfahren zur Polypenlokalisierung; absteigende Reihenfolge in Bezug auf die erreichten Genauigkeiten (alle Angaben in Prozent).

Verfahren	Gen	σ_{Gen}	Spez	σ_{Spez}	Sens	σ_{Sens}
Gaborfilterbasierte Aktive Konturen	80,70	11,89	94,22	6,34	61,04	22,34
Chan-Vese-Verfahren	61,54	16,41	85,55	16,25	48,14	20,51
Template Matching	58,72	23,26	98,09	4,48	30,43	25,50
Aktive Strahlen	57,69	22,85	96,80	6,23	31,51	24,41
Generalisierte Hough Transformation	47,65	23,41	99,31	2,25	9,30	11,45
Parametrische Aktive Konturen	45,37	23,11	99,89	0,50	3,31	2,58

Polypens, d.h. eine niedrigere Sensitivität, ist dafür unter der Annahme, dass die detektierte Polypenoberfläche repräsentative Merkmale aufweist, wesentlich unproblematischer. Abbildung 1 präsentiert einen visuellen Vergleich des Chan-Vese-Verfahrens [4] mit den Gaborfilterbasierten Aktiven Konturen. Für beide Ergebnisbilder gilt $\mu = 1$ und eine Iterationszahl von 250. Während das Chan-Vese-Verfahren in Abbildung 1(b) nur die Regionenhomogenität der Intensitätswerte berücksichtigt, reagieren die Gaborfilterbasierten Aktiven Konturen (Abbildung 1(c)) auf Texturen und erlauben eine deutlich bessere Polypensegmentierung.

Literaturverzeichnis

1. Robert Koch Institut (ed). Krebs in Deutschland 2005/2006: Häufigkeiten und Trends. Robert Koch Institut und Gesellschaft der epidemiologischen Krebsregister in Deutschland e.V.; 2010.
2. Tischendorf JJW, Wasmuth HE, Koch A, et al. Value of magnifying chromoendoscopy and narrow band imaging (NBI) in classifying colorectal polyps: A prospective controlled study. Endoscopy. 2007;39(12):1092–6.
3. Gross S, Palm S, Behrens A, et al. Segmentierung von Blutgefäßstrukturen in koloskopischen NBI-Bilddaten. Proc BVM. 2011; p. 13–7.
4. Breier M, Gross S, Behrens A. Chan-Vese-Segmentation of Polyps in Colonoscopic Image Data. Proceedings of the 15th International Student Conference on Electrical Engineering POSTER 2011. 2011.
5. Gross S, Kennel M, Stehle T, et al. Polyp Segmentation in NBI Colonoscopy. Proc BVM. 2009; p. 252–6.
6. Osher S, Sethian JA. Fronts propagating with curvature-dependent speed: Algorithms based on Hamilton-Jaccobi Formulation. Journal of Computational Physics. 1988;79:12–49.
7. Hoang MA, Geusebroek JM, Smeulders AWM. Color texture measurement and segmentation. Signal Process. 2005;85:265–75.
8. Sagiv C, Sochen NA, Zeevi YY. Integrated Active Contours for Texture Segmentation. IEEE Trans Image Process. 2006;15(2):1633–46.

Greedy Projection Access Order for SART
Simultaneous Algebraic Reconstruction Technique

Sylvia Kiencke[1], Yulia M. Levakhina[1,2], Thorsten M. Buzug[1]

[1]Institute of Medical Engineering, University of Lübeck
[2]Graduate School for Computing in Medicine and Life Sciences, University of Lübeck
kiencke@imt.uni-luebeck.de

Abstract. The projection access order in which the projections are used in the Simultaneous Algebraic Reconstruction Technique (SART) has great influence on the convergence rate and the quality of the reconstructed image. It is a well known fact that the correlation between the used projections should be as small as possible. Common methods achieve a small correlation based on the projection angles by applying special angle schemes. In this paper, we present a novel Greedy Projection Access Order (GPAO). GPAO is an angle-independent method, which is based on the structural information of the object itself. We create a projection-based information vector for each angle. By using the pairwise correlation of these vectors, a Greedy algorithm finds a short path through all projections. In this order the SART uses the projections to reconstruct the image. As the simulation results show, the performance of GPAO is similar to the performance of a random order. Advantageously, GPAO is robust and adapted to the object. Potentially, more complex path finding algorithms will show better results than the Greedy solution.

1 Introduction

Computed tomography (CT) is a medical imaging technique based on X-rays, which is widely used for clinical diagnostics. In tomography, the chosen reconstruction algorithm affects the quality of the reconstructed image. There are two main techniques for reconstruction, namely analytical and iterative methods. Since iterative reconstruction can produce images with less noise and artefacts than the conventional filtered backprojection, the focus of this work is the Simultaneous Algebraic Reconstruction Technique (SART). SART has been proposed by Andersen and Kak [1]. The order in which the SART algorithm accesses the projections has a great influence on the convergence rate and the quality of the reconstructed image [2]. The simplest way to determine a projection access order is the Sequential Access Scheme (SAS), however, it is known that SART with SAS has a slow convergence rate. A scheme, which results in a fast convergence is the Random Projection Scheme (RPS). On the other hand, RPS is unpredictable and highly chaotic. Numerous scientists have used alternative schemes in the attempt to produce predictable results with the same or

H.-P. Meinzer et al. (Hrsg.), *Bildverarbeitung für die Medizin 2013*, Informatik aktuell,
DOI: 10.1007/978-3-642-36480-8_18, © Springer-Verlag Berlin Heidelberg 2013

better quality than RPS. Herman and Meyer used an access scheme based on the Prime Number Decomposition of the number of projections [3]. Guan and Gordon developed the angle-based Multi Level Scheme for local angle optimisation [4], which shows the best results when the number of projections is to the power of two. The Weighted-Distance Scheme, a global angle optimisation, was introduced by Mueller et al. [5]. It takes more than the nearest neighbouring projection into account. The primary function of the above angle-based schemes is to minimise the correlation between used projections. This is because a lower correlation leads to a higher quality of image reconstruction within less iterations [3, 4]. Based on a software-based simulation we present the results of a novel angle-independent Greedy Projection Access Order (GPAO) taking into account, not only the angular information, but also the information based on the data itself.

2 Materials and methods

2.1 SART

Object representation as a discrete grid of pixels allows us formulating the reconstruction problem as a system of linear equations

$$\sum_{j=1}^{N_{\text{pixel}}} l_{i,j} \cdot f_j = p_i \quad 1 \le i \le N_{\text{total}} \tag{1}$$

where N_{pixel} is the number of grid pixels, N_{total} the total number of projections with N_γ projection directions, and N_{det} detector element measurements per direction ($N_{\text{total}} = N_\gamma \cdot N_{\text{det}}$), p_i is the i-th projection value and f_j is the gray value of the j-th pixel in the grid. There are different methods to weight the passing of a ray through a pixel. We use the length of the passing through a pixel [6]. In order to approximate the weighting factor $l_{i,j}$ in a better way we use an oversampling of R rays per detector element measurement ($R \in \mathbb{N}$). Factor $l_{i,j}$ is the mean value of the sum of weighting factors for each ray. The linear equation system is solved iteratively by the SART. The SART equation for updating a pixel in the q-th iteration step for the current projection image P_γ can be written as

$$f_j^{(q)} = f_j^{(q-1)} + \lambda \cdot \frac{\sum_{p_i \in P_\gamma} \left(\frac{p_i - \sum_{n=1}^{N_{\text{pixel}}} l_{i,n} \cdot f_n^{(q-1)}}{\sum_{n=1}^{N_{\text{pixel}}} l_{i,n}} \right) \cdot l_{i,j}}{\sum_{p_i \in P_\gamma} l_{i,j}} \tag{2}$$

where λ is a relaxation factor within the interval (0,2].

2.2 Data-based projection access order

The proposed GPAO approach consists of two steps. Firstly, a correlation matrix using the projection data is generated. Secondly, a path through these projections that leads to minimal total correlation is determined. The resulting path is the projection access order for the SART reconstruction.

Correlation matrix. The $N_\gamma \times N_\gamma$ correlation matrix is calculated based on the pairwise correlation between vectors containing projection-related information. The correlation $\varrho_{u,v}$ between two vectors u and v of length N can be written as

$$\varrho_{u,v} = \frac{\frac{1}{N-1} \cdot \sum_{n=1}^{N}(u_n - \mu_u) \cdot (v_n - \mu_v)}{\sigma_u \cdot \sigma_v} \tag{3}$$

where μ_u and μ_v are the mean values and σ_u and σ_v are the standard derivations of the vectors. We propose three ways in which to use projection data to calculate the vectors for the correlation matrix:

1. The unmodified sinogram column for each direction γ.
2. The simple backprojection (SBP) for each direction γ.
3. The masked SBP for each direction γ.

A backprojection view B_γ is a result of the SBP for one direction γ

$$B_\gamma = \text{SBP}(p_\gamma) \tag{4}$$

A masked backprojection view takes the object support into account. Using a threshold related to the maximum value of the simple backprojected binary sinogram (for this a more simple thresholding was taken by setting all values about the value of the background to one) we get a binary mask m. The data outside the object support mask are removed from vector B_γ

$$B_\gamma^{\text{masked}} = B_\gamma(m := 1) \tag{5}$$

As well as removing irrelevant information, this method also saves calculation time and storage space by using this particular SBP. The extent of the saved time and storage space depends on the size of the object or more specifically the object support mask.

Greedy algorithm. In order to find the minimal correlation path it is necessary to solve the Travelling Salesmen Problem (TSP). Here a greedy method is used. Firstly, the algorithm searches for the smallest value ϱ_{i_1,i_2} in the correlation matrix. The two corresponding projection indices (i_1, i_2) are used as the first two entries of the projection access order vector. Then the algorithm searches for the next smallest correlation coefficient ϱ_{i_2,i_3} for projection of index i_2, and add i_3 to the vector. After each index has been used once, the result represents the GPAO vector for the SART reconstruction.

2.3 XCAT phantom and CT-scanner setting

Noiseless projections of a chest slice from XCAT-phantom have been simulated using parallel beam geometry [7]. The slice also was used as a reference for the evaluation of the quality of reconstruction. The number of directions is 1200 with equidistant spacing of 0.3°, the number of detector elements 1024 with 0.39 mm element size and the reconstructed image has a size of 512×512 pixels with 0.78 mm pixel size.

2.4   Evaluation

To compare the GPAO-based reconstruction methods with the SAS- and RPS-based methods two different error measures were used. The first one $\varepsilon_{1,q}$ is the arithmetic mean of the absolute gray value differences between the original data f^{ref} (Fig. 1(a)) and the reconstructed data $f^{(q)}$ of the q-th iteration divided by the maximal difference of possible gray values in percent

$$\varepsilon_{1,q} = \frac{\sum_{j=1}^{N_{\mathrm{pixel}}} |f_j^{\mathrm{ref}} - f_j^{(q)}|}{|\mathrm{max(gray\ value)\text{-}min(gray\ value)}|} \cdot 100 \tag{6}$$

The second quality measure $\varepsilon_{2,q}$ is the correlation coefficient between the two images. It describes the similarity of the two images

$$\varepsilon_{2,q} = \frac{\frac{1}{N_{\mathrm{pixel}}-1} \cdot \sum_{j=1}^{N_{\mathrm{pixel}}} (f_j^{\mathrm{ref}} - \mu_{f^{\mathrm{ref}}}) \cdot (f_j^{(q)} - \mu_{f^{(q)}})}{\sigma_{f^{\mathrm{ref}}} \cdot \sigma_{f^{(q)}}} \tag{7}$$

2.5   Simulation

The following itemisation describes the simulation in a chronological order:

1. Simulate the projection for the given XCAT-phantom slice shown in Fig. 1(a) by the above described scanner parameters.
2. Process the sinogram information with unmodified sinogram column, SBP and masked SBP for each direction.
3. Calculate the correlation matrix for each preprocessed dataset.
4. Produce the GPAO for each correlation matrix.
5. Reconstruction by SART with SAS, RPS, and GPAOs.
6. Produce the reconstructions from one to five iterations ($q = 1, ..., 5$) to evaluate the convergence rate.

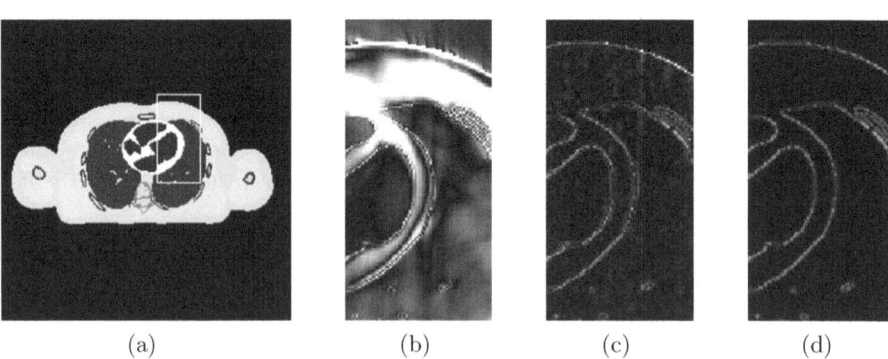

(a)   (b)   (c)   (d)

Fig. 1. Cutout of the absolute difference between the original image (a) and the reconstructed image for one iteration with (b) SAS, (c) the GPAO with correlation data from the masked SBP and (d) RPS (error scale $0 - 0.05\frac{1}{\mathrm{cm}}$, black equals $0\frac{1}{\mathrm{cm}}$ and white $0.05\frac{1}{\mathrm{cm}}$ or higher).

7. Calculate the errors $\varepsilon_{1,q}$ and $\varepsilon_{2,q}$ in reference to the original XCAT-phantom slice.

3   Results

Fig. 2(a) represents the results from subsection 2.5, showing the arithmetic mean of the absolute difference of gray values between the original data and the reconstructioned images of Fig. 1(a) for one to five iterations with SAS, RPS and GPAO with sinogram, SBP and masked SBP. In Fig. 2(b) the correlation curves between the reconstructed and the original image are shown. To get an impression of the quality after one iteration for selected reconstructions (SAS, GPAO with masked SBP and RPS) in Fig. 1 the absolute difference between the reconstruction and the reference image is visualised.

4   Discussion

In this paper, we presented a new data-based approach for pre-ordering projections for SART with a Greedy method. We used three projection-based information processing methods to prepare correlation matrices on which the Greedy algorithm was applied. In Fig. 2 we can see that our three GPAOs show an error behaviour between SAS and RPS, with SAS having the worst error behaviour and RPS having a better error behaviour. The GPAO behaviour highly depends on the projection-based information we used to calculate the correlation matrix. Since the GPAO is based on a projection information vector, there is no need for a special angle scheme. Equidistant as well as non-equidistant angles can be used to create GPAO. We should note that angle information is not necessary to calculate GPAO, however, it is highly useful to add it indirectly by simple BP for each direction. This is archived through the effect of

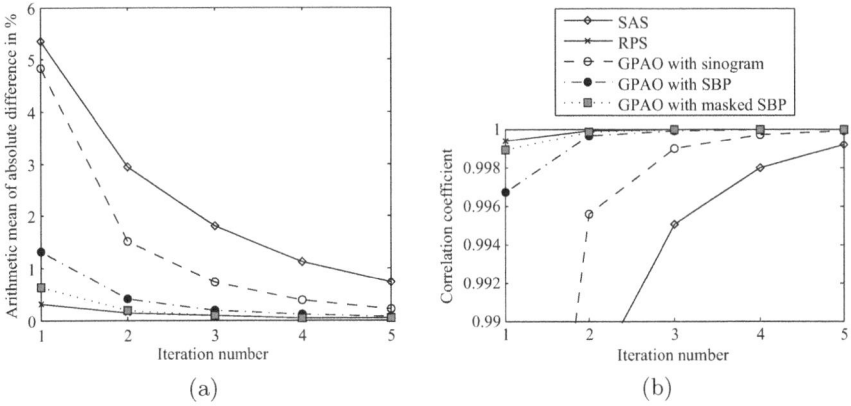

Fig. 2. Arithmetic mean of the absolute difference of gray values between original and reconstruction data (a) and correlation between them from one to five iterations with SAS, RPS and GPAO with sinogram, SBP and masked SBP (b).

smearing up the information of one projection over the image in a characteristic direction. Nevertheless, the GPAO with masked SBP shows better results than GPAO with SBP (Fig. 2). The SBP for each direction causes an error for the whole region around the object transferred to the correlation matrix. This error has a negative effect on the GPAO. In order to suppress this error and still keep the indirect angle information, an object supported mask was added to the SBP for each direction. Through binary masking we can focus on the object itself and get similar results in comparison to RPS. Looking at the visualised absolute differences between the reference image and the reconstructions of SAS (Fig. 1(b)), GPAO with masked SBP (Fig. 1(c)) and RPS (Fig. 1(d)) gives the same visual impression. We can notice that the errors for RPS are concentrated at the object edges, whereas GPAO errors can be found, not only toward the edges, but within the object itself. Comparing the computing time SAS has no preprocessing, RPS takes the time to permute the sequence of angles once and for GPAO the preprocessing time for calculating the correlation matrix depends on the method and the object. GPAO with masked SBP needs an additional time for calculating a mask. Finding a projection access order by the Greedy algorithm has the same processing time for each of the three GPOA methods. At this point the efficiency should be considered less than the benefit by the robustness and the angle-independence. We see huge potential for the data-based optimisation of projection access order. Although SART with GPAO does not result in the optimal solution, it has shown promising results in the reconstruction of images. Future work will focus on different solutions for the TSP and build on the potential of region supported masking, as well as consider data with noise and compare the methods with angle-based approaches.

References

1. Andersen AH, Kak AC. Simultaneous algebraic reconstruction technique (SART): a superior implementation of the art algorithm. Ultrason Imaging. 1984;6(1):81–94.
2. Herman GT. Image reconstruction from projections: the fundamentals of computerized tomography. New York: Academic Press; 1980.
3. Meyer LB, Herman GT. Algebraic reconstruction techniques can be made computationally efficient. IEEE Trans Med Imaging. 1993;12(3):600–9.
4. Guan H, Gordon R. A projection access order for speedy convergence of ART (algebraic reconstruction technique): a multilevel scheme for computed tomography. Phys Med Biol. 1994;39(11):2005–22.
5. Mueller K, Yagel R, Cornhill JF. The weighted-distance scheme: a globally optimizing projection ordering method for ART. IEEE Trans Med Imaging. 1997;16(2):223–30.
6. Siddon RL. Fast calculation of the exact radiological path for a three-dimensional CT array. Med Phys. 1985;12(2):252–5.
7. Mueller J, Kaiser F, Levakhina YM, et al. An open database of metal artifacts cases for clinical CT imaging. Proc of the second international conference on image formation in X-Ray CT. 2012; p. 210–3.

ROI Selection for Remote Photoplethysmography

Georg Lempe[1], Sebastian Zaunseder[1], Tom Wirthgen[2], Stephan Zipser[2], Hagen Malberg[1]

[1]Institut für Biomedizinische Technik, TU Dresden
[2]Fraunhofer IVI, Dresden
georg.lempe@tu-dresden.de

Abstract. Camera-based remote photoplethysmography (rPPG) is a technique that can be used to measure vital signs contactlessly. In order to optimize the extraction of photoplethysmographic signals from video sequences, we investigate the spatial dependence of the photoplethysmographic signal. For an evaluation of the suitability of various regions of interest for rPPG measurements, we conducted a study on 20 healthy subjects. We analysed the videos using a refined pulse amplitude mapping approach. Our results show that the signal-to-noise ratio of rPPG signals can be improved by limiting the region of interest to certain regions of the face.

1 Introduction

Photoplethysmography (PPG) is a technique used to non-invasively determine blood volume changes at a measurement site by measuring the absorption of light. In a clinical setting PPG is used to measure oxygen saturation, but cardiac and respiratory activity can be derived from PPG signals as well. Remote photoplethysmography (rPPG) makes use of optical imaging sensors to measure subtle skin-color changes resulting from blood volume changes in near-surface vessels [1]. The contactless measurement principle makes rPPG an interesting technology in applications outside the clinical environment where traditional biomedical monitoring is not feasible today. The decreasing prices and the abundant availability of digital cameras and processing power over the last years have contributed to a growing number of rPPG related publications.

However, the image and signal-processing methods used today are not yet robust enough to allow for a reliable monitoring of cardiac activity in everyday situations. Common artifacts due to movement or changes in illumination can surpass the signal by orders of magnitude and pose the main problem that hinders rPPG. Several signal processing approaches to improve the quality of rPPG signals were therefore proposed in the past [2, 3].

Another aspect of the signal extraction, the selection of the region of interest (ROI), has received little attention. In recent publications most commonly the entire face or static areas within are being used as ROI. Poh et al. determine the ROI using face detection. Hereby the rectangle enclosing the detected face is shrunk and then used as ROI [2]. Sun et al., Lewandowska et al. and Takano et al. use rectangular ROIs centered on the forehead and the cheeks [4, 3, 5]. While in the latter cases the selection was done manually, Lewandowska et al. also propose a method to geometrically determine a ROI on the forehead in relation to the position of the eyes. Verkruysse as well as Hülsbusch and Blažek have shown that not all parts of the skin's surface undergo the same amount of color change [6, 7]. Even though these phenomena have been described qualitatively, no quantitative analyses have been conducted yet.

2   Materials and methods

We hypothesize that it is possible to improve the rPPG signal's quality by determining a well-suited ROI. Building upon the aforementioned studies by Hülsbusch, Blažek and Verkruysse we investigate whether it is possible to define an optimized ROI using Lewandowska's approach of defining landmarks in the face. To achieve this we apply Verkruysse's method of pulse amplitude mapping [6], extending it by using precise reference signals.

2.1   Measurement setup

We conducted a study on 20 healthy subjects (age: 26.5 ± 4 years, sex: 8 female, 12 male). The subjects were asked to lie down on a tilt table and to hold still during the measurement. The camera (IDS uEye 5240 CP-C) was mounted 1 m above the table's surface, in front of the face. The videos were recorded synchronously with data of conventional, contacting medical sensors. We recorded RGB videos of 3 minutes length with a color depth of 10 Bit per channel, a resolution of 300×200 px and a frame rate of 100 Hz. The subject was illuminated frontally by four fluorescent tubes (NARVA LT 58 W/025 universalwhite). The distance between the lamps and the subject's face was 1.5 m. The lamps were equipped with electronic ballast circuits that drive the tubes with a frequency of 40 kHz avoiding the flickering with the line frequency. As ground truth reference

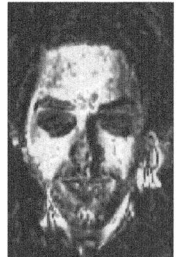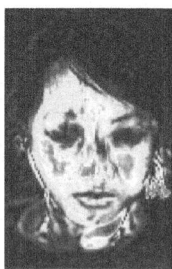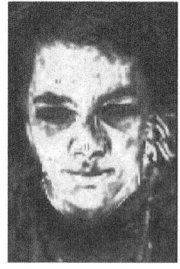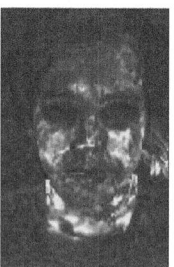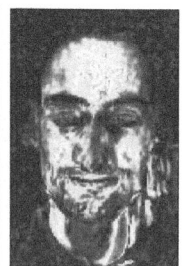

Fig. 1. Pulse amplitude maps showing the distribution of the rPPG signal's quality. Blue stands for a low value of the signal quality, red for a high value.

we recorded a PPG from an ear clip on the subjects right earlobe as well as an electrocardiogram (ECG) with clamp electrodes with a sampling frequency of 1 kHz. An ADInstruments PowerLab 16/35 was used to record the output of these sensors.

2.2   Mapping the signal quality

For the following analyses only the green color channel was considered, since this channel contains the strongest rPPG signal. The videos were scaled down by a factor of 4 by averaging spatially over neighborhoods of 16 px. By evaluating the signal quality of each pixel of the scaled video, maps can be created that show the spatial distribution of the signal quality (Fig. 1). In this context we defined the signal quality based on the spectral features of the rPPG signal x_r

$$q = \frac{A_{hr}}{\sum_{i=0}^{N/2} \mathcal{F}\{x_r(i)\}} = \frac{\mathcal{F}\{x_r(i_{hr})\}}{\sum_{i=0}^{N/2} \mathcal{F}\{x_r(i)\}} \tag{1}$$

where A_{hr} is the signal's amplitude at the heart rate f_{hr} and $\mathcal{F}(x)$ is the discrete Fourier transform (Fig. 2). The heart rate is determined using the reference

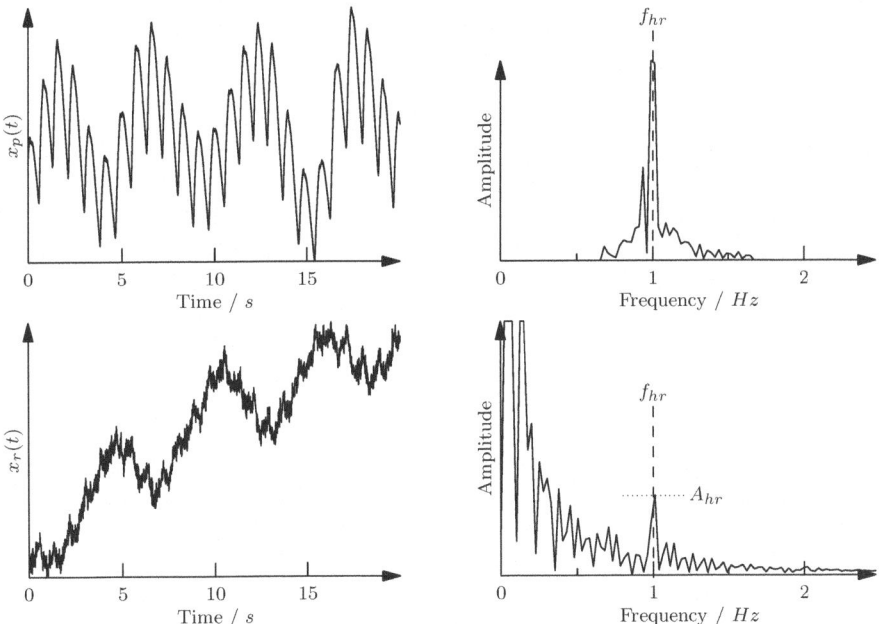

Fig. 2. Time signals and spectra of the reference PPG (top) and the rPPG (bottom) signals. The rPPG was derived using a 16 px neighborhood as ROI. The high frequent noise visible in its time signal is due to the comparatively small ROI, the flickering of the light source and the short exposure times / high sampling rates.

PPG. For each subject a total of 100 partially overlapping windows with a length of 20 seconds each were analysed in terms of Eq. 1.

2.3   Comparison of ROIs

In order to determine favorable ROIs we compared average signal qualities. As a reference, we manually labeled an ROI containing the subject's face. We also manually labeled landmarks whose coordinates were used to construct several square ROIs within the face. Fig. 3 shows the position of the landmarks and the ROIs. We determined each ROI's signal quality by averaging the values of the signal quality maps within the ROI. By applying this method to all windows of each measurement and averaging over all the results we determined one single signal quality parameter μ_q for each ROI.

3   Results

The methods described earlier lead to the generation of maps of the signal qualities as depicted in Fig. 1. These maps show a non uniform distribution of the signal quality. The averaged signal qualities μ_q of the single ROIs, as well as their standard deviations are shown in Fig. 3. It can be seen that similar ROIs show a similar signal quality. Comparing the highest and lowest signal quality the results show an improvement of 50 percent.

4   Discussion

In this article we have shown that the choice of the ROI has a significant influence on the quality of the rPPG signal. The resulting signal qualities suggest the

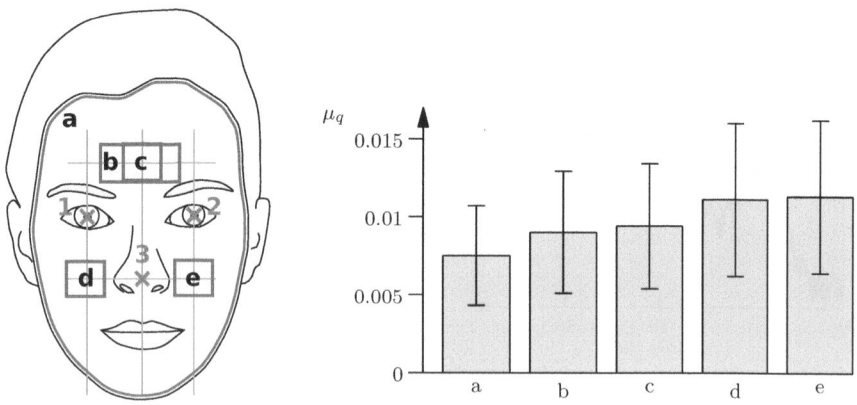

Fig. 3. Left: Position of the ROIs (green) and landmarks (red) within the face. Right: Mean signal quality μ_q and standard deviation for all measurements and windows. The cheeks, ROIs d and e, show the highest mean signal quality.

selection of the cheeks as ROIs for the extraction of rPPG signals. This is favorable since practical considerations support the use of the cheeks as ROIs as well. They are rarely covered by clothing or facial hair. We conclude that the selection of the entire face as an ROI, as it is used in state of the art publications, is not the optimal base for the extraction of rPPG signals. Using only parts of the face, such as the cheeks, for the signal extraction however introduces additional challenges. In future work segmentation algorithms capable of robustly tracking the desired ROIs have to be designed and tested for their applicability to rPPG. It has to be noted that these conclusions are valid for uniform illumination. The application of rPPG in everyday situations may require dynamic ROI selection in order to adapt the signal extraction to unfavorable lighting.

References

1. Blazek V, Wu T, Hoelscher D. Near-infrared CCD imaging: possibilities for non-invasive and contactless 2D mapping of dermal venous hemodynamics. Proc SPIE. 2000;3923:2.
2. Poh MZ, McDuff DJ, Picard RW. Advancements in noncontact, multiparameter physiological measurements using a webcam. Biomed Eng. 2011;58(1):7–11.
3. Lewandowska M, Nowak J. Measuring pulse rate with a webcam. J Med Imaging Health Inform. 2012;2(1):87–92.
4. Sun Y, Hu S, Azorin-Peris V, et al. Motion-compensated noncontact imaging photoplethysmography to monitor cardiorespiratory status during exercise. J Biomed Opt. 2011;16:077010.
5. Takano C, Ohta Y. Heart rate measurement based on a time-lapse image. Med Eng Phys. 2007;29(8):853–7.
6. Verkruysse W, Svaasand LO, Nelson JS. Remote plethysmographic imaging using ambient light. Opt Expr. 2008;16(26):21434–45.
7. Huelsbusch M, Blazek V. Contactless mapping of rhythmical phenomena in tissue perfusion using PPGI. Proc SPIE. 2002;4683:110.

Scaling Calibration in the ATRACT Algorithm

Yan Xia[1], Andreas Maier[1], Frank Dennerlein[2], Hannes G. Hofmann[1],
Joachim Hornegger[1,3]

[1]Pattern Recognition Lab (LME), Friedrich-Alexander-University
Erlangen-Nuremberg, Erlangen, Germany
[2]Healthcare Sector, Siemens AG, Erlangen, Germany
[3]Erlangen Graduate School in Advanced Optical Technologies (SAOT),
Friedrich-Alexander-University Erlangen-Nuremberg, Erlangen, Germany
yan.xia@cs.fau.de

Abstract. Recently, a reconstruction algorithm for region of interest (ROI) imaging in C-arm CT was published, named Approximated Truncation Robust Algorithm for Computed Tomography (ATRACT). Even in presence of severe data truncation, it is able to reconstruct images without the use of any explicit extrapolation or prior knowledge. However, this method suffers from a scaling artifact in the reconstruction. In this paper, we have investigated a calibration applied in the projection domain to compensate this scaling problem. The proposed correction method is evaluated by using six clinical datasets in presence of different artificial truncation. The results shows that a relative root mean square error (rRMSE) of up to 0.9% is achieved by the corrected ATRACT method.

1 Introduction

For three-dimensional (3D) X-ray imaging during the interventions, changes of the examined patient are often restricted to a small part of the field of view (FOV), e.g. cochlear implants, and needle biopsies. This suggests region of interest (ROI) imaging by irradiating the diagnostic interest area only. However, the corresponding 3D ROI reconstruction from laterally truncated projections poses a challenge to the conventional tomographic reconstruction algorithms and can result in a noticeable degradation of image quality.

So far various truncation correction methods have been proposed to overcome the effect of truncation artifact [1, 2, 3, 4]. Recently, a novel method for ROI reconstruction of highly truncated projection data with neither the use of prior knowledge nor any explicit extrapolation has been suggested [5, 6]. This method (ATRACT) is based on a decomposition of the standard ramp filter within FDK (Feldkamp, Davis, and Kress algorithm [7]) into a local and a non-local filtering step, where the local step is a 2D Laplace operator and the non-local step is a 2D Radon-based filtering that can be converted into a 2D convolution-based filtering [8]. The ATRACT method can provide satisfactory reconstruction results even in presence of severe data truncation. But it suffers from a global scaling

H.-P. Meinzer et al. (Hrsg.), *Bildverarbeitung für die Medizin 2013*, Informatik aktuell,
DOI: 10.1007/978-3-642-36480-8_20, © Springer-Verlag Berlin Heidelberg 2013

and bias problem in the reconstruction. It is therefore our goal to compensate this problem in the projection domain by searching projection calibration parameters.

2   Materials and methods

The ATRACT algorithm discussed here is an optimized version, where the non-local operation corresponds a 2D convolution-based filter. This significantly increases computational performance compared to Radon-based filtering [8].

2.1   ATRACT algorithm

We focus on the circular cone-beam imaging geometry shown in Fig. 1. Then, the ATRACT algorithm can be written as follows:

– *Step 1:* Cosine- and Parker-like weighting of projection data to obtain $g_1(\lambda, u, v)$

$$g_1(\lambda, u, v) = \frac{Dm(\lambda, u)}{\sqrt{D^2 + u^2 + v^2}} g(\lambda, u, v) \tag{1}$$

– *Step 2:* 2D Laplace filtering to obtain projection data $g_2(\lambda, u, v)$

$$g_2(\lambda, u, v) = \left(\frac{\partial^2}{\partial u^2} + \frac{\partial^2}{\partial v^2}\right) g_1(\lambda, u, v) \tag{2}$$

– *Step 3:* 2D convolution-based filtering to get filtered projection data

$$g_F(\lambda, u, v) = \frac{1}{4\pi^2} \frac{R}{D} \int\limits_{u_1}^{u_2} \int\limits_{v_1}^{v_2} g_2(\lambda, u - u', v - v') \frac{|v'|}{u'^2 + v'^2} du' dv' \tag{3}$$

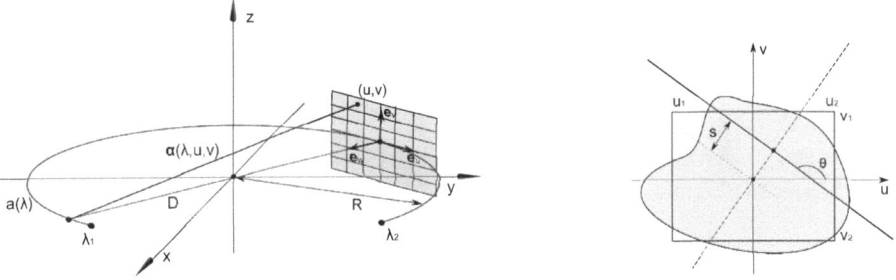

Fig. 1. Cone-beam geometry and associated notation: The curve $\mathbf{a}(\lambda) = (R\cos\lambda, R\sin\lambda, 0)$ describes the trajectory of the X-ray source, with the scan radius R and the rotation angle λ. The planar detector is parallel to the unit vectors $e_u(\lambda)$ and $e_v(\lambda)$ and at distance D from the source. $e_w(\lambda)$ is the detector normal. (θ, s) represent Radon-based coordinates. We use the function $g(\lambda, u, v)$ to describe the projection data at the point (u, v) acquired at angle λ.

– *Step 4:* 3D cone-beam backprojection to get $f^{(\text{ATRACT})}(x, y, z)$

$$f^{(\text{ATRACT})}(x, y, z) = \int_{\lambda_1}^{\lambda_2} \frac{RD}{[R - (x, y, z) \cdot \mathbf{e}_w(\lambda)]^2} g_F(\lambda, u, v) d\lambda \qquad (4)$$

2.2   Scaling correction in ATRACT

In the ATRACT algorithm, we remove the singularities at the edges of lateral data truncation after Laplace filtering. This causes a loss of the information on the thickness of the object. The following residual filtering of truncated projections will result in a offset with respect to the FDK filtering of non-truncated projection, as illustrated in Fig. 2(a). In the previous literature, a correction of scaling and bias was manually performed in the final reconstructed volume for each dataset, to align the value range between the reference and ATRACT.

In this paper, we compensate the scaling problem by calibrating the projection-related parameters. The scheme is formulated as follows

$$g_F^{\text{corrected}}(\lambda, u, v) = g_F(\lambda, u, v) + \text{offset}(\lambda) \qquad (5)$$

$$\text{offset}(\lambda) = A \cdot \sum_{u_1}^{u_2} \sum_{v_1}^{v_2} g(\lambda, u, v) + B + C \cdot (u_2 - u_1) \cdot (v_2 - v_1) \qquad (6)$$

where $g_F(\lambda, u, v)$ and $g_F^{\text{corrected}}(\lambda, u, v)$ denote the filtered projections by ATRACT without and with the scaling correction.

The attenuation-related linear parameters A and B were determined by comparing the difference between the filtered projections by ATRACT and by the full FOV FDK. The last term in (6) is a compensation factor in case that truncation size is too small. The corresponding parameter C was determined in the

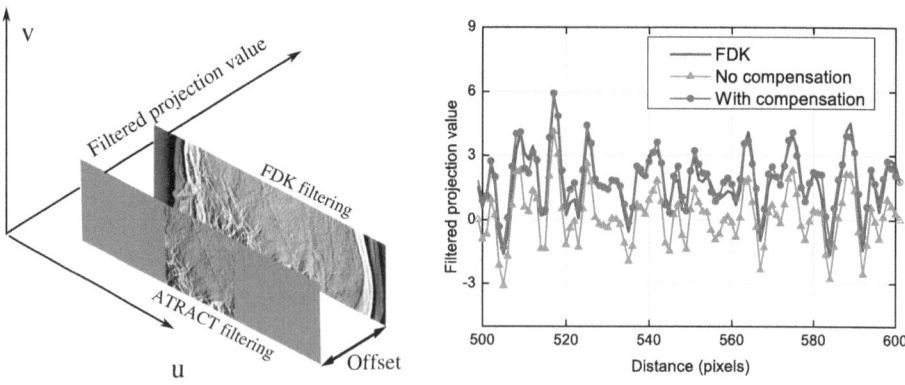

Fig. 2. Offset problem in ATRACT filtering of a truncated projection (left) and line profiles of the filtered projection by the corrected and uncorrected ATRACT and by FDK (right).

small truncation case. Fig. 2(b) shows the line profiles of ATRACT filtering of the truncated projection with and without correction as well as FDK filtering of the truncation-free projection. Note that in the following evaluation parameters A, B and C are fixed in all datasets and calibration has to be performed only once for a given acquisition scenario.

2.3   Experiment setup

To validate and evaluate the new scaling correction, six clinical datasets of patient heads were employed. All datasets were acquired on a C-arm system (Artis Zee, Siemens AG) from St. Luke's Episcopal Hospital (Houston, TX, USA). All scans containing 496 projection images (1240×960) with the resolution of 0.308 mm / pixel were acquired on a $200°$ short-scan circular trajectory. The calibration parameters were determined using the dataset 1 with $A = -3.68E - 7$, $B = 1.78$ and $C = -6.76E - 7$.

Three experiment setups were considered. In Setup 1, no collimation was applied, yielding the non-truncated projection data. In Setup 2 and 3, the data sets were virtually collimated (by setting the outside to zero) to the two different levels (FOV: 104 mm and 72 mm), so that only the desired FOV was kept.

All clinical data were reconstructed onto a Cartesian grid ($512 \times 512 \times 350$) with sampling spacing $\triangle x = \triangle y = \triangle z = 0.4$ mm in Setup 1 and 2 and with different sampling spacing $\triangle x = \triangle y = \triangle z = 0.2$ mm in Setup 3. The standard FDK reconstruction of Setup 1, i.e. non-truncated projection was used as the reference in each clinical case. The truncated datasets were reconstructed by the corrected and uncorrected ATRACT algorithm. The quantitative evaluation for the six clinical datasets was carried out by using the relative root mean squared error (rRMSE) and the correlation coefficient within the entire ROIs.

3   Results

The reconstruction results of the clinical dataset 1 and 4 from all three setups are presented in Fig. 3 and Fig. 4, respectively. In the visual inspection, no significant difference is observed in the same grayscale window between the corrected ATRACT-based ROI reconstructions and the reference reconstructions from non-truncated data, even in presence of different truncation levels. However, for visualizing the reconstructions from the uncorrected ATRACT, totally different display windows are applied. Also note that the incorrect scaling and bias in the reconstructed volume might cause difficulties for any volume-based post-processing algorithm in different stages of the imaging pipeline. Here, for instance, we can observe that the ring artifact reduction algorithm does not produce proper results (marked by the arrows) if no correction is applied.

A summary of the quantitative evaluation from the reconstructions of all six clinical datasets are shown in Tab. 1. The corrected ATRACT reduces the rRMSE of up to 0.92% compared to the rRMSE of 3.29% for uncorrected one. Also, it is clear that the new scaling calibration performs nicely in all evaluated

108   Xia et al.

datasets with the same calibration parameters A, B and C. Note that due to the fact that the correlation coefficient is independent to the scaling and bias problem in the reconstruction, no significant difference is observed for these values between the corrected ATRACT and the uncorrected one. Improvements emerge only from the improved ring correction.

4 Discussion

In this paper, we presented a calibration that can be applied on an existing truncation correction using ATRACT. The average RMSE was reduced by 7 times using the corrected ATRACT method. A potential limitation of this study is

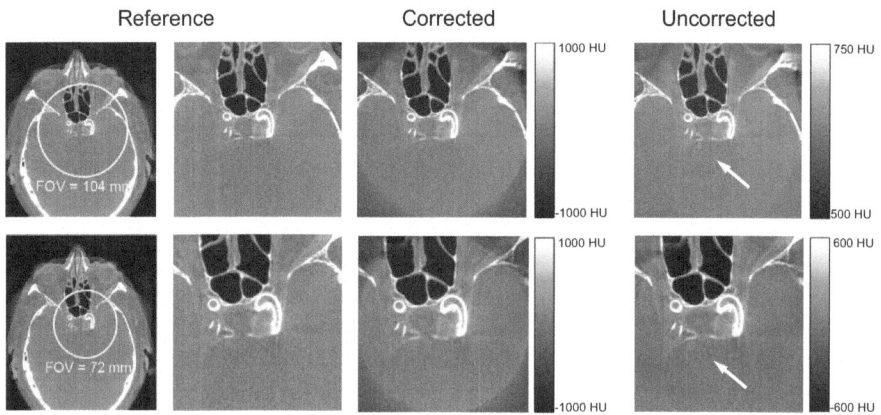

Fig. 3. Reconstruction results of the clinical dataset 1 by the ATRACT algorithm. From left to right: The FDK reconstructions of non-truncated data, zoomed FDK reconstructions, the corrected ATRACT reconstructions, the uncorrected ones.

Fig. 4. Homogeneous area of the clinical dataset 4 reconstructed by the corrected ATRACT algorithm in a compressed display window (C:0 HU, W:200 HU). The first row: the reference with slice thickness 0.4 mm, the ROI reconstruction by the corrected ATRACT from Setup 2 (FOV:104mm). The bottom row: the reference with slice thickness 0.2 mm, the ROI reconstruction by the corrected ATRACT from Setup 3 (FOV:72mm).

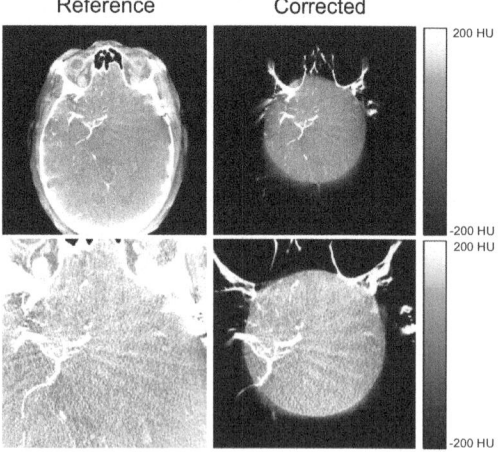

Table 1. Summary of the quantitative evaluation computed from the reconstructions of the six patient head datasets by means of the corrected and uncorrected ATRACT.

Dataset	FOV (mm)	rRMSE (%) Uncorrected	Corrected	Correlation Uncorrected	Corrected
1	104	7.56	0.922	0.989	0.990
	72	3.29	0.923	0.981	0.982
2	104	10.4	1.72	0.984	0.984
	72	9.58	1.49	0.990	0.992
3	104	7.72	1.55	0.974	0.976
	72	11.4	2.54	0.970	0.970
4	104	9.78	2.10	0.985	0.985
	72	12.6	1.99	0.990	0.991
5	104	20.6	1.36	0.951	0.953
	72	22.0	2.04	0.982	0.989
6	104	15.5	1.48	0.985	0.985
	72	15.7	1.53	0.994	0.994

that only patient head datasets were employed. Differences between the anatomy of the patient are likely to result in variations in calibration parameters.

References

1. Hsieh J, Chao E, Thibault J, et al. A novel reconstruction algorithm to extend the CT scan field-of-view. Med Phys. 2004;31(9):2385–91.
2. Defrise M, Noo F, Clackdoyle R, et al. Truncated Hilbert transform and image reconstruction from limited tomographic data. Inverse Probl. 2006;22(3):1037–53.
3. Kolditz D, Kyriakou Y, Kalender WA. Volume-of-interest (VOI) imaging in C-arm flat-detector CT for high image quality at reduced dose. Med Phys. 2010;37(6):2719–30.
4. Maier A, Scholz B, Dennerlein F. Optimization-based extrapolation for truncation correction. 2nd CT Meeting. 2012; p. 390–4.
5. Dennerlein F. Cone-beam ROI reconstruction using the Laplace operator. Proc Fully 3D 2011. 2011; p. 80–3.
6. Dennerlein F, Maier A. Region-of-interest reconstruction on medical C-arms with the ATRACT algorithm. Proc SPIE. 2012; p. 83131B.
7. Feldkamp LA, Davis LC, Kress JW. Practical cone beam algorithm. J Opt Soc Am. 1984;1(6):612–9.
8. Xia Y, Maier A, Dennerlein F, et al. Efficient 2D filtering for cone-beam VOI reconstruction. Proc IEEE NSS/MIC. 2012;To appear.

Improvement of an Active Surface Model by Adaptive External Forces

Tony Pilz, Eduard Fried, Stefan van Waasen, Gudrun Wagenknecht

Multimodal Image Processing Group, Electronic Systems, ZEA-2,
Forschungszentrum Jülich GmbH
t.pilz@fz-juelich.de

Abstract. Deformable models still suffer from deficiencies for objects with weak features, which is, e.g., the case in subcortical areas. In this work, an extension of a deformable model is presented, which improves the situation by introducing object appearance information into the model. This information is obtained by exploiting a partial object definition, which is provided by the user in advance to initialize the 3D deformable model. The effectiveness of the presented method is demonstrated in the context of a combined 2D live wire–3D active surface model (2DLW-3DASM) approach, which is applied to a set of phantoms. It is shown that the method improves the segmentation results significantly.

1 Introduction

Medical imaging methods, such as MRI and PET, provide in vivo structural and functional information on biological tissue. In order to process this information quantitatively, a segmentation of the desired objects to be processed (volumes of interest (VOIs)) is mandatory. Deformable models are used widely in the field of medical image segmentation because of their beneficial properties [1]. Various improvements have been proposed to adjust the initial approach by Kass, Witkin, and Terzopoulos (1987) [2] to other applications and to tackle aspects not covered sufficiently in its initial formulation. One of the most important aspects concerns the improvement of an input-derived vector field, which is a common part in all deformable models. The vector field is used to deform an initial contour/surface until a stable state is reached. The vector field properties addressed most are capture range, convergence speed, computational effort, noise, and accuracy. A comprehensive survey of vector field improvements can be found in [3].

In this work, we propose a new method for vector field adaptation. The overall approach is to introduce object appearance information into the feature image from which the vector field is computed. The required appearance information is obtained in advance from a partial object definition provided by the user.

2 Materials and methods

The method is integrated in a combined semi-automatic 2D live wire–3D active surface model (2DLW-3DASM) approach [4], summarized in this paragraph and

H.-P. Meinzer et al. (Hrsg.), *Bildverarbeitung für die Medizin 2013*, Informatik aktuell,
DOI: 10.1007/978-3-642-36480-8_21, © Springer-Verlag Berlin Heidelberg 2013

shown in Fig. 1. This approach requires the user in a first step to partially segment the 3D object of interest on a set of 2D sample slices using the 2DLW. With
these 2D regions of interest (ROIs), the 3DASM is initialized, which automatically segments the complete 3D object by moving the initial surface under the
influence of internal and external forces. The internal forces have a smoothing
effect on the object shape [5], and the external forces, calculated by the generalized gradient vector flow (GGVF) approach [6], move the shape towards high
gradient magnitudes assuming that the object borders coincide with strong image edges. This assumption often does not hold, especially in medical imaging.
For example, in T1-weighted MR images of the brain, strong edges are to be
found at liquor-white matter borders but to a lesser extent at subcortical region
borders.

Motivated by this, an extended adaptive method has been implemented to
mitigate the assumption by adapting the feature image to the actual object
(Fig. 1). This is achieved by employing the user-defined partial object segmentation to create a model of the object surface, which is then used to create
an adaptive feature image. In this adaptive feature image, high voxel values
represent a high similarity to the object and low voxel values a low similarity.
The adaptive feature image is used within the 3DASM to steer the deformation
process (Fig. 1).

The adaptive features were inspired by the training algorithm of the live-wire
approach [7]. The main idea is to first create a model of the object surface using
all user-segmented ROI contour voxels and then to extrapolate the model to
other image voxels.

Let the input image I be defined over a set of discrete voxels $\mathcal{P} \subset \Re^3$. Then
a set of features

$$f_P(x) = G_{\sigma_f}(x) * I(x) \qquad \text{(smoothed pixel value)} \qquad (1)$$

$$f_D(x) = |\nabla G_{\sigma_f}(x) * I(x)| \qquad \text{(smoothed gradient magnitude)} \qquad (2)$$

$$f_I(x) = G_{\sigma_f}(x) * I(x + s \cdot n(x)) \quad \text{(smoothed inside pixel value)} \qquad (3)$$

$$f_O(x) = G_{\sigma_f}(x) * I(x - s \cdot n(x)) \quad \text{(smoothed outside pixel value)} \qquad (4)$$

can be derived from I using the convolution operator $*$, the Gaussian func-
tion G_{σ_f}, the constant s and the gradient direction $\mathbf{n} = \nabla I / |\nabla I|$. Let $C = \{\mathbf{c}_1, \ldots, \mathbf{c}_m\}$ with $C \subseteq \mathcal{P}$ be a contour.

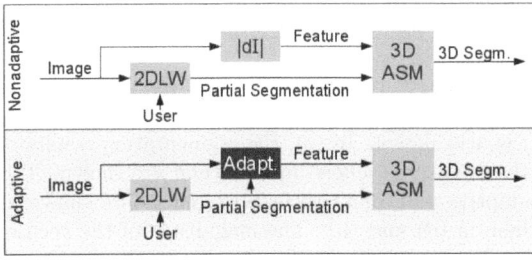

Fig. 1.   Scheme of the combined 2DLW-3DASM approach
(top) and its extension by
an adaptive model (bottom).
The box with "|dI|" stands for
the nonadaptive feature computation and the box with
"Adapt." refers to the adaptive
computation.

For each voxel $\mathbf{c}_k$ of the contour C a local histogram

$$h_{\mathbf{c}_k,f}(u) = \sum_{\{1 \leq j \leq m | \mathbf{c}_j \in C_f(u)\}} w_h(|k-j|) \tag{5}$$

can be computed along the contour, where f denotes the features to be used, $C_f(u) \subseteq C$ denotes the set of voxels which fall into the same histogram bin

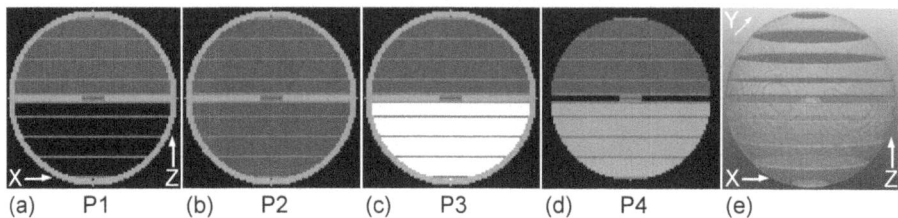

(a)   P1   (b)   P2   (c)   P3   (d)   P4   (e)

Fig. 2. In (a-d), Y-plane 67 of the four base phantoms is shown, overlaid in red by sample slices of the ground truth object which are 9 voxels apart. In (e), the sample slices are shown together with the transparent ground truth object. All base phantoms were generated using the PhantomDesigner [8].

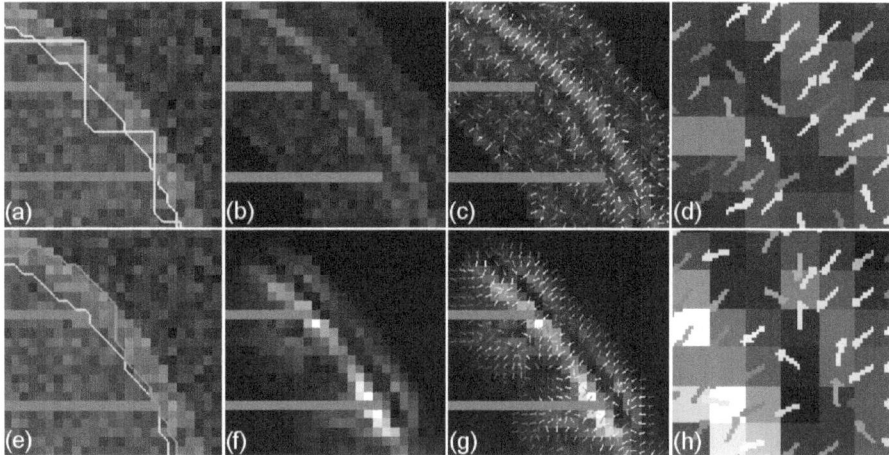

Fig. 3. In (a-h), the same right upper part of Y-plane 67 of the P3 phantom with Gaussian noise 42.5 and Z-directed quadratic 40% inhomogeneity is shown superimposed by object sample slices (red bars) which are used as 2D input segmentation. The background of (a,e) contains gray values. The background of (b-d) contains nonadaptive, and of (f-h) adaptive feature values. In (a), the initial surface of the 3DASM (green) and the ground truth object (cyan) is also shown. In (e), the segmentation results of the nonadaptive (purple line) and the adaptive (yellow line) method are shown. The vector fields derived from the nonadaptive and adaptive feature images are shown in (c) and (g) and close-up views of them in (d) and (h). The magnitude of the vectors is indicated by the color ranging from blue (low) to red (high).

as feature value u does, and $w_h(.)$ is a weighting function. We use $w_h(i) = \min(a; \max(0; b - i)) \cdot z$, with normalization z so that $\sum_{|C|} w_h = 1$. The user-defined values a and b reflect the extent of local properties along the contour. Thus, for each voxel in C, a histogram is filled with w_h-weighted elements of C.

Let the set of all user-segmented ROIs be denoted by $\mathcal{C}$ and let $\hat{h}_{c,f}$ be a Gaussian-smoothed version of $h_{c,f}$. Then, a histogram value for an arbitrary image voxel not contained in $\mathcal{C}$ can be computed by extrapolating the known histograms in $\mathcal{C}$. For this, a weighted sum is used

$$H_{\mathcal{C},f}(x) = \sum_{C \in \mathcal{C}} \sum_{c_j \in C} w_H(|x - c_j|) \cdot \hat{h}_{c_j,f}(f(x)) \tag{6}$$

with weights w_H chosen to be a Gaussian function with $\sigma = d(\mathcal{C}, x)$ being the Euclidean distance between x and the closest voxel in $\mathcal{C}$. The weights w_H are normalized, so that the sum of the coefficients is one. The interpolated histogram value is additionally weighted with a decreasing, distance-dependent function $\hat{H}_{\mathcal{C},f}(x) = H_{\mathcal{C},f}(x) \cdot \max(0; 1 - d(\mathcal{C}, x)/d_{\max})$, where the user-defined constant $d_{\max}$ relates to the distance between the contours in $\mathcal{C}$. Now, the features f_D, f_P, f_I, and f_O can be transformed by applying the above-defined histogram function

$$\hat{H}_{\mathcal{C}}(x) = \omega_D \cdot \hat{H}_{\mathcal{C},f_D}(x) + \omega_P \cdot \hat{H}_{\mathcal{C},f_P}(x) + \omega_I \cdot \hat{H}_{\mathcal{C},f_I}(x) + \omega_O \cdot \hat{H}_{\mathcal{C},f_O}(x) \tag{7}$$

with the user-defined weighting parameters ω_P, ω_D, ω_I, and ω_O.

As a result, the function $\hat{H}_{\mathcal{C}}$ maps a voxel x to a higher value, the closer it is to $\mathcal{C}$, and the more similar its features $f_D(x)$, $f_P(x)$, $f_I(x)$, and $f_O(x)$ are to the features of the nearby voxels in $\mathcal{C}$.

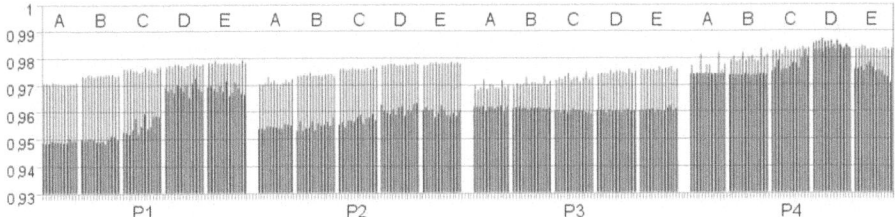

Fig. 4. The diagram shows the Dice similarity coefficients obtained from the comparison of the adaptive (orange) and nonadaptive (blue) phantom segmentations and the ground truth. The four base phantoms are separated by the big gaps and the small gaps separate the different noise levels of each base phantom: noiseless (A), 21.25 (B), 42.5 (C), 63.75 (D), 85 (E). No gaps are in between the different inhomogeneities at each noise level: L2X (left), L2Z, L2S, L4X, L4Z, L4S, Q2X, Q2Z, Q2S, Q4X, Q4Z, Q4S (right) with L = linear, Q = quadr., 2 = 20%, 4 = 40%, and direction S = XYZ.

3 Results

256 phantoms with known ground truth objects were segmented by applying the 2DLW-3DASM approach with and without adaptive features. The segmented objects were then compared to the true objects using the Dice coefficient.

The phantom data sets consist of four different base types (Fig. 2 a-d) modified by four different noise levels and 12 inhomogeneities. The four base types were chosen to simulate different real world situations found at subcortical regions, i.e., VOIs with different gradient magnitudes at their borders (e.g., nucleus caudatus) and higher gradient magnitudes at their surrounding structures (e.g., cortex close to putamen). The intensity values are as follows: The background of all phantoms is set to value 85, and the upper hemispheres of all objects are set to 170. The value of the neighborhood region in P1, P2, and P3 is set to 255. The lower hemispheres of the objects have the values 85 (P1), 170 (P2), 595 (P3), and 255 (P4). The additive Gaussian noise with sigma values 21.25, 42.5, 63.75, and 85 is cut off at zero. The linear (20%, 40%) and quadratic (20%, 40%) inhomogeneities change the image values along the directions X, Z, and XYZ and were applied before adding the noise. The object spheres of all phantoms have a radius of 40 voxels and a slit height of three. The neighborhood object spheres of the P1, P2, and P3 phantoms have a radius of 43 voxels, and the volume of the whole phantom has a size of $135 \times 135 \times 135$ voxels. The live-wire segmentation is simulated using a set of sample slices of the ground truth object (Fig. 2e).

User-adjusted parameters for the adaptive method were: $\sigma_f = 1$, $s = 2$, $\sigma_{\tilde{h}} = 1$, $a = 25$, $b = 50$, $d_{\max} = 10$, $\omega_P = \omega_D = \omega_I = \omega_O = 1$. To accelerate the computation, we used only the 20 nearest contour voxels for the sums in (6). The following 3DASM parameters were used for both methods: 50 GGVF diffusion iterations, 0.01 as GGVF diffusion factor, GGVF gradient sigma $\sigma = 1$, and 0.8 as a parameter to compute the locally adaptive weighting factor of internal forces.

The average computational time for the nonadaptive 3DASM was 290 sec per phantom and for the adaptive 3DASM 530 sec, measured on a PC with a 2.3 GHz Intel Xeon CPU and with nonoptimized code.

Fig.3 e illustrates a typical segmentation result with and without adaptive features. It can be seen that the segmented surface of the nonadaptive approach is partly attracted to the neighborhood, whereas the surface of the adaptive approach does not exhibit this behavior. The reason for this lies in the different feature images used (Fig. 3 b,f), where the nonadaptive method assigns a much higher value to the neighborhood than to the actual object since the gradient magnitude is higher there. This leads to the vector field shown in Fig. 3 c,d which caused the segmentation errors in the nonadaptive method. The adaptive feature method on the other hand assigns lower values to the neighborhood and higher ones to the actual object border, yielding a more suitable vector field (Fig. 3 g,h). Thus, better segmentation is achieved.

4   Discussion

Fig. 4 shows the resulting Dice coefficients for the whole data set. It can be seen that the adaptive method yields higher values than the nonadaptive method. The only exception can be found at some P4 phantoms with Gaussian noise of 63.75. This has two reasons. The first reason lies in the phantom itself. It has no attracting neighborhood structures (Fig. 2 d) producing good nonadaptive feature images and, therefore, high score levels for all phantoms of this type. However, the problem persists at the central slit of the sphere, which is why the adaptive method still generally performs a bit better. Adding Gaussian noise with $\sigma = 63.75$ changes this by distracting the attraction process just enough to mitigate the problem at the central slit, which leads to equal and in some cases slightly better results for the nonadaptive method.

To conclude, the segmentation results in Fig. 4 show that the adaptive approach is significantly and reliably better than the nonadaptive approach in most cases. In the remaining cases, the adaptive method produces comparable results.

Furthermore, we want to point out that the presented method is not specifically tailored to be used within the 2DLW-3DASM approach, and that it can be applied to all deformable models which have prior access to a partial object definition. Ongoing work is investigating the evaluation on real world data.

Acknowledgement. This work was supported by BMBF (grant no. 01EZ0822) and the Helmholtz-Validierungsfond (grant no. HVF-0012).

References

1. Hegadi R, Kop A, Hangarge M. A survey on deformable model and its applications to medical imaging. Int J Comput Appl. 2010;2:64–75.
2. Kass M, Witkin A, Terzopoulos D. Snakes: active contour models. Int J Computer Vis. 1988;1(4):321–31.
3. Amarapur B, Kulkarni PK. External force for deformable models in medical image segmentation: a survey. Signal Image Process. 2011;2(2):82–101.
4. Wagenknecht G, Poll A, Losacker M, et al. A new combined live wire and active surface approach for volume-of-interest segmentation. IEEE Nucl Sci Conf R. 2009 11; p. 3688–92.
5. Taubin G. A signal processing approach to fair surface design. Proc SIGGRAPH. 1995; p. 351–8.
6. Xu C, Prince JL. Generalized gradient vector flow external forces for active contours. Signal Process. 1998;71(2):131–9.
7. Mortensen EN, Barrett WA. Intelligent scissors for image composition. Proc SIGGRAPH. 1995; p. 191–8.
8. Hamo O, Nelles G, Wagenknecht G. A design toolbox to generate complex phantoms for the evaluation of medical image processing algorithms. Proc BVM. 2010; p. 256–60.

Assisting the Machine
Paradigms for Human-Machine Interaction in Single Cell Tracking

Nico Scherf[1], Michael Kunze[2], Konstantin Thierbach[1], Thomas Zerjatke[1],
Patryk Burek[2], Heinrich Herre[2], Ingmar Glauche[1], Ingo Roeder[1]

[1]Institute for Medical Informatics and Biometry, TU Dresden
[2]Institute for Medical Informatics, Statistics and Epidemiology, University of Leipzig
nico.scherf@tu-dresden.de

Abstract. Single cell tracking emerged as one of the fundamental experimental techniques over the past years in basic life science research. Though a large number of automated tracking methods has been introduced, they are still lacking the accuracy to reliably track complete cellular genealogies over many generations. Manual tracking on the other hand is tedious and slow. Semi-automated approaches to cell tracking are a good compromise to obtain comprehensive information in feasible amounts of time. In this work, we investigate the efficacy of different interaction paradigms for manual correction and processing of pre-computed tracking results and present a respective tool that implements those strategies.

1 Introduction

Single cell tracking is a vital field of research in biology and experimental medicine. It covers a broad spectrum of analyses, ranging from migration patterns in cell cultures to comprehensive genealogical information for developing organisms. Different biological questions require different degrees of tracking accuracy and reliability. For migration studies, a centroid position for each cell is sufficient and valuable information can be extracted even from imperfect tracking results. Studies focusing on cellular genealogies [1, 2] however, require a higher accuracy since a single error can lead to large deviations in the resulting lineage trees. Though manual tracking is tedious and time consuming for larger numbers of cells and experiments, it is still more reliable than automated tracking in many cases due to the superior abilities of the human cognitive system. Typical tools for manual tracking are ImageJ/FIJI [3, 4],TTT [5, 1, 2], or ICY [6].

Automated tracking on the other hand can handle arbitrary numbers of cells and long image sequences in a very time-efficient manner if the tracking problem is relatively straightforward. In case of more problematic situations (high cell densities, low frame rates, low contrast) automated methods are likely to fail. A good compromise is to combine both approaches in a semi-automated framework. That is, partial cell tracks are computed in an automated manner and the human expert can correct and validate the results in a post-processing step to obtain the complete information. There are several approaches that use this idea [6, 7].

However, as there seems to be no single best approach to automated track-ing, there might also be no single superior paradigm for semi-automated cell tracking. In this paper we will explore a few different paradigms for manual human-machine interaction and quantify their performance. We will further-more present an implementation of a platform-independent tool providing sev-eral of these options that can be chosen flexibly during tracking depending on the actual situation.

2   Materials and methods

In the following we will briefly introduce some important parts of the semi-automated analysis framework.

2.1   Automated tracking

Since we rely on manual correction of errors anyway, we use a conservative nearest neighbor tracking (termed naive tracking in [8]). The method does not resolve ambiguous situations by itself, but rather marks the problematic positions for later manual correction.

2.2   Data model

To keep the different parts of the processing modular, a common data structure is needed. This would further facilitate the exchange of data between different tools and groups. Unfortunately, no such standard is available for single cell tracking datasets to date. One step into this direction has been presented by

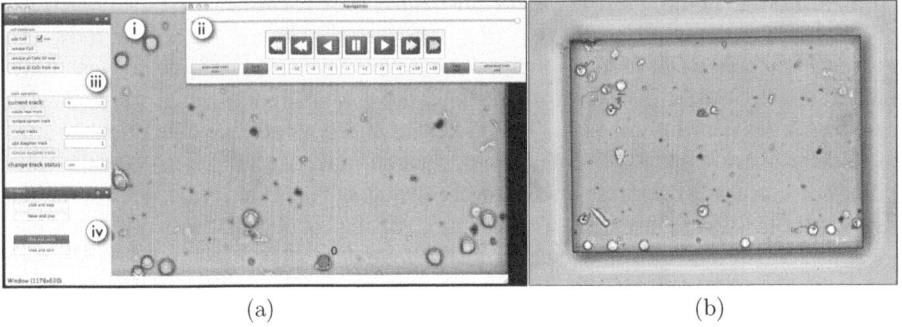

(a)   (b)

Fig. 1. CellTracker program and sample sequence. Screenshot (a) with (i) main win-dow showing the processed movie with detected cell masks as blue overlays, (ii) tem-poral controls, (iii) tools to process the tracks, and (iv) selection window for different interaction strategies. (b) Sample data used for evaluation. Cell tracks are shown as colored lines.

Herre et al. [9]. They introduced an ontology-based format to annotate and exchange single cell tracking data [10]. The tool presented in this work uses a data format based on these principles. We use the respective naming conventions to distinguish between different levels of the tracking process. A single observation of a cell at a certain point in time is called a *presential cell*. Corresponding observations of presential cells in consecutive images are connected by a *succession link*, that can be annotated by e.g. probability or confidence of matching. A partial cell track, i.e. a series of presential cells with respective succession links is called a *processual cell* (the term *tracklet* is also quite common). A fully annotated processual cell with a defined endpoint, e.g. cell division or apoptosis is a *cell*. Briefly, the underlying data structures are:

- raw data as an image sequence
- meta information per image, containing the automated detection results. For each presential cell we store:
  - coordinates of the cell centroids,
  - coordinates of the polygonal outline of each cell (alternatively a pixel based cell mask),
  - coordinates of the bounding box of each cell (optional),
  - a unique ID.
- for each processual cell (or tracklet), we store an adjacency list (the succession links) containing all presential cells

The data structures are stored in a human-readable XML format that allows for a subsequent integration into an ontology framework. The data generated by the automated tracking part is imported into the tracking tool for further processing.

2.3   User interface

The application window is divided into several parts (Fig. 1a). The main panel (i), containing the image for the current time point together with a color-coded overlay of the detected cell shape (e.g. processed cells are shown in red). To navigate the image sequence, temporal controls (ii) are available to e.g. play, pause, fast forward. To facilitate faster tracking, all functions are linked with respective keyboard shortcuts. The general tracking controls (iii) allow to manipulate the processed cell tracks (e.g. create new tracks, delete certain time points of a track, annotate a cell division event etc.). Different tracking modes are available (iv). They are suitable for different situations depending on e.g. local cell density, or motility of cells. These modes are discussed in more detail in the following. The tracking tool is implemented in C++ using the Qt framework to allow for platform independent use.

2.4   Tracking modes

Providing different modes of tracking allows to pick the best option for the current situation. While it might be necessary to control each step of the tracking in areas of high local cell densities where tracking errors are likely to occur, it is far too time-consuming for other parts of the movie, where cells are distributed rather sparse. The proposed tool provides the following paradigms:

- *Click-and-step.* The cell of interest is clicked in each image, added to the track and the movie is advanced to the next time point. This standard is available in virtually all available tracking methods [3], and serves as the baseline algorithm here.
- *Click-and-jump.* Since the automated tracking already provides partial cell tracks, it is easier to selectively move to the positions where a cell was lost (or the respective cell succession link was ambiguous) and correct these parts of the movie. Thus, the number of required interactions (i.e. clicks) are greatly reduced, yielding a faster tracking. The user just clicks the desired presential cell and the movie jumps to the last known position. At this point, the user can select one of the alternative continuations of the cell track. This is repeated until the cell is completely tracked or the movie ends. At the present state, the program also stops at cell divisions, to let the user manually create and label the respective daughter cells.
- *Hover-and-step.* This method is designed to further reduce the number of clicks. It allows to track the presential cells by simply moving the mouse over the respective cell. The succession links are created and the movie is advanced in time in an automated manner. Thus, one can simply follow the cell with the mouse. This strategy can be very efficient if the local cell density is high. Under these circumstances, the automated tracking is likely to produce a number of errors due to touching or partially overlapping cells. This would result in a tedious step-wise selection of cells for the other tracking modes.

2.5   Experiments

The performance of the different tracking paradigms was quantified by means of a short sequence of an in vitro culture of human hematopoietic stem and progenitor cells. The sequence shows 15 cells exhibiting different migration patterns. In this rather short test sequence, only one cell division occurs. The entire sequence consists of 100 images (692x520 px, 50 sec between frames). An overview of the used test sequence is provided in Fig. 1b. Each cell was tracked using manual tracking provided by FIJI [3] as a baseline result, and subsequently with each of the methods described above. The total amount of time required for tracking each cell was recorded to facilitate a quantitative comparison. The sequence was completely tracked by an expert user, experienced with cell tracking and the presented tool.

3   Results

The empirical distributions of tracking times per cell are shown in Fig. 2a. To further dissect these results, the time needed to track each individual cell is depicted in Fig. 2b. All results are normalized relative to the baseline results for the manual tracking by the FIJI plugin (black line). Finally, Fig. 2c visualizes the total amount of time needed to track the whole sequence.

As is apparent from the quantitative tests, there is no real gain in processing speed for using manual per step tracking of the preprocessed data. However, it should be noted that while for most manual tracking tools only the centroid position is recorded, an automated cell detection step yields additional information per cell (e.g. cell shape, area etc.). The other two tracking modes result in statistically significant 5 to 6-fold reduction in median processing time (up to 20 fold decrease for some cells). While the hover-and-step mode usually takes a bit longer per cell as compared to the click-and-jump setting in normal situations, this is reversed in more complicated cases where erroneous detections or exchanges of cell identities are frequent. Overall, the different modes facilitate the generation of manually validated results in reasonable amounts of time. A mix of strategies further reduced total processing time by about 30% as indicated by the yellow bar in Fig. 2c.

4   Discussion

For a number of underlying biological questions where complete genealogical trees are necessary, high quality, human assisted tracking results are still needed. An optimized strategy for human interaction with pre-computed cell tracking results can considerably improve the performance of manual correction of single cell data. Thus, depending on the experimental setting, different degrees of automation can be necessary. Ideally, one could freely mix automated tracking and manual processing to varying degrees depending on the given context. The proposed interaction paradigms have their own advantages and drawbacks. Being able to choose the respective paradigm according to the given situation can significantly decrease the time needed to analyze an experiment and is thus, crucial to analyze the given data in its full extents.

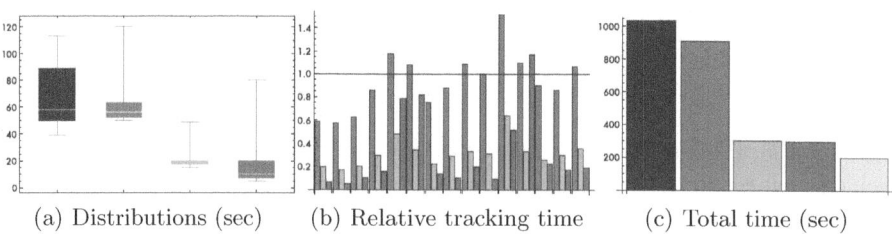

(a) Distributions (sec)   (b) Relative tracking time   (c) Total time (sec)

Fig. 2. Results. Distribution of processing times (Box-Whisker plots) for each method (click-and-step blue, hover-and-step pink, click-and-jump red, and reference manual FIJI plugin black) (a); The relative performance of each tracking mode for each cell, the FIJI plugin serves as baseline (black line) (b); Total amount of time needed for the whole sequence. Same color scheme as (a). The yellow bar indicates the performance of a mixed, optimal strategy (c).

To assess the advantages for realistic applications in more detail, a comprehensive validation will be done in the future. We further argue that it is crucial to ultimately set up a standard data format for single cell tracking to facilitate exchange and the creation of standard datasets. The use of existing frameworks such as ImageJ/FIJI is very attractive and the establishment of a baseline tracking tool on this platform, where different modes of manual interaction can be integrated (e.g. within a plugin structure) is a desirable goal for future work. This will render the analysis of single cell tracking experiments more efficient, reproducible and comparable.

Acknowledgement. This research was supported by the the BMBF-grant on Medical Systems Biology HaematoSys (BMBF-FKZ 0315452), and the Human Frontier Science Program (HFSP-grant RGP0051/2011).

References

1. Eilken HM, Nishikawa SI, Schroeder T. Continuous single-cell imaging of blood generation from haemogenic endothelium. Nature. 2009;457(7231):896–900.
2. Rieger MA, Hoppe PS, Smejkal BM, et al. Hematopoietic cytokines can instruct lineage choice. Science (New York). 2009;325(5937):217–8.
3. Schindelin J, Arganda-Carreras I, Frise E, et al. Fiji: an open-source platform for biological-image analysis. Nat Methods. 2012;9(7):676–82.
4. Schneider CA, Rasband WS, Eliceiri KW. NIH image to ImageJ: 25 years of image analysis. Nat Methods. 2012; p. 671–5.
5. Schroeder T. Long-term single-cell imaging of mammalian stem cells. Nat Methods. 2011;8(4s):S30–5.
6. de Chaumont F, Dallongeville S, Chenouard N, et al. Icy: an open bioimage informatics platform for extended reproducible research. Nat Methods. 2012;9(7):690–6.
7. Klein J, Leupold S, Biegler I, et al. TLM-Tracker: software for cell segmentation, tracking and lineage analysis in time-lapse microscopy movies. Bioinformatics. 2012;28(17):2276–7.
8. Rapoport DH, Becker T, Madany Mamlouk A, et al. A novel validation algorithm allows for automated cell tracking and the extraction of biologically meaningful parameters. PLoS ONE. 2011;6(11):e27315.
9. Burek P, Herre H, Roeder I, et al. Towards a cellular genealogy ontology. IMISE Reports. 2010;2:59–63.
10. Poli R, Healy M, Kameas A, editors. Theory and Applications of Ontology: Computer Applications. Dordrecht: Springer Netherlands; 2010.

Co-Registration of Intra-Operative Photographs and Pre-Operative MR Images

Benjamin Berkels[1], Ivan Cabrilo[2], Sven Haller[2], Martin Rumpf[1], Carlo Schaller[2]

[1]Institut für Numerische Simulation, Rheinische Friedrich-Wilhelms-Universität Bonn
[2]Hôpitaux Universitaires de Genève
benjamin.berkels@ins.uni-bonn.de

Abstract. Brain shift, the change in configuration of the brain after opening the dura mater, is a key problem in neuronavigation. We present an approach to co-register intra-operative microscope images with pre-operative MRI data to adapt and optimize intra-operative neuronavigation. The tools are a robust classification of sulci on MRI extracted cortical surfaces, guided user marking of most prominent sulci on a microscope image, and the actual variational registration method with a fidelity energy for 3D deformations of the cortical surface combined with a higher order, linear elastica type prior energy. Furthermore, the actual registration is validated on an artificial testbed and on real data of a neuro clinical patient.

1 Introduction

The development of medical imaging in the last decades quickly triggered intense interest from the medical world to translate this progress on the imaging side to clinical diagnostics and treatment planning. In that respect image registration and in particular recently also the fusion of 2D and 3D image data is a fundamental task in image–guided medical intervention. In [1] 2D photographs of human faces are registered with a triangulated facial surface extracted from MRI data using rigid deformations. A registration method for sparse but highly accurate 3-D line measurements with a surface extracted from volumetric planning data based on the consistent registration idea and higher order regularization is introduced in [2].

The matching of photographic images with pre-operative MRI data is a particular challenge in cranial neuronavigation. The photograph to MRI registration problem in the context of intracranial electroencephalography has been investigated via a control point matching approach in [3]. Recently, normalized mutual information has been applied for the rigid transformation co-registration of brain photographs and MRI extracted cortical surfaces [4]. A major limitation of note, however, is that due to the brain shift the surgeon's view of the operating site is not in a rigid transformation correspondence to pre-operative images. Indeed, standard intracranial neuronavigation devices do not correct for this movement

H.-P. Meinzer et al. (Hrsg.), *Bildverarbeitung für die Medizin 2013*, Informatik aktuell,
DOI: 10.1007/978-3-642-36480-8_23, © Springer-Verlag Berlin Heidelberg 2013

of brain [5]. The main contributions of this paper are a novel classification method for crease pattern such as sulci on implicit (cortical) surfaces and the actual 2D-3D registration method, where a non-rigid 3D deformation of the cortical surface is identified based on user marked sulci on photographs and the camera parameters.

2   Materials and methods

The aim of this paper is to register a photograph of the exposed human cortex with the cortex geometry extracted from an MRI data set (Fig. 1) using the sulci

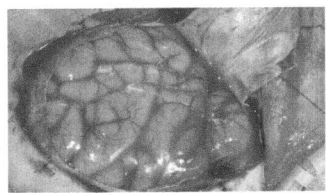 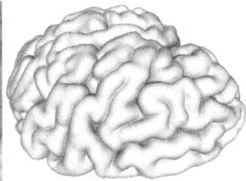

Fig. 1.   Input photograph and MRI graph surface.

as fiducials. The main ingredients of the proposed approach are a sulci classification on the cortex geometry (Sect. 2.1) and on the photograph (Sect. 2.2), as well as a model that uses the two classifications to register photograph and cortical geometry (Sect. 2.3). The 2D digital photographs were taken intra-operatively after supratentorial craniotomy and durotomy, and before corticotomy, using a digital camera with 10 mega pixel resolution positioned 20 cm above the craniotomy. The MR imaging was performed on a 3T MRI scanner. A T1-weighted MP2RAGE sequence ($1 \times 1 \times 1$ m^3, $256 \times 256 \times 176$ matrix) was segmented into gray and white matter using BrainVoyager QX [6] and then converted into a signed distance function of the cortical surface using a fast marching method.

2.1   Sulci classification on MRI data

We now describe how to classify creases on the contour surface of a 3D object $\mathcal{B} \subset \Omega$ represented via its signed distance function $d : \Omega \to \mathbb{R}$ on a computational domain Ω. In the application the object is a brain volume and the creases are the sulci on the cortical surface. We aim for a moment based analysis of the (cortical) surface $\mathcal{C} := \partial \mathcal{B}$ and define the zero moment shift of the implicit surface $\mathcal{C}$ as follows $M_\epsilon^0[\mathcal{B}](x) = \frac{1}{|B_\epsilon(x)|} \int_{B_\epsilon(x)} d(y)(y - x) \mathrm{d}y$ which returns larger values in flat regions of $\mathcal{C}$ than in edge regions and even smaller near corners (a related moment-based classification on explicit surfaces is given in [7]). We define the scalar classification $\mathbf{C}(x) = g_\beta \left(\|M_\epsilon^0[\mathcal{B}](x)\|/\epsilon^2 \right)$, where $g_\beta(t) = \frac{1}{1+\beta t^2}$. Fig. 2 illustrates the behavior of the classifier $\mathbf{C}$ on three simple shapes and a cortical surface extracted from an MRI using a white-green-blue-red color coding. We observe a robust distinction for a single set of parameters ($\beta = 20$ and $\epsilon = 8h$ or $4h$, where h denotes the grid width).

Fig. 2. Moment-based classification.

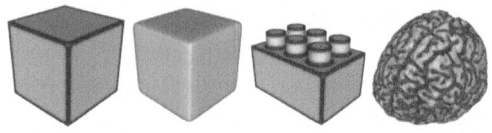

Fig. 3. Cortex photograph and dictionary based pre-classification.

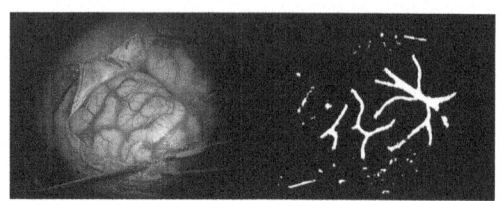

2.2   Generation of annotated cortex photographs

Essential problems for the classification of sulci on photographs are additional structures and their misinterpretation. Most prominent are cortical veins, which in addition partially occlude sulci (these veins are almost invisible in MRI in the used MP2RAGE sequence). On this background we here confine to a still manual marking of sulci by an expert who is supported by the results of a prior automatic pre-classification of sulci based on learned discriminative dictionaries (Fig. 3) using the method from [8].

2.3   Registration of photograph and cortex geometry

The co-registration of an MRI extracted cortical surface $\mathcal{C} \subset \mathbb{R}^3$ and a photograph to compensate for effects such as the brain shift is based on a co-registration of the sulci classifiers on $\mathcal{C}$ and the photograph. To this end, we suppose $\mathcal{C}$ to be described as a graph

$$\mathcal{C} = \{(x, z(x)) \in \mathbb{R}^3 | x \in \omega\}$$

with parameter domain $\omega \subset \mathbb{R}^2$ and graph function $z : \omega \to \mathbb{R}$. We are interested in a local registration described by the craniotomy, where such a graph representation can be easily derived from the signed distance function used in Section 2.1. Furthermore, let $g \in L^2(\Omega)$ denote the sulci classifier on the photograph domain Ω (Sect. 2.2), and $f \in L^2(\omega)$ the corresponding classifier on the cortical surface given as a function on the parameter domain ω, obtained by a suitable clamping of $\mathbf{C}$ and rescaling of the values to the unit interval $[0, 1]$ (Sect. 2.1). Both classifiers are supposed to be close to 1 in the central region of the sulci and small outside. Finally, we denote by $P : \mathbb{R}^3 \to \Omega$ the projection of points in $\mathbb{R}^3$ onto the image plane Ω derived from known camera parameters. Let us remark that we thereby implicitly rule out self occlusions of the graph surface $\mathcal{C}$ under the image plane projections. Now, we ask for a deformation $\Psi : \omega \to \mathbb{R}^3$ defined on the parameter domain ω of the graph function z that matches $\mathcal{C}$ to its deformed configuration represented under the projection P in the photograph. Thereby, matching is encoded via the coincidence of the surface classifier $f(x)$ on the MRI described cortical surface and the image classifier $g(P(\psi(x)))$ evaluated at the projected deformed position $P(\psi(x))$ for all x on the parameter domain ω. Thus, proper matching can be encoded via the minimization of the matching energy

$$E_{\mathrm{match}}[\psi] = \frac{1}{2}\int_\omega [g(P(\psi(x))) - f(x)]^2 A(x)\mathrm{d}x \qquad (1)$$

based on a surface integral over $\mathcal{C}$ with the area element $A(x) = (1 + |\nabla z(x)|^2)^{\frac{1}{2}}$, to consistently reflect the cortex geometry (Fig. 4). In the overall variational approach the matching energy is complemented by a suitable elastic regularization energy, which acts as a prior on admissible deformations ψ. Here, we consider the second order, elastic energy

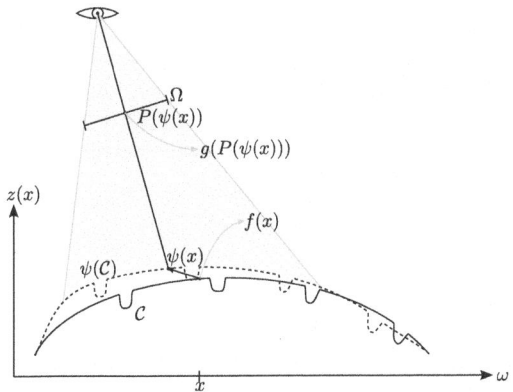

Fig. 4. Geometric configuration.

$$E_{\mathrm{reg}}[\psi] = \frac{1}{2}\int_\omega |\Delta\psi_1(x)|^2 + |\Delta\psi_2(x)|^2 + |\Delta\psi_3(x) - \Delta z(x))|^2 \mathrm{d}x \qquad (2)$$

Note that a simple first order regularization like the Dirichlet energy of the displacement $\psi - (\cdot, z(\cdot))$ is not sufficient since matching information is mostly given on a low dimensional subset where proper nonlinear extrapolation is required and bending modes play an important role. Obviously, E_{reg} is rigid body motion invariant [9]. Finally, we combine the matching energy E_{match} and the regularization energy E_{reg} to the total energy functional $E[\psi] = E_{\mathrm{match}}[\psi] + \lambda E_{\mathrm{reg}}[\psi]$ on deformations ψ encoding the deformation of the cortical surface $\mathcal{C}$, where λ is a positive constant controlling the strength of the regularization.

To minimize the objective functional we use a time discrete regularized gradient descent taking into account a suitable step size control combined with a cascadic descent approach to handle the registration in a coarse to fine manner. The first variation necessary for the descent algorithm is

$$\langle E'[\psi], \zeta \rangle = \int_\omega [g(P(\psi(x))) - f(x)]\nabla g(P(\psi(x))) \cdot DP(\psi(x))\zeta(x)A(x)\mathrm{d}x$$

$$+ \lambda \int_\omega (\Delta^2\psi_1, \Delta^2\psi_2, \Delta^2(\psi_3 - z)) \cdot \zeta\mathrm{d}x \qquad (3)$$

where the natural boundary conditions $\partial_\nu \Delta\psi = \Delta\psi = 0$ on $\partial\omega$ for the normal ν on $\partial\omega$ are considered and ψ is initialized as the identity on $\mathcal{C}$, i.e. $\psi(x) = (x, z(x))$. For the spatial discretization we consider bilinear Finite Elements on a rectangular mesh overlaying ω and Ω, and approximate the bi-Laplacian Δ^2 by the squared standard discrete Laplacian $\Delta_h^2 = M^{-1}LM^{-1}L$. Here, M and L denote the standard (lumped) mass and stiffness matrices, respectively.

3   Results

We have applied our registration approach both to test data and to real data. For the test data a cortical surface segmented on a 3D MRI data set has been taken as input together with an image generated from this surface via a given projection concatenated with an additional 3D nonrigid deformation. Then on the projected image selected sulci have been marked by hand. Furthermore, we considered a photograph of the brain surface seen through a left fronto-temporo-parietal craniotomy performed in a patient before placement of a subdural electrode grid for investigation of drug-resistant cryptogenic epilepsy (Fig. 5).

4   Discussion

We have proposed a novel method for the registration of photographs (2D) of the brain with the cortical surface extracted from 3D MRI data. The method turns out to be effective and robust both on test and on real data. It can be considered as an alternative to intra-operative MRI allowing subsequent co-registration with neuronavigation [10]. Currently, we aim for a validation study with an increased number of cases considering also data of patients with substantially smaller craniotomies.

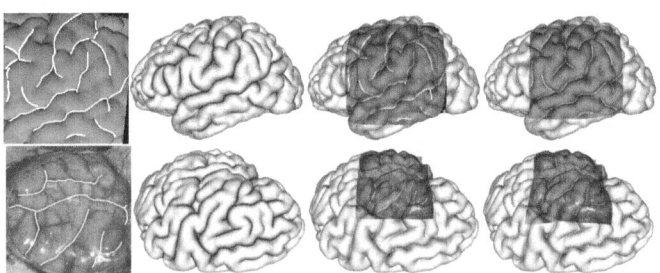

Fig. 5. Both for the test data (top row) and the pair of a true photograph and an MRI extracted cortical surface (bottom row) we show (from left to right) the input image with marked sulci (computed image and real photograph respectively), the sulci classification on the 3D cortical surface segmented from MRI data, the initial misfit of the sulci marking on the 2D image projected on the cortical surface overlaying the cortical surface itself, and the final registration result.

Furthermore, there is potential, that the iterative 2D/3D surface registration of digital images together with morphological 3D MRI data sets will enable to build up a "dictionary" of brain surface features. Ultimately, the creation of such a dictionary might, to a certain extent, permit "intelligent" automatic recognition of brain surface features, where the 2D brain surface, seen through the intra-operative microscope standardly used during intra-cerebral procedures, would directly be co-registered to pre-interventional 3D MRI data.

As already discussed, the sensitivity of MRI and photography is substantially different for different anatomic structures, veins are very prominent on images yet not on the MRI modality used here. One could incorporate multiple MRI sequences and fuse vein sensitive images with the present images to improve the registration results. Finally, let us remark that one could also consider stereo photographs of the deformed surface to improve the methods performance. In that respect our approach can easily be adapted summing over copies of the matching energy.

References

1. Clarkson MJ, Rueckert D, Hill DLG, et al. Using photo-consistency to register 2D optical images of the human face to a 3D surface model. IEEE Trans Pattern Anal Mach Intell. 2001;23(11):1266–80.
2. Bauer S, Berkels B, Ettl S, et al. Marker-less reconstruction of dense 4-D surface motion fields using active laser triangulation from sparse measurements for respiratory motion management. Proc MICCAI. 2012;7510:414–21.
3. Dalal SS, Edwards E, Kirsch HE, et al. Localization of neurosurgically implanted electrodes via photograph–MRI–radiograph coregistration. J Neurosci Methods. 2008;174(1):106–15.
4. Wang A, Mirsattari SM, Parrent AG, et al. Fusion and visualization of intraoperative cortical images with preoperative models for epilepsy surgical planning and guidance. Comput Aided Surg. 2011;16(4):149–60.
5. Reinges MHT, Nguyen HH, Krings T, et al. Course of brain shift during microsurgical resection of supratentorial cerebral lesions: limits of conventional neuronavigation. Acta Neurochir (Wien). 2004;146(4):369–77.
6. Fischla B, Serenob MI, Dalea AM. Cortical Surface-Based Analysis: II: Inflation, Flattening, and a Surface-Based Coordinate System. Neuroimage. 1999;9(2):195–207.
7. Clarenz U, Rumpf M, Telea A. Robust feature detection and local classification for surfaces based on moment analysis. IEEE Trans Vis Comput Graph. 2004;10(5):516–24.
8. Berkels B, Kotowski M, Rumpf M, et al. Sulci detection in photos of the human cortex based on learned discriminative dictionaries. Lect Notes Computer Sci. 2011.
9. Modersitzki J. Numerical Methods for Image Registration. Oxford University Press; 2004.
10. Kuhnt D, Bauer MH, Nimsky C. Brain shift compensation and neurosurgical image fusion using intraoperative MRI: current status and future challenges. Crit Rev Biomed Eng. 2012;40:175–85.

Depth-Layer-Based Patient Motion Compensation for the Overlay of 3D Volumes onto X-Ray Sequences

Jian Wang[1,2], Anja Borsdorf[2], Joachim Hornegger[1,3]

[1]Pattern Recognition Lab, Friedrich-Alexander-Universität Erlangen-Nürnberg
[2]Healthcare Sector, Siemens AG, Forchheim
[3]Erlangen Graduate School in Advanced Optical Technologies (SAOT)
jian.wang@cs.fau.de

Abstract. A novel depth-layer based patient motion compensation approach for 2D/3D overlay applications is introduced. Depth-aware tracking enables automatic detection and correction of patient motion without the iterative computation of digitally reconstructed radiographs (DRR) frame by frame. Depth layer images are computed to match and reconstruct 2D features into 2D+ space. Using standard 2D tracking and the additional depth information, we directly estimate the 3D rigid motion. The experimental results show that with about 30 depth layers a 3D motion can be recovered with a projection error below 2 mm.

1 Introduction

In interventional radiology, a typical scenario is that real-time information (e.g. projection position of a catheter tip) is provided by 2D X-ray sequences acquired by the C-arm system. The pre-interventional 3D volume is overlaid to augment the 2D images with additional spatial information, noted as 2D/3D overlay. Over decades, different 2D/3D registration methods were developed [1]. In nowaday clinical practice, 2D/3D overlay can achieve high accuracy at the beginning of a procedure as well as after the correction of misalignments due to patient motion during the procedure. However, patient motion needs to be detected by the physician and the correction is manually triggered in most of state-of-the-art applications. Our goal is to achieve automatic patient motion detection and real-time compensation. State-of-the-art 2D/3D registration methods [1] commonly depend on the expensive iterative computation of DRR images of the 3D volume. Meanwhile, standard tracking based motion detection/compensation methods are not optimal for X-ray sequences, due to the fact that structures from different depths overlap each other in the X-ray projection sequences.

In this paper, a novel approach of 2D/3D registration for rigid patient motion compensation is introduced. Instead of iteratively computing DRRs frame by frame, we introduce the concept of depth layer images for recovering depths of the 2D features. Then a standard tracking method is employed to find 2D correspondences between neighboring frames. 3D rigid motion is directly estimated from the depth-aware correspondences.

H.-P. Meinzer et al. (Hrsg.), *Bildverarbeitung für die Medizin 2013*, Informatik aktuell,
DOI: 10.1007/978-3-642-36480-8_24, © Springer-Verlag Berlin Heidelberg 2013

2   Materials and methods

The proposed approach takes the advantage of depth information from the initially registered 3D volume, and estimates the rigid 3D motion from depth-aware tracking. As illustrated in Fig. 1, it starts with an initially registered 2D/3D overlay, based on which depth layer images are generated (2.1) and compared to the initial frame for 2D+ reconstruction of 2D patches (2.2). A standard tracker is then employed to track patches over time. The rigid 3D motion is estimated taking into account depth information (2.3), which is then applied to the 3D volume for motion compensation.

2.1   Depth layer generation

Depth information is lost in the X-ray projections, which is one of the reasons of using 2D/3D overlay. Given a registered 2D/3D overlay, depth of the overlaid 3D can be encoded in color to improve the depth perception [2]. This leads to the idea of recovering depth information of 2D X-ray features from the initially registered 3D volume. We divide the 3D volume into a stack of depth layer volumes $V_{d_i}, i = 1, ..., n$ (n is the number of depth layers), in the way that all subvolumes are uniformly divided along the principal ray direction (Fig. 2), which can be rendered independently to generate depth layer images D_i.

One advantage of this concept is that depth layers decompose the overlapping structures into certain depth intervals. Another advantage is that the windowing and volume rendering technique can be specifically selected according to the registration content. For example, in our work bone structures are rendered as the structure of interest due to the fact that bones are almost rigid during the intervention and can represent the rigid patient motion. Contour enhanced volume rendering is used for the purpose of 2D/3D matching. Since the patient motion during the procedure is relative small, the depth layer generation is done only once as an initialization for a specific working position.

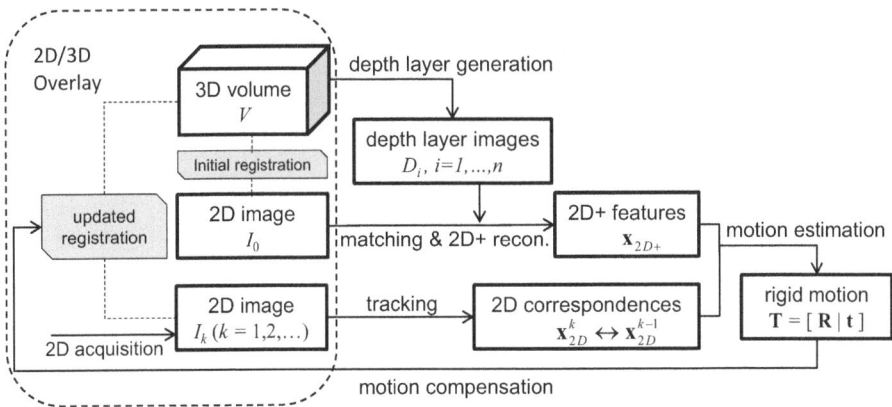

Fig. 1. Flow chart of depth layer based 2D/3D registration for motion compensation.

2.2   2D/3D matching and 2D+ reconstruction

Given the depth layers generated from the initially registered 3D volume, the 2D/3D matching procedure is performed between the X-ray image I_0 and the depth layer image D_i $(i = 1, ..., n)$. As distinctive boundaries of structures in 3D image correspond to strong intensity gradients in the 2D image, our matching strategy is gradient-based: volumetric contour rendering technique [3] is employed to generate the depth layers, and the 2D gradient magnitude map $(|\nabla I_0|)$ is used.

The matching is done by patchwise similarity measurement. 2D grids are applied to $|\nabla I_0|$ and D_i to generate 2D patches $p^k_{|\nabla I_0|}$ and $p^k_{D_i}$ from the images $(k = 1, ..., K$, where K is the number of patches in a 2D image). In our case, $|\nabla I_0|$ and D_i with the size of 800×800 pixels have the patch size of 8×8 pixels. Normalized cross correlation (NCC) [4] is employed as the similarity measure, and the similarity between $p^k_{|\nabla I_0|}$ and $p^k_{D_i}$ is weighted by

$$w^k_i = NCC(p^k_{D_i}, p^k_{|\nabla I_0|}) \cdot \left(\sum_{j=1}^{n} NCC(p^k_{D_j}, p^k_{|\nabla I_0|}) \right)^{-1} \tag{1}$$

The weight w^k_i indicates the matching probability of $p^k_{I_0}$ (the kth patch of the X-ray image I_0) with a certain depth d_i. The weight w^k_i is normalized over all depths d_i $(i = 1, ..., n)$ for the same patch position k.

Then the 3D position of the 2D feature patches $\{p^k_{I_0}, k = 1, ..., K\}$ with high matching weight (e.g. for $w^k_i \geq 0.5$) are estimated by 2D+ reconstruction. Since the depth values of the 2D patches associated with D_i are all estimated as the center depth d_i of V_{d_i}, we call the procedure 2D+ reconstruction.

The reconstruction procedure is based on the back-projection of points to rays [5]. In homogeneous coordinates, a 2D point $\mathbf{x}_{2D} \in \mathbb{R}^3$ can be back projected to a ray $\mathbf{r}(\lambda) = \mathbf{P}^+\mathbf{x}_{2D} + \lambda\mathbf{c}$, that passes through the X-ray source $\mathbf{c}$ and the point

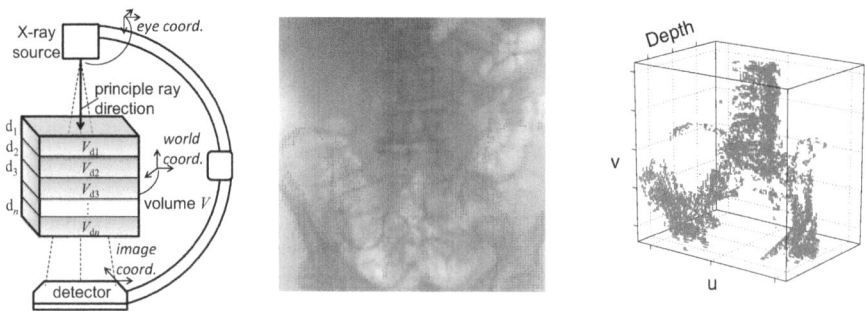

Fig. 2.   Matching & reconstruction. Left: Depth layer volumes in C-arm geometry; middle: Matching patches with high weights; right: 2D+ reconstructed matching patches.

$\mathbf{x}_r = \mathbf{P}^+\mathbf{x}_{2D}$ ($\mathbf{P}^+$ is the pseudo-inverse of the projection matrix $\mathbf{P} \in \mathbb{R}^{3\times4}$). And the 2D+ reconstruction $\mathbf{x}_{2D+}$ of $\mathbf{x}_{2D}$ in depth d_i can be determined by

$$\mathbf{x}_{2D+} = \mathbf{x}_r + \lambda(d_i)\mathbf{c} \qquad (2)$$

In the eye coordinate system (Fig. 2), the origin is at the X-ray source $\mathbf{c}$ and the z-axis is aligned with the principal ray direction. Therefore, we have $\mathbf{c} = (0,0,0,1)^{\mathrm{T}}$ and $z_{2D+}/\omega_{2D+} = d_i$, where $\mathbf{x}_{2D+} = (x_{2D+}, y_{2D+}, z_{2D+}, \omega_{2D+})^{\mathrm{T}}$. Together with 2, we have $\lambda(d_i) = (z_{\mathbf{x}_r} - d_i\omega_{\mathbf{x}_r})/d_i$, which is used to determine entries of $\mathbf{x}_{2D+}$. The results can be transformed to world coordinate system using the projection parameters of C-arm system. The center points of 2D patches with high weights (above) are reconstructed in 2D+ space (below).

2.3   Tracking and motion estimation

After the reconstruction procedure, motion in 3D is estimated by depth-aware tracking. Kanade-Lucas-Tomasi (KLT) Feature Tracker [6] is employed to find 2D correspondences $\mathbf{x}'_{2D} \leftrightarrow \mathbf{x}_{2D}$ between neighboring frames. Our goal is to estimate the motion of the patient between two frames. This motion can be expressed as the inverse of the relative motion of the C-arm, which is considered as a perspective camera. The projection matrix $\mathbf{P}$ can be represented as $\mathbf{P} = \mathbf{K}[\mathbf{R}|\mathbf{t}]$, where $\mathbf{K} \in \mathbb{R}^{3\times3}$ contains the intrinsic parameters, rotation $\mathbf{R} \in \mathbb{R}^{3\times3}$ and translation $\mathbf{t} \in \mathbb{R}^3$ give the rigid camera motion $\mathbf{T} = [\mathbf{R}|\mathbf{t}] \in \mathbb{R}^{3\times4}$.

Non-linear optimization is applied to recover the parameters of rotation and translation. The following error function is minimized between two frames

$$\arg\min_{\mathbf{T}} \left(\sum w \cdot \mathrm{dist}(\hat{\mathbf{x}}_{2D}, \mathbf{x}'_{2D}) \right) \qquad (3)$$

where $dist(\cdot, \cdot)$ is the Euclidean distance and $\hat{\mathbf{x}}_{2D} = \mathbf{K} \cdot \mathbf{T} \cdot \mathbf{x}_{2D+}$. The projection errors are weighted by the matching weights w (calculated in (1)) so that points with higher w contributes more to the results and vise versa.

3   Results

3.1   Point-based simulation experiment (quantitative)

The aim of the experiment is to answer the following questions: (i) how accurate the algorithm can be, (ii) how many depth layers are needed and (iii) how robust is the method with respect to noise. The projection parameters of a real C-arm system (detector pixel size 0.308 mm) is used in the experiment. 3D point sets (20 sets, 50 points per set) were randomly generated in 3D space where the patient is usually laid. Two projections of the 3D points (without and with rigid motion) were generated as two neighboring frames.

The experiment results of 5 examples are shown in Tab. 1. Four motions (pure translation(motion 1), in-plane motion(motion 2), pure rotation(motion 3) and general motion(motion 4)) were tested without 2D corresponding noise. 2D

Table 1. Experiment results of projection errors. The general case refers to motion 4 with 2D noise.

	motion 1	motion 2	motion 3	motion 4	general
translation (mm)	(6, 4, 4)	(6, 0, 4)	(0, 0, 0)	(6, 4, 4)	(6, 4, 4)
rotation (°)	(0, 0, 0)	(0, 9, 0)	(-9, 9, 4.5)	(-9, 9, 4.5)	(-9, 9, 4.5)
ϵ_{ref}(mm)	2.78	4.74	6.15	6.45	6.45
# depth layers	projection errors after registration ϵ_{reg}(mm)				
15	0.12 ± 0.05	0.11 ± 0.05	3.39 ± 1.58	3.20 ± 1.48	3.22 ± 2.01
25	0.08 ± 0.03	0.06 ± 0.03	1.47 ± 1.46	1.90 ± 0.93	2.70 ± 0.79
35	0.06 ± 0.03	0.05 ± 0.02	1.69 ± 0.92	1.56 ± 0.85	2.08 ± 1.23

correspondence noise (± 2 pixels or ± 0.62 mm) was added in the general motion case. The mean 2D offsets (ϵ_{ref}) caused by the motions vary from 2.78 mm to 6.45 mm. The projection errors after registration (ϵ_{reg}) with 15, 25 and 35 depth layers are shown. In the non-noise case, the projection error ϵ_{reg} decreased below 2 mm using 25 depth layers. In the pure translation and the in-plane motion cases, the motions were better corrected. Using 35 depth layers, ϵ_{reg} was around 2 mm in the general motion case with noise.

In Fig. 3, the estimation errors of the motion components are plotted with all tested depth resolutions (motion 4 with noise). The rotation errors were bounded within $\pm 1°$ after 10 depth layers. The in-plane rotation (ΔR_y) was better estimated then off-plane rotation (ΔR_x and ΔR_z). The translation errors also stabilized after 20 to 30 depth layers. These results show that our approach is capable of recovering 3D motion by using depth-aware 2D correspondences, even for the stronger motion (motion 4) under 2D correspondence noise.

3.2   Preliminary tracking-based experiment (qualitative)

In the tracking-based experiment, the X-ray sequence was simulated by DRR computation from a clinical CT volume with a rigid motion sequence. KLT tracking method was employed for 2D tracking. An example of the results is shown in Fig. 4. The initial registered 2D/3D overlay (left), which is the starting point of our approach. Using our depth-layer based motion compensation, the overlay was corrected using the estimated motion from frame to frame. The

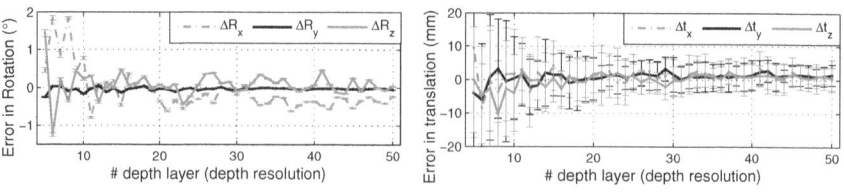

Fig. 3. Simulation experiment: general motion case (motion 4, with 2D noise).

Fig. 4. Tracking based experiment. Left: Initially registered 2D/3D overlay (red); middle: Depth layer based motion compensation (green); right: Overlay with (green) and without (red) motion compensation.

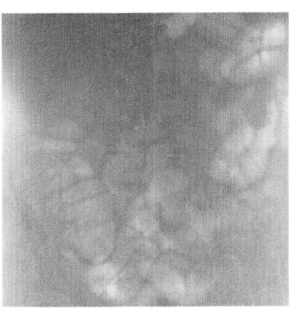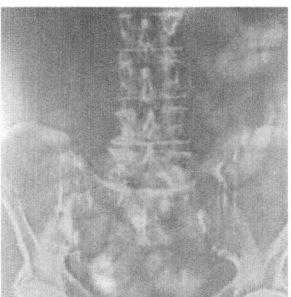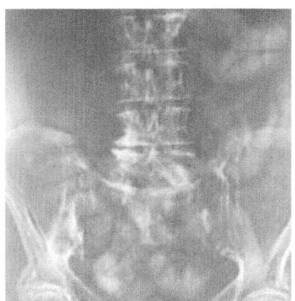

preliminary result shows the potential of our depth-aware tracking based approach towards real-time rigid motion compensation.

4   Discussion

We have presented a novel depth-layer based 2D/3D registration approach. The experimental results show that our approach is capable to estimate the rigid 3D motion by 2D tracking and depth-aware motion estimation. With depth layers ($n \in [25, 35]$) the 3D motion can be recovered with a projection error below 2 mm. The method was tested for its robustness against noise in 2D tracking. Furthermore, the method is computationally very efficient, because we do not rely on frame-by-frame iterative DRR computation. This shows the high potential of our approach for robust and real-time compensation of patient motion for 2D/3D overlay.

References

1. Markelj P, Tomaževič D, Likar B, et al. A review of 3D/2D registration methods for image-guided interventions. Med Image Anal. 2012;16(3):642–61.
2. Wang J, Fallavollita P, Wang L, et al. Augmented reality during angiography: integration of a virtual mirror for improved 2D/3D visualization. Proc IEEE Int Symp Mixed Augment Real. 2012; p. 257–64.
3. Csébfalvi B, Mroz L, Hauser H, et al.; Wiley Online Library. Fast visualization of object contours by non-photorealistic volume rendering. Proc Comput Graph Forum. 2002;20(3):452–60.
4. Penney G, Weese J, Little J, et al. A comparison of similarity measure for use in 2D–3D medical image registration. IEEE Trans Med Imaging. 1998;17(4):586–95.
5. Hartley R, Zisserman A. Multiple view geometry in computer vision. 2nd ed. Cambridge Univsersity Press; 2003.
6. Tomasi C, Kanade T. Detection and tracking of point features. Tech Report: CMU-CS; 1991.

4D-MRT-basierte Simulation der Lungenbewegung in statischen CT-Daten

Mirko Marx[1], Jan Ehrhardt[1], René Werner[1], Heinz-Peter Schlemmer[2],
Heinz Handels[1]

[1] Institut für Medizinische Informatik, Universität zu Lübeck
[2] Abteilung Radiologie, DKFZ Heidelberg
marx@imi.uni-luebeck.de

Kurzfassung. In diesem Beitrag wird ein Modell vorgestellt, dass die durchschnittliche atembedingte Lungenbewegung patientenspezifisch für die Dauer eines Atemzyklus zeitkontinuierlich beschreibt. Die Modellgenerierung erfolgt auf Basis von thorakalen 4D-MRT-Bilddaten, aus denen die Bewegungsinformationen gewonnen und Atemphasen zugeordnet werden. Das generierte Bewegungsmodell repräsentiert die durchschnittliche intraindividuelle Lungenbewegung für die Dauer eines Atemzyklus mittels periodischer B-Spline-Kurven. Das so erhaltene Bewegungsmodell wird auf eine statische CT-Aufnahme desselben Patienten übertragen und so die Simulation atembewegter CT-Daten ermöglicht. Hierzu wird eine affine Koordinatentransformation auf das Modell angewandt.

1 Einleitung

Atembedingte Organ- und Tumorbewegungen sind ein zentrales Problem der Strahlentherapie. Ziel ist es eine ausreichende Strahlendosis auf den Tumor zu applizieren, die Strahlenexposition für das gesunde Gewebe jedoch zu minimieren. In der konventionellen Bestrahlungsplanung erfolgt die Berechnung der Dosisverteilung und die Risikoabschätzung auf Basis von 3D-CT-Aufnahmen. Da diese nur Momentaufnahmen darstellen, ist die Bewegungsvariabilität atembewegter Tumoren nur schwer einzuschätzen. Eine besondere Relevanz besitzt dieses Problem bei der Bestrahlungsplanung von Lungentumoren, weshalb in verschiedenen Arbeiten 4D-CT-Daten verwendet wurden, um die Bewegung von Lungentumoren zu erfassen [1]. Die 4D-CT hat jedoch den Nachteil einer hohen Strahlenbelastung für den Patienten, weshalb sie nur zur Erfassung eines oder einiger weniger Atemzyklen eingesetzt wird. Dank moderner 4D-MRT-Bildgebungstechniken ist es möglich geworden, Organbewegungen über viele Atemzyklen ohne einer Strahlenexposition mit einer zeitlichen Auflösung von 0.5 s zu erfassen. Zunehmende Bedeutung in der Strahlentherapie erlangt die modellbasierte Schätzung von atembedingten Organ- und Tumorbewegungen.

In diesem Beitrag werden 4D-MRT-Daten verwendet, um ein Modell der individuellen durchschnittlichen atembedingten Lungenbewegung zu erstellen. Hierbei wird die Idee aufgegriffen, die mittlere Bewegung jedes Voxels durch

H.-P. Meinzer et al. (Hrsg.), *Bildverarbeitung für die Medizin 2013*, Informatik aktuell,
DOI: 10.1007/978-3-642-36480-8_25, © Springer-Verlag Berlin Heidelberg 2013

eine B-Spline-Kurve für die Dauer eines Atemzyklus zu beschreiben [2]. In einem zweiten Schritt wird das so generierte Bewegungsmodell auf einen statischen 3D-CT-Datensatz desselben Patienten übertragen. Dadurch kann die atembedingte Lungenbewegung zeitkontinuierlich beschrieben und so das übertragene Modell zur 4D-Strahlentherapieplanung und Dosisberechnung verwendet werden [3].

2 Material und Methoden

Das Verfahren teilt sich in zwei Schritte. Der erste Schritt ist die Modellgenerierung, welche auf Basis von thorakalen 4D-MRT-Bilddaten erfolgt. Der zweite Schritt ist die Übertragung des Modells von MRT-Koordinaten auf die Bildkoordinaten eines statischen 3D-CT-Bildes desselben Patienten.

2.1 Modellgenerierung

Ausgangsdaten für die Modellgenerierung bilden thorakale 4D-MRT-Bilddaten eines Patienten, welche aus N 3D-MRT-Bildern bestehen und die atembedingte Lungenbewegung über mehrere (ca. 20) Atemzyklen (Atemzyklus definiert von Ausatmung über Einatmung zur nächsten Ausatmung) erfassen.

Zunächst werden Bewegungsinformationen extrahiert, indem jedes MRT-Bild auf ein MRT-Referenzbild registriert wird. Dabei wird das in [1] beschriebene intensitätsbasierte nichtlineare symmetrisch-diffeomorphe Registrierungsverfahren eingesetzt. Das Ergebnis sind N Bewegungsfelder

$$\varphi_j(\boldsymbol{x}) = \boldsymbol{x} + \boldsymbol{u}_j(\boldsymbol{x}) \qquad j = 1, \dots, N \qquad (1)$$

Nun soll jedes Bewegungsfeld φ_j bzw. jedes Verschiebungsfeld $\boldsymbol{u}_j$ mit einer Atemphase $p_j \in [0, 1]$ verknüpft werden. Die Berechnung der Atemphasen p_j erfordert die Analyse des zugehörigen Atemsignals. Im vorliegenden Fall ist ein Atemsignal nicht verfügbar, sodass es mittels eines Surrogatparameters (Lungenvolumen) aus den MRT-Aufnahmen geschätzt wird. Zur Berechnung der

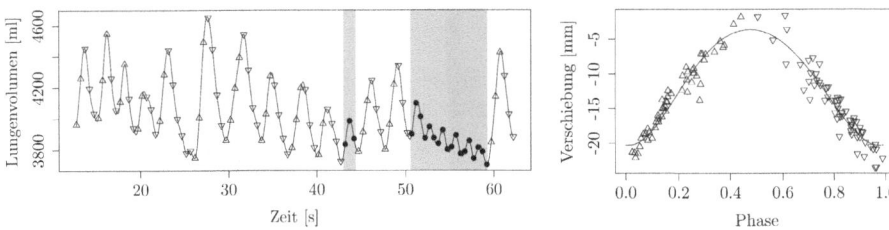

Abb. 1. Ausschnitt eines aus den Lungenvolumina rekonstruierten Atemsignals (links) und zugehörige berechnete Bewegungskurve eines bewegungsintensiven Lungenvoxels nahe des Zwerchfells in Superior-Inferior-Richtung (rechts). MRT-Aufnahmen in anormalen Atemzyklen (schwarze Kreise in den grauen Bereichen) sind unberücksichtigt.

Lungenvolumina wird für den Referenzzeitpunkt (max. Einatmung) eine Lungensegmentierung (unter Einsatz eines Volumenwachstumsverfahrens inklusive manueller Vorsegmentierung) erstellt und mittels der Bewegungsfelder auf alle anderen Zeitpunkte übertragen. Die Lungenvolumina lassen sich nun über der Zeitachse der einzelnen Aufnahmezeitpunkte abtragen. Anschließend wird das Atemsignal zu den 4D-MRT-Daten mittels einer Lanczos-Interpolation rekonstruiert (Abb. 1, links). Zur Bestimmung der zugehörigen Atemphasen wird ein amplitudenbasierter Ansatz verwendet, wobei anormale Atemzyklen automatisch detektiert und von der weiteren Analyse ausgeschlossen werden.

Nach der Berechnung der Atemphasen können die Bewegungsfelder in einen Atemzyklus eingeordnet werden. Die zugehörigen Verschiebungsfelder $\boldsymbol{u}_j$ werden dann voxelweise durch periodische B-Spline-Kurven dritten Grades über der Atemphase approximiert (Abb. 1, rechts). Das so generierte Modell beschreibt die zeitkontinuierliche Bewegung der Voxel in den MRT-Daten und besitzt nun die mathematische Form

$$\boldsymbol{\varphi}^{\mathrm{MRT}}\left(\boldsymbol{x}^{\mathrm{MRT}},p\right) = \boldsymbol{x}^{\mathrm{MRT}} + \sum_{i=1}^{7} \boldsymbol{c}_i^{\mathrm{MRT}}\left(\boldsymbol{x}^{\mathrm{MRT}}\right) N_{i,3}(p) \tag{2}$$

wobei $N_{i,3}(p)$ die B-Spline-Basisfunktionen und $\boldsymbol{c}_i^{\mathrm{MRT}}\left(\boldsymbol{x}^{\mathrm{MRT}}\right)$ die B-Spline-Kontrollpunkte für Voxel $\boldsymbol{x}^{\mathrm{MRT}}$ in den MRT-Koordinaten darstellen.

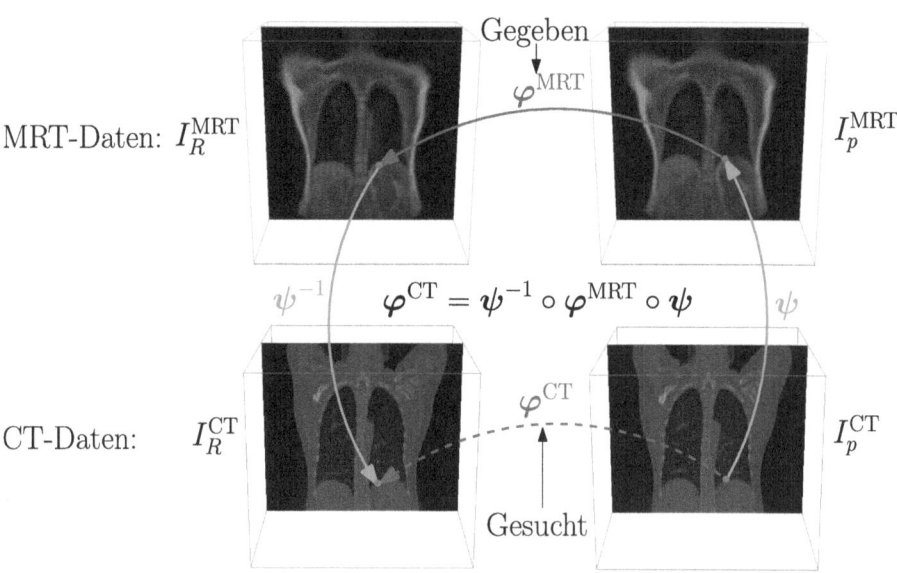

Abb. 2. Modellübertragung durch eine Koordinatentransformation.

2.2 Modellübertragung

Um die Simulation der Lungenbewegung nun auch in statischen CT-Daten in Form eines zeitkontinuierlichen Bewegungsmodells φ^{CT} zu ermöglichen, wird eine Koordinatentransformation zur Übertragung des Modells durchgeführt [4] (Abb. 2). Hierbei wird davon ausgegangen, dass eine statische 3D-CT-Aufnahme desselben Patienten zur korrespondierenden Atemphase des MRT-Referenzbildes vorliegt. Die räumliche Korrespondenz zwischen MRT- und CT-Daten wird durch eine affine Transformation ψ beschrieben. Zur Bestimmung der Transformation ψ wird zunächst eine automatische Segmentierung [5] der Lunge im statischen CT-Bild durchgeführt und die Oberflächenmodelle der Lunge von MRT- und CT-Bild mittels des ICP-Algorithmus affin registriert [6].

Das CT-basierte Bewegungsmodell

$$\varphi^{\mathrm{CT}}\left(\boldsymbol{x}^{\mathrm{CT}}, p\right) = \boldsymbol{x}^{\mathrm{CT}} + \sum_{i=1}^{7} \boldsymbol{A}^{-1} \boldsymbol{c}_i^{\mathrm{MRT}} \left(\boldsymbol{A}\boldsymbol{x}^{\mathrm{CT}} + \boldsymbol{b}\right) N_{i,3}(p) \tag{3}$$

resultiert dann aus der Koordinatentransformation über die Konkatenation der affinen Transformation $\psi\left(\boldsymbol{x}^{\mathrm{CT}}\right) = \boldsymbol{A}\boldsymbol{x}^{\mathrm{CT}} + \boldsymbol{b}$ mit den B-Spline-Kontrollpunkten des MRT-basierten Bewegungsmodells. Dabei stellt $\boldsymbol{x}^{\mathrm{CT}}$ einen Voxel in CT-Koordinaten dar. Somit kann das Modell zur Generierung zeitkontinuierlicher 4D-CT-Aufnahmen eingesetzt werden.

2.3 Evaluation

Für die Evaluation standen MRT- und CT-Daten drei verschiedener Patienten (mit jeweils einem Tumor im rechten Lungenflügel) zur Verfügung, welche beim DKFZ in Heidelberg aufgenommen wurden. Die 4D-MRT-Daten besitzen eine Auflösung von $128 \times 36 \times 128$ Voxel mit einer Voxelgröße von $3.91 \times 10 \times 3.91$ mm und einer zeitlichen Auflösung von 157 Zeitschritten mit einem Abstand von 0.5 s. Sie wurden unter freier Atmung aufgenommen und zeigen die atembewegte Lunge über mehrere Atemzyklen hinweg. Die 3D-CT-Daten besitzen eine Auflösung von $512 \times 512 \times \{94, 125, 235\}$ Voxel mit einer Voxelgröße von $0.98 \times 0.98 \times 3$ mm.

In einer ersten Evaluation wurden die Abweichungen der modellgenerierten mittleren Bewegungsfelder von den berechneten Bewegungsfeldern der originären MRT-Daten bestimmt. Es wurde hierzu $\frac{1}{N} \sum_j \left\| \boldsymbol{\varphi}_j(\cdot) - \boldsymbol{\varphi}^{\mathrm{MRT}}(\cdot, p_j) \right\|$ berechnet, wobei p_j die dem j-ten MRT-Bild zugeordnete Phase ist.

In einer zweiten Evaluation wurde die Genauigkeit der affinen Übertragung des Modells von MRT-Koordinaten auf die Bildkoordinaten eines statischen 3D-CT-Bildes quantitativ bewertet. Da nur 3D-CT-Daten der Patienten zur Verfügung standen, war ein Vergleich des übertragenen MRT-basierten Modells mit einem CT-basierten Modell nicht möglich.

3 Ergebnisse

Die Evaluation zur Genauigkeit der MRT-basierten Modellbeschreibung lieferte (gemittelt über alle 3 Patienten und alle Lungenvoxel) eine durchschnittliche

Tabelle 1. Vergleich der Ergebnisse dreier Patienten zur Bewertung der affinen Registrierung der Lunge in den MRT-Daten an die Lunge in den CT-Daten. Vergleichsmaße: Dice-Koeffizient C_{Dice}, Hausdorff-Distanz H, mittlere Oberflächendistanz $\bar{D}$.

| Lungenflügel | Patient 1 | | | Patient 2 | | | Patient 3 | | |
	C_{Dice}	$H\,[\text{mm}]$	$\bar{D}\,[\text{mm}]$	C_{Dice}	$H\,[\text{mm}]$	$\bar{D}\,[\text{mm}]$	C_{Dice}	$H\,[\text{mm}]$	$\bar{D}\,[\text{mm}]$
beide	0.936	11.36	2.13	0.907	21.93	3.33	0.915	15.68	2.78
gesund	0.937	11.36	1.38	0.909	11.18	2.06	0.915	15.17	2.35

Abweichung der modellierten Bewegung von 1.39 ± 0.75 mm. Die maximale aufgetretene Abweichung betrug dabei $5.07/5.13/7.46$ mm für Patient $1/2/3$.

Um die Modellübertragung zu bewerten, wurden die berechneten affinen Transformationen auf die MRT-Lungensegmentierungen angewandt und mittels Überlappungsmaße und Oberflächenabstände mit den CT-Lungensegmentierungen verglichen. Die Ergebnisse sind in Tab. 1 für alle drei Patienten dargestellt. Dabei wurde die Registrierung sowohl auf beiden Lungenflügeln (obere Zeile) als auch nur auf den gesunden Lungenflügeln (untere Zeile) durchgeführt. Wie aus der Tabelle hervorgeht, konnten dabei auf den gesunden Lungenflügeln bessere Registrierungsergebnisse erzielt werden.

4 Diskussion

In diesem Beitrag wurde ein Modell vorgestellt, dass die durchschnittliche patientenspezifische Lungenbewegung zeitkontinuierlich für die Dauer eines Atemzyklus beschreibt. Das Modell wird auf Basis von MRT-Daten gewonnen, die über mehrere Atemzyklen aufgenommen sind. Das generierte Modell kann über eine affine Koordinatentransformation auf statische CT-Bilddaten übertragen werden, um so 4D-CT-Bilddaten zu simulieren. Gegenüber direkt akquirierten 4D-CT-Daten haben diese simulierten Daten den Vorteil, dass sie einen mittleren Atemzyklus repräsentieren, sowie zeitkontinuierlich und frei von den üblichen

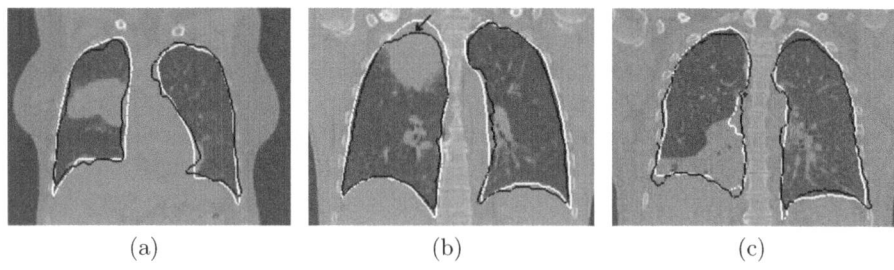

(a)   (b)   (c)

Abb. 3. Koronale Schichten der Lunge in den CT-Bildern der drei Patienten. Die Lungenkonturen der registrierten MRT-Referenzbilder sind schwarz und die der CT-Bilder weiß eingezeichnet. Starke Abweichungen sind im Bereich des Tumors vorhanden (schwarzer Pfeil in b)).

Artefakten sind. Die Modellerstellung und -übertragung wurde auf der Basis von Bilddatensätzen drei verschiedener Patienten evaluiert.

Eine Evaluation zur Genauigkeit des MRT-basierten Bewegungsmodells hat gezeigt, dass das Modell die durchschnittliche Lungenbewegung der Patienten gut abbildet. So wurden, obwohl die rekonstruierten Atemsignale der Patientendaten auch größere Variationen im Atemverhalten aufwiesen, im Modell durchschnittliche Abweichungen von lediglich 1.39 mm beobachtet.

In einer zweiten Evaluation wurde die affine Modellübertragung bewertet. Hierbei konnte gezeigt werden, dass affine Transformationen geeignet sind, um geometrische Unterschiede zwischen korrespondierenden MRT- und CT-Bilddaten desselben Patienten zu beschreiben. Jedoch ist die Qualität der Registrierung aufgrund des eingesetzten ICP-Algorithmus maßgeblich auch von der Qualität der Lungensegmentierungen in den MRT- und CT-Bilddaten abhängig. Abweichungen zwischen den Segmentierungen in CT- und MRT-Daten sind sowohl auf unterschiedliche Auflösung und Kontraste als auch auf Fehlsegmentierungen im Bereich des Tumors zurückzuführen (Abb. 3). Patient 2 und Patient 3 weisen festgewachsene Tumoren an den Lungenrändern auf, wodurch eine präzise Segmentierung erschwert wird (Abb. 3b,) und Abweichungen zwischen der CT-Segmentierung und der übertragenen MRT-Segmentierung entstehen.

Weitergehende Aussagen zur Robustheit und Genauigkeit der entwickelten Methoden sind nach Analysen weiterer Bilddatensätze zu erwarten. In weiterführenden Arbeiten wird eine vollautomatische gekoppelte formbasierte Segmentierung der MRT- und CT-Daten angestrebt, um möglichst gleiche Lungensegmentierungen beider Datensätze zu gewährleisten. Außerdem soll das Modell um eine Möglichkeit zur Skalierung der Lungenbewegung erweitert werden, um auch patientenspezifische Variationen der Atmung besser abbilden zu können.

Literaturverzeichnis

1. Ehrhardt J, Werner R, Schmidt-Richberg A, et al. Statistical modeling of 4D respiratory lung motion using diffeomorphic image registration. IEEE Trans Med Imaging. 2011;30(2):251–65.
2. McClelland J, Blackall J, Tarte S, et al. A continuous 4D motion model from multiple respiratory cycles for use in lung radiotherapy. Med Phys. 2006;33(9):3348–58.
3. Werner R, Ehrhardt J, Schmidt-Richberg A, et al. Towards accurate dose accumulation for IMRT: Impact of weighting schemes and temporal image resolution on the estimation of dosimetric motion effects. Z Med Phys. 2012;22:109–22.
4. Rao A, Chandrashekara R, Sanchez-Ortiz GI, et al. Spatial transformation of motion and deformation fields using nonrigid registration. IEEE Trans Med Imaging. 2004;23(9):1065–76.
5. Wilms M, Ehrhardt J, Handels H. A 4D statistical shape model for automated segmentation of lungs with large tumors. Proc MICCAI. 2012; p. 347–54.
6. Besl PJ, McKay ND. A method for registration of 3-D shapes. IEEE Trans Pattern Anal Mach Intell. 1992;14(2):239–56.

Image-Based Palpation Simulation With Soft Tissue Deformations Using Chainmail on the GPU

Dirk Fortmeier[1,2], Andre Mastmeyer[1], Heinz Handels[1]

[1]Institute of Medical Informatics, University of Lübeck [2]Graduate School for Computing in Medicine and Life Sciences, University of Lübeck

fortmeier@imi.uni-luebeck.de

Abstract. Virtual reality surgery simulation can provide an environment for the safe training of medical interventions. In many of these interventions palpation of target organs is common to search for certain anatomical structures in a first step. We present a method for visuo-haptic simulation with tissue deformation caused by palpation solely based on CT data of a patient. Generation of haptic force feedback involves a force parameter image based on distances to the patient's skin and bone. To create a deformed version of the patient's image data, the ChainMail method is applied; bone structures are considered to be undeformable. The simulation can be used to palpate the iliac crest and spinous processes for the preparation of a lumbar puncture or for palpation of the ribcage.

1 Introduction

Finding anatomical structures for the preparation of medical interventions is an aspect of recent visuo-haptic surgery simulator frameworks. In [1], optical markers have been placed in the scene to indicate the location of the iliac crest and spinous processes. In a real intervention, these are palpated before performing a lumber puncture.

The frameworks of [2, 3] use haptic devices to simulate the palpation of the femoral artery to prepare the steps necessary for the Seldinger technique. In these simulations, soft tissue is rendered using triangular surfaces. To display deformations of these surfaces, several methods such as finite element methods or mass-spring models can be used. Another approach is to compute deformed volumetric images based on data obtained by imaging procedures as computed tomography (CT) and visualize these by direct volume rendering. In [4], this was demonstrated for the deformations occurring in a needle insertion simulator. Rendering and calculation of deformations directly on the image data can reduce or circumvent a time-consuming segmentation process that is normally needed for the creation of virtual patients.

In this paper, we present (1) an image-based haptic algorithm for palpation simulation and (2) a ChainMail implementation on graphics hardware based on

H.-P. Meinzer et al. (Hrsg.), *Bildverarbeitung für die Medizin 2013*, Informatik aktuell, DOI: 10.1007/978-3-642-36480-8_26, © Springer-Verlag Berlin Heidelberg 2013

the work of [5, 6] to visualize the deformations occurring in a palpation only using the CT data of virtual patients. The methods presented can be used to palpate the iliac crest and spinous processes for the preparation of a lumbar puncture or for palpation of the ribcage using a Phantom Omni haptic device.

2 Methods and Materials

Visuo-haptic systems rely on two components: Visualization and the simulation of haptic force-feedback. In the following, we present a method for simulation of haptic force-feedback based on a force parameter image and a visualization scheme for rendering of the deformations occuring during the palpation.

2.1 Palpation Simulation

Palpation is simulated by a proxy based volume haptic rendering approach [7]. Here, instead of haptic rendering of the image data, a force parameter image $\mathbf{F} : \mathbb{N}^3 \rightarrow \mathbb{R}$ is created based on the original CT image $\mathbf{I} : \mathbb{N}^3 \rightarrow \mathbb{R}$ in a preprocessing step. Similar to the work of [8], distance maps are used to calculate the values of the force parameter image. Here, these depend on the distance to the patient's skin surface and proximity to bone structures. It is obtained as follows: Using a thresholding operation, bone structures are segmented. For the patient's surface, region growing is used to mask each voxel outside of the patient (giving binary mask $\mathbf{C}$). From these binary masks, euclidean distance maps $\mathbf{A}$ and $\mathbf{B}$ are created (for bone and surface resp.), which assign to each voxel the distance to the nearest voxel of the masks. These are combined together with the binary mask for the body ($\mathbf{C}$) to obtain the force parameter image

$$\mathbf{F} = \alpha \frac{\mathbf{C}}{\beta + \mathbf{A}} + \gamma \mathbf{B} \qquad \alpha, \beta, \gamma \in \mathbb{R} \tag{1}$$

Parameter settings for eq. (1) have been adjusted manually (e.g. for the rib cage scenario, $\alpha = \frac{200}{3}$, $\beta = 2$, $\gamma = \frac{1}{60}$ yielded good results). An example of a slice of a force parameter image can be seen in Fig. 1. Based on the force parameter image and the the current position of the haptic device $\mathbf{x}$, a proxy position $\mathbf{p}$ is computed

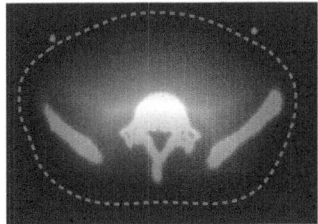 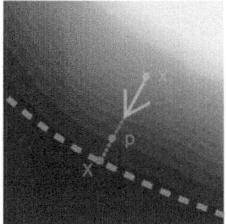

Fig. 1. Left: Force parameter image for the computation of palpation. The patients skin is indicated by a red line. Right: Computation of the proxy $\mathbf{p}$ and surface point $\mathbf{X}$ based on the device tip $\mathbf{x}$ and the normalized gradient of the force parameter image.

$$p = x + \frac{\nabla F(x)}{||\nabla F(x)||} F(x) \qquad (2)$$

The proxy position and position of the haptic device is then connected by a virtual spring that is used to calculate the force feedback $f = k(x-p)$ by Hooke's law. To simulate friction, the new proxy position is interpolated linearly with the old proxy position.

Furthermore, the surface point X is computed by finding the intersection of the skin and the line defined by x and p (Fig. 1). This point is needed for the visualization of the deformation in the following.

2.2   Visualization of Deformations

The deformations in our simulator are computed by the ChainMail algorithm optimized for the processing with graphics hardware [5]. The main idea is to consider each element of the image as an element in a chainmail-like structure and restrict the positions of each element based on the positions of the neighbors. These restrictions are enforced iteratively until no further elements have been moved. In each iteration, each element checks if one of its six neighbors has been moved. If this is true, and the restrictions are violated, the restrictions are enforced and the element itself is considered as moved in the next iteration.

In Fig. 2 the restrictions imposed by a left neighbor on an element are illustrated. The parameters defining the restricted area are the minimum and maximum distance to the neighbor element and the maximum sheer distance (minDist, maxDist and maxSheer).

We further modify the algorithm in a way that bone structures (elements with a Houndsfield value higher than a certain threshold) are not considered: Each element that is classified as bone omits the enforcement of the restrictions imposed by its neighbors. For the relaxation step, we use a diffusive approach together with a material function [4] to regulate the diffusion rate. Here, a continuous approximation of the Heaviside function with the step at the bone threshold is used to restrict the diffusion to non-bone structures. Now, to calculate and display a deformed image J based on the undeformed image I, several steps have to be performed (Fig. 3). We implemented these steps on the GPU using NVidia CUDA. First, the surface point X and the haptic device position x are used as undeformed and deformed position of the first moved element for the ChainMail computations. The deformed image is then created by relaxation

Fig. 2. Restrictions of the movement of the white element imposed by the left neighbor (gray) and bottom neighbor (dashed) as done by [5].

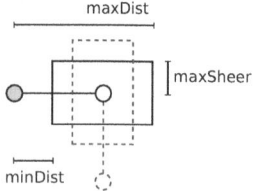

	Average ± Std dev	min	max
1. ChainMail	5.58 ± 2.06	0.22	11.53
2. Relax	52.27 ± 5.02	36.72	65.39
3. Invert	2.55 ± 0.25	1.68	3.26
4. Copy to PBO	0.17 ± 0.02	0.14	0.32
5. Update texture	0.75 ± 0.17	0.56	2.38
6. Reset	3.57 ± 0.19	0.90	4.15
total+overhead	65.07 ± 6.75	44.24	82.23

Table 1. Measured times for the parts of the algorithm in ms. The average is shown together with the corresponding standard deviation.

and inversion of the deformation field. For better performance, each of the steps is only calculated in a cubic volume of interest (VOI) around **x** with a fixed edge length. A pixel buffer object (PBO) is then used as the interface between an OpenGL 3D texture and the CUDA data.

Afterwards, the 3D texture can be rendered by a conventional volume renderer (we use the vtkGPUVolumeRayCastMapper provided by the open source Visualization Toolkit). For all results presented in the following, a NVidia GTX 680 has been used.

3   Results

In Fig. 4, a simple cube object and a cube surrounded by bone are deformed by the ChainMail algorithm. Different parameter settings are demonstrated: (p_1) minDist $= 0.5$, maxDist $= 1.5$, maxSheer $= 0.5$; $(p2)$ minDist $= 0.25$, maxDist $= 1.5$, maxSheer $= 1.0$. In the first two columns, no relaxation is applied. In the other two 20, resp. 40, iterations of the diffusive relaxation are used. The figure demonstrates that bone is not deformed neither by the ChainMail algorithm nor by the diffusive relaxation.

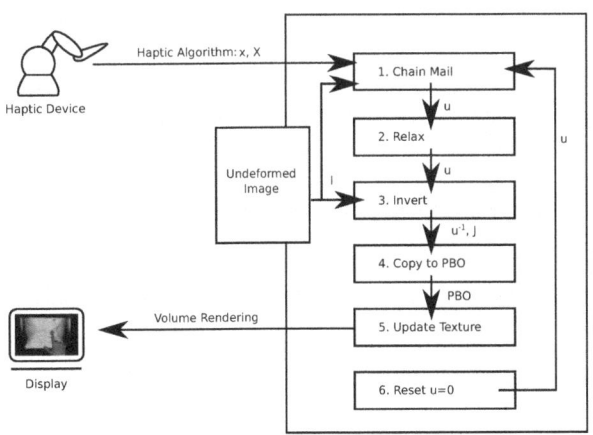

Fig. 3. Data transfer from each part of the deformation visualization algorithm on the GPU. The initial displacement calculated by the haptic algorithm $(\mathbf{X}, \mathbf{x})$ is transfered to the GPU based calculation of deformations. After computation of the deformed image, it is rendered via a volume renderer.

Table 2. Measured mean runtimes t_i in ms and number of moved elements n_i for the ChainMail algorithm with parameter setting p_i and initial moved distance d (in voxel edge length). The parameters used are p_1 = (minDist = 0.5, maxDist = 1.5, maxSheer = 0.5) and $p2$ = (minDist = 0.25, maxDist = 1.5, maxSheer = 1.0).

d	t_1	n_1	t_2	n_2
3	0.22	230	0.22	56
5	0.40	1158	0.39	259
10	1.23	9918	1.08	2120
20	5.98	82238	4.71	17309
30	18.04	280958	13.88	58898

A screenshot of the simulator is presented in Fig. 5. At the tip of the virtual finger, deformed tissue can be seen in a 3D volume rendering and slices of the deformed volume. For a virtual patient with image data consisting of $256 \times 256 \times 236$ elements and a VOI size of 64^3 elements, an interactive total frame rate of 11.50 ± 1.52 Hz has been achieved.

Tab. 1 shows times for each of the components of the visual deformation algorithm. The average processing times with standard deviation and minimum/maximum processing times were measured during a normal use of the simulator. Obviously, the diffusive relaxation is the most time consuming subtask (80% of the total time needed for the whole deformation algorithm). Runtimes of only the ChainMail subtask with parameter settings p_1 and p_2 are displayed in tab. 2: One element has been moved a distance d and the time necessary and the total number of moved elements is shown.

Haptic forces enable the user to distinguish ribs and the space between them in a ribcage palpation scenario. Furthermore, in a lumbar puncture scenario, the iliac crest and spinous processes can be palpated using the methods presented.

4   Discussion

A visual deformation algorithm together with a haptic rendering component have been presented in a simulator framework for the palpation of virtual patients. The effectiveness of the ChainMail algorithm on the GPU using CUDA has

Fig. 4. Several test cases with varying ChainMail parameter settings (p_1, p_2) and relaxation steps (20 resp. 40 in the two columns on the right side).

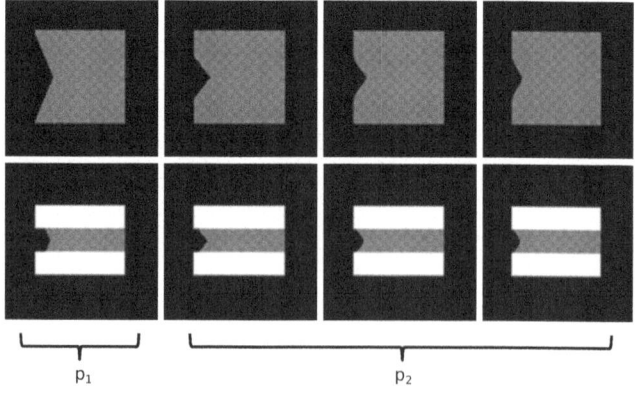

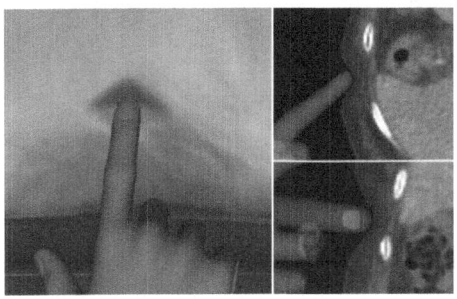

Fig. 5.   Screenshot of a simulated palpation of the ribcage. The diamond-shaped deformation caused by the ChainMail algorithm can be seen clearly. On the right, slices of the deformed CT data are shown.

been confirmed, several thousand elements can be computed in just a few milliseconds. Relaxation is the most time consuming part due to the relatively high number of iterations needed to produce smooth deformations (here, 20 iterations were applied). Even with this high number of iterations, the diamond-shaped deformation caused by the limitations of the ChainMail algorithm cannot be compensated completely. Thus, in future work, improvements in this area are desired. Further work has to include a study of face validity, user acceptance and portability to other patients and scenarios. A comparison of the deformations and forces of the haptic simulation to ground truth data (e.g. aquired with a finite element simulation) should be done to verify the realism of the models.

Acknowledgement. This work is supported by the German Research Foundation (DFG HA 2355/10-1) and the Graduate School for Computing in Medicine and Life Sciences funded by Germany's Excellence Initiative (DFG GSC 235/1).

References

1. Färber M, Hummel F, Gerloff C, et al. Virtual Reality Simulator for the Training of Lumbar Punctures. Methods Inf Med. 2009;48(5):493–501.
2. Coles TR, John NW, Gould D, et al. Integrating Haptics with Augmented Reality in a Femoral Palpation and Needle Insertion Training Simulation. IEEE Trans Haptics. 2011;4(3):199–209.
3. Ullrich S, Kuhlen T. Haptic Palpation for Medical Simulation in Virtual Environments. IEEE Trans Vis Comput Graph. 2012;18(4):617–25.
4. Fortmeier D, Mastmeyer A, Handels H. GPU-based Visualization of Deformable Volumetric Soft-Tissue for Real-time Simulation of Haptic Needle Insertion. In: Bildverarbeitung für die Medizin. Berlin: Springer; 2012. p. 117–22.
5. Rössler F, Wolff T, Ertl T. Direct GPU-based Volume Deformation. In: Proceedings of Curac 2008. Leipzig; 2008. p. 65–8.
6. Gibson SF. 3D Chainmail: A Fast Algorithm for Deforming Volumetric Objects. In: Proc Interactive 3D Graphics. New York: ACM; 1997. p. 149–ff.
7. Lundin K, Ynnerman A, Gudmundsson B. Proxy-based Haptic Feedback from Volumetric Density Data. In: Eurohaptics Conference. United Kingdom: University of Edinburgh; 2002. p. 104–9.
8. Bartz D, Gürvit. Haptic Navigation in Volumetric Datasets. In: Proc PHANToM Users Research Symposium. Konstanz: Hartung-Gorre; 2000. p. 43–7.

Simulation mammographischer Brustkompression zur Generierung von MRT-Projektionsbildern

Julia Krüger[1], Jan Ehrhardt[1], Arpad Bischof[2], Heinz Handels[1]

[1]Institut für Medizinische Informatik, Universität zu Lübeck
[2]Klinik für Radiologie und Nuklearmedizin, Universitätsklinikum Schleswig-Holstein
krueger@imi.uni-luebeck.de

Kurzfassung. Um die Brustkrebsdiagnose zu unterstützen, kann zusätzlich zu einer Mammographie ein MRT-Bilddatansatz akquiriert werden. Die kombinierte Analyse der Bilddaten wird erschwert durch die unterschiedliche Dimensionalität und Kontrastwerte sowie eine unterschiedliche Lage und Deformation der Brust während der Untersuchungen. Die hier vorgestellte Methode liefert einen Ansatz, die Korrespondenzanalyse zwischen 2D-Mammographie und 3D-MRT erheblich zu erleichtern. Der starke Deformationsunterschied wird durch eine oberflächenbasierte 3D/3D-Registrierung ausgeglichen. Anschließend wird ein MRT-Projektionsbild simuliert. Eine erste Evaluation zeigt, dass die Analyse korrespondierender Strukturen deutlich verbessert werden kann.

1 Einleitung

Aufgrund der überlagerungsbehafteten Darstellung von Strukturen und des geringen Kontrasts zwischen Tumor- und gesundem Drüsengewebe, ist die Auswertung von Mammographie-Daten herausfordernd. Daher können weitere Modalitäten zur genaueren Abklärung der Diagnose eingesetzt werden, wie zum Beispiel die kontrastverstärkte Magnetresonanztomographie (MRT), die neben 3D-Bilddaten auch Informationen über die Fuktionalität zur Verfügung stellt. Im Gegensatz zur Mammographie, wird ein MR-Bild ohne Brustkompression akquiriert. Um die Informationen der Bilddaten beider Modalitäten kombiniert zu analysieren und auszuwerten, muss der untersuchende Radiologe korrespondierende Strukturen in den Bilddaten lokalisieren. Diese Aufgabe wird erschwert durch (1) die unterschiedliche Dimensionalität und Auflösung der Daten, (2) die unterschiedlichen Kontrastwerte zwischen den verschiedenen Gewebstypen und (3) der unterschiedlichen Lage und Deformation der Brust der Patientin während der Untersuchung.

Bei bisher veröffentlichten Arbeiten wurde das Problem der unterschiedlichen Brustdeformation mittels biomechanischer Finite Element Modellierungstechniken (FEM) gelöst [1, 2]. Diese Methoden sind jedoch teilweise manuell, zeitaufwändig und schwierig in die klinische Routine zu integrieren. Werden nach Deformation weitere Anpassungen an die vorliegende Mammographie

H.-P. Meinzer et al. (Hrsg.), *Bildverarbeitung für die Medizin 2013*, Informatik aktuell,
DOI: 10.1007/978-3-642-36480-8_27, © Springer-Verlag Berlin Heidelberg 2013

durchgeführt, erfolgt dies meist durch 2D/2D-Registrierung zwischen Mammographie und MRT-Projektion [3, 4]. Mertzanidou et. al führen eine 2D/3D-Registrierung zwischen Mammographie und MRT mithilfe einer affinen Transformation durch [5]. Diese bietet jedoch nur eine grobe Approximation der Weichgewebedeformation. Im Gegensatz dazu stellt die B-Spline-Transformation eine flexiblere Deformation bereit.

2 Methoden

Die vorgestellte Methode der 2D/3D-Korrespondenzanalyse zwischen Mammographie und MRT-Aufnahmen unterteilt sich in vier Schritte (Abb. 1), die im Folgenden genauer beschrieben werden.

2.1 Vorverarbeitung

Da die Bilddaten unter sehr unterschiedlichen Bedingungen (Kompression, Kontrast) akquiriert wurden, müssen die Daten im ersten Schritt einander angeglichen werden. Zuerst werden sowohl in der 2D-Mammographie als auch im 3D-MRT mithilfe von Schwellwertverfahren das Brustgewebe vom Hintergrund getrennt und die Brustoberfläche bzw. Brustkontur mit Marching Cubes/Squares extrahiert. Anschließend wird jeweils die Mamillenposition als anatomisch eindeutiger Punkt bestimmt und im MRT die Grenzen zwischen linker und rechter Brust ermittelt (Abb. 2(a)).

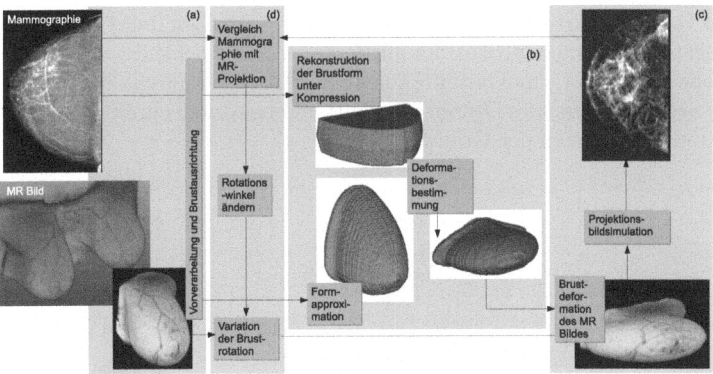

Abb. 1. Übersicht des Workflows: (a) Vorverarbeitung der Bilddaten: Segmentierung des interessierenden Brustbereiches mit anschließender Ausrichtung der MRT-Daten zu den Mammographie-Daten und Segmentierung von Drüsen- und Fettgewebe. (b) Bestimmung der 3D-Deformation zwischen 3D-MRT-Brustoberfläche und rekonstruierter 3D-Brustoberfläche unter Mammographie-Kompression. (c) Projektion der deformierten MRT-Daten mit anschließendem (d) Vergleich der MRT-Projektion und der Mammographie und daraus resultierender Korrektur der MRT-Brustausrichtung.

Da in der Mammographie dichte Strukturen, Gefäße und Drüsengewebe hell erscheinen, wohingegen diese Strukturen im T1-gewichteten MRT dunkel erscheinen, ist ein direkter Vergleich der Grauwerte der Bilddaten nicht sinnvoll. Daher wird im MRT eine Segmentierung von Drüsen- und Fettgewebe durchgeführt, die bei der MRT-Projektionssimulation zur Anwendung kommt (Abb. 2(b)).

2.2   Bestimmung der zu registrierenden Oberflächen

Im Gegensatz zu früheren Ansätzen, wie FEM-Modellierung oder 2D/3D- Registrierung, schlagen wir eine oberflächenbasierte 3D/3D-Registrierung vor. Hierfür ist es zuerst notwendig, die beiden zu registrierenden Oberflächen zu rekonstruieren (Abb. 3, ausführlicher in [6]).

Durch die stark unterschiedliche Lage der Brust in beiden Aufnahmen ist eine initiale Ausrichtung beider Oberflächen in 3D nötig. Hierfür wird die Mamillenposition beider Aufnahmen als gemeinsamer fixer Punkt gewählt. Weiterhin wird

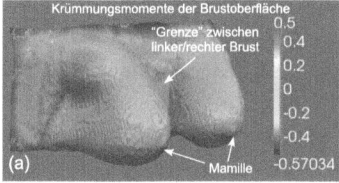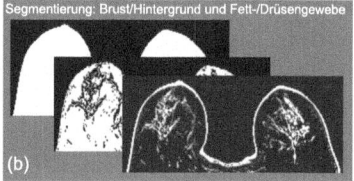

Abb. 2. Vorverarbeitung der MRT-Daten: (a) Krümmungsmomente der Brustoberfläche zur automatischen Bestimmung der Mamillenposition (größte Krümmung (orange/rot) im vorderen Brustbereich) und der „Grenze"zwischen linker und rechter Brust (größte negative Krümmung (blau) im mittleren Brustbereich). (b) Segmentierung von Brustgewebe und Hintergrund mithilfe eines Schwellwertverfahrens auf den Grauwerten und grobe Segmentierung des Drüsen- und Fettgewebes durch ein Schwellwertverfahren auf den Gradientenwerten der Grauwerte.

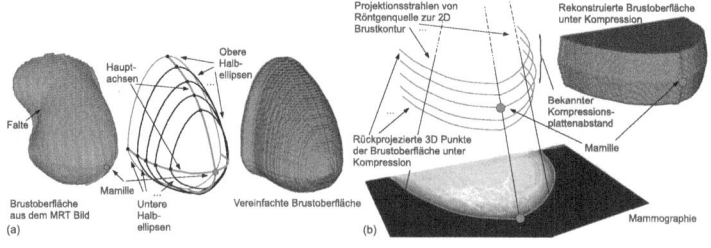

Abb. 3. Rekonstruktion der zu registrierenden 3D-Brustoberflächen: (a) Die MRT-Oberfläche wird aus den MRT-Daten generiert. Hierbei wird die Brustform durch Ellipsen schichtweise approximiert, um während der Aufnahme entstandene Faltungen zu eliminieren. (b) Bei der Mammographie wird aus der 2D-Brustkontur mithilfe der bekannten Röntgenquellenposition und des bekannten Abstandes der Kompressionsplatten die wahrscheinliche Form der komprimierten 3D-Brust rückprojiziert.

die MRT-Aufnahme rotiert, sodass die Schwerpunkte beider von den Oberflächen umschlossenen Brustformen im Brustwandbereich übereinstimmen (Abb. 4).

2.3   Approximation der Deformation

Für die Registrierung der approximierten MRT-Oberfläche und der rückprojizierten Mammographie-Oberfläche wurde eine ICP-basierte B-Spline-Methode entwickelt, die in [6] genauer beschrieben ist.

2.4   Projektionssimulation

Um die Mammographie mit den deformierten MRT-Daten vergleichen zu können, wird ein Projektionsbild der MRT-Daten simuliert. Hierfür wird die bekannte Geometrie der Röntgenquelle verwendet und das segmentierte Drüsengewebe (siehe Vorverarbeitung) in die Mammographie-Ebene projiziert. Daher erscheint

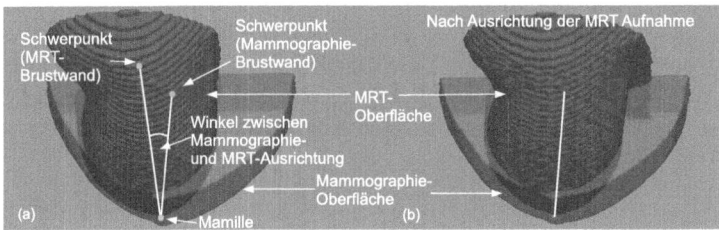

Abb. 4. Rotation der MRT-Aufnahme zur initialen Ausrichtung: Der Rotationswinkel ist bestimmt durch die Abweichung der Schwerpunkte der MRT- (rot) und der Mammographie-Brustform (grün) im Bereich der Brustwand. Die Mamille wird in beiden Brustformen als fixer Punkt (Rotationszentrum) gewählt.

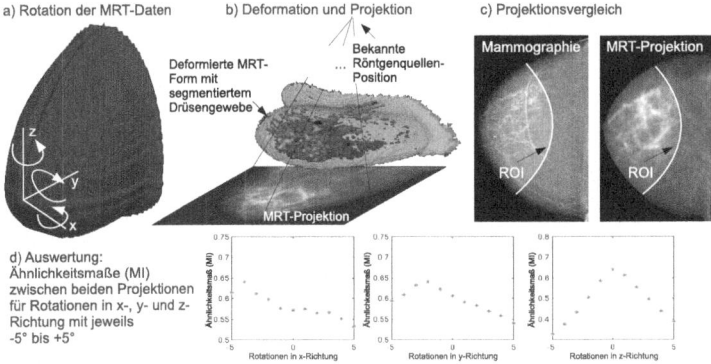

Abb. 5. Vergleich der Mammographie und der MRT-Projektion: a) Variation der Ausrichtung der MRT-Daten, b) Deformation der rotierten und segmentierten MRT-Daten mit anschließender Projektion auf die Mammographie-Ebene, c) Vergleich der Projektionen innerhalb einer ROI im vorderen Brustbereich, d) Winkelbestimmung.

sowohl in der Mammographie als auch in der MRT-Projektion dichtes Gewebe und Drüsengewebe hell.

2.5 Korrektur der Ausrichtung

Da es sich bei der mammographischen Komprimierung der Brust um eine sehr starke Deformation handelt, ist diese Deformation und damit auch die resultierende Projektion stark abhängig von der initialen Lage der Brust vor der Deformation. Daher ist es sinnvoll, diese Lage zu variieren, um die optimale Brustausrichtung zu ermitteln. Abb. 2.3 stellt das Vorgehen bei der hierfür genutzten Projektionsauswertung dar, wobei mithilfe der Mutual Information (MI) die Winkel, die zu der höchsten übereinstimmung zwischen Mammographie und MRT-Projektion führen, ausgewählt werden.

2.6 Evaluation

Für eine erste Evaluation wurden sechs Mammographien von zwei Patientinnen genutzt (Patientin 1: rechts/links, CC/MLO, Patientin 2: rechts, CC/MLO). Der Effekt der Deformation und Ausrichtung der MRT-Daten wurde evaluiert, indem korrespondierende Strukturen in der Mammographie und der MRT-Projektion manuell markiert wurden und der mittlere Abstand der Skelette dieser Strukturen vor und nach Deformation sowie nach Ausrichtung der MRT-Daten bestimmt wurde (Abb. 2.3).

3 Ergebnisse

Abb. 2.3(d) zeigt beispielhaft für eine Mammographie die MI in Beziehung zur Winkelvariation in x-, y- und z-Richtung der MRT-Daten vor der Deformation. Dabei ist ersichtlich, dass die Rotation in y- und z-Richtung einen Einfluss auf die Güte der MRT-Projektion hat und der Einfluss der Rotation in x-Richtung (in Projektionsrichtung) geringer ist. Tab. 1 zeigt, dass sich der Abstand korrespondierender Strukturen nach Deformation der MRT-Daten deutlich reduziert hat und dass eine weitere Verbesserung nach Ausrichtung der MRT-Daten erreicht werden konnte.

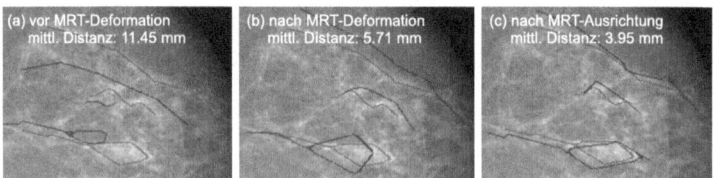

Abb. 6. überlagerung der Skelette von leicht zu identifizierenden Strukturen wie Gefäße oder Drüsenkanäle in der Mammographie (grün) und der MRT-Projektion (rot): (a) ohne Deformation mit großen Abständen zwischen den korrespondierenden Strukturen, (b) nach Deformation mit wesentlich geringeren Abständen und (c) nach Ausrichtung der MRT-Daten.

Tabelle 1. Mittlere Distanzen zwischen den Skeletten korrespondierender Strukturen in Mammographie und MRT-Projektion.

MRT	Mammographie	vor Deformation	nach Deformation	nach Ausrichtung
1	CC re.	14.08 mm	6.46 mm	6.47 mm
1	CC li.	11.45 mm	5.71 mm	3.95 mm
1	MLO re.	35.61 mm	9.88 mm	5.30 mm
1	MLO li.	37.35 mm	21.06 mm	10.94 mm
2	CC re.	24.69 mm	11.26 mm	7.39 mm
2	MLO re.	23.22 mm	16.35 mm	6.09 mm

4 Diskussion

Der vorgestellte Workflow erleichtert die Korrespondenzanalyse zwischen 2D-Mammographie und 3D-MRT. Zum einen wird der starke Deformationsunterschied durch eine oberflächenbasierte 3D/3D-Registrierung ausgeglichen, bei der nicht nur die MRT-Informationen (wie bei FEM-Modellen), sondern auch die 3D-rückprojizierten Mammographie-Daten mit einfließen. Dies ermöglicht es, initial die Daten 3D auszurichten. Die unterschiedliche Dimensionalität der beiden Modalitäten wird durch die Simulation eines MRT-Projektionsbildes kompensiert.

Die Ergebnisse zeigen, dass durch Deformation und Ausrichtung der MR-Daten eine Korrespondenzanalyse zwischen Mammographie und simulierter MR-Projektion deutlich verbessert werden kann, was die Grundlage für eine möglichst genaue Punkt-zu-Linien-Korrespondenz zwischen 2D-Mammographie und deformiertem Projektionsstrahl im 3D-MRT-Datensatz darstellt. Weitergehende Aussagen über die Genauigkeit der Verfahren sind nach einer Analyse einer größeren Anzahl an Datensätzen zu erwarten.

Literaturverzeichnis

1. Ruiter NV, Müller TO, Stotzka R, et al. Registration of X-ray mammograms and MR-volumes of the female breast based on simulated mammographic deformation. Proc IWDM. 2004.
2. Tanner C, White M, Guarino S, et al. Large breast compressions: observations and evaluation of simulations. Med Phys. 2011;38(2):682–90.
3. Behrenbruch C, Marias K, Yam M, et al. The use of magnetic resonance imaging to model breast compression in X-ray mammography for MR/X-ray data fusion. Proc IWDM. 2000.
4. Martí R, Zwiggelaar R, Rubin CME, et al. 2D-3D correspondence in mammography. Cybernet Syst. 2004;35(1):85–105.
5. Mertzanidou T, Hipwell J, Cardoso MJ, et al. MRI to X-ray mammography registration using a volume-preserving affine transformation. Med Image Anal. 2012;16(5):966–75.
6. Krüger J, Ehrhardt J, Bischof A, et al. Breast compression simulation using ICP-based B-spline deformation for correspondence analysis in mammography and MRI datasets. Proc SPIE. 2013;(accepted).

Automated Image Processing to Quantify Cell Migration

Minmin Shen[1], Bastian Zimmer[2], Marcel Leist[2], Dorit Merhof[1]

[1]Interdiscipinary Center for Interative Data Analysis, Modelling and Visual Exploration (INCIDE), University of Konstanz [2]The Doerenkamp-Zbinden Chair of in-vitro Toxicology and Biomedicine, University of Konstanz

minmin.shen@uni-konstanz.de

Abstract. Methods to evaluate migration capacity of stem cells and the inhibition by chemicals are important for biomedical research. Here, we established an automated image processing framework to quantify migration of human neural crest (NC) cells into an initially empty, circular region of interest (ROI). The ROI is partially filled during the experiment by migrating cells. Based on an image captured only once at the end of the biological experiment, the framework identifies the initial ROI. The identification worked also, when the distribution of surrounding cells showed large heterogeneity. After segmentation, the number of migrated cells was identified. The image processing framework was capable of efficiently quantifying chemical effects on cell migration.

1 Introduction

Safety assessment of chemicals with new stem cell-based in vitro methods requires not only new biological test systems, but also technical and computer science solutions that allow for high throughput and for unbiased observer-independent data analysis. Manual scoring and manipulation of cells requires intensive, time-consuming training of operators and easily introduces bias into the data. This is particularly important for image-based methods that require quantification and classification of cells in time and/or space.

For detection of environmental toxicants that may adversely affect human development, a screening strategy based on the use of stem cells has been worked out [1]. Within this approach, a test system evaluating the migration capacity of human neural crest (NC) cells has been established.

In a new, technically optimized version of the assay (Fig. 1), cells are seeded onto the culture plates, with stoppers inserted to block cell adhesion in circular areas within a cell culture dish. After removal of the stopper, a defined cell-free area is created (the ROI). The cells are then incubated for 48 h with cell culture medium either containing no test chemicals, or containing different potential neurodevelopmental toxicants (C1-C5). At the end of the experiment, the cells are stained, and images of the culture dish are taken to determine how many cells migrated into the ROI. Different manual and semiautomatic scoring methods have been used in the past. For instance, the area where the stopper had been placed may be defined mechanically, on the basis of the recorded x, y coordinates. However, this requires additional manipulation steps, and a second imaging step. Moreover, the inaccuracy of positioning and of relocating the coordinates (e.g. 0.1 mm) often introduces noise into the data. Therefore, a new method is required which automatically identifies the ROI after a single imaging step at the end of the experiment, and then scores the number of migrated cells operator-independently.

To quantify cell migration, it is required to localize the ROI. However, it would be difficult to determine its exact location before acquiring cell images by manual operations, e.g. putting stamps inside or under the cell cultures. And a small mismatch would cause rather low precision due to the small size of a stopper (its diameter is 2 mm). For this reason, the location of the ROI needs to be estimated using automated image processing approaches.

In this paper, an image processing framework is presented for automated cell migration analysis in response to this need. The acquisition of image data and the image processing framework are elaborated in Section 2. The results are shown in Section 3 to demonstrate the validity of the proposed framework.

2   Material and methods

2.1   Experimental setup

Oris plates (Platypus technologies, Madison, WI) were used to perform migration experiments into an area initially generated by a stopper. The cell source were human-embryonic stem cells derived NC cells [1]. They were stained with two fluorescent dyes and imaged on an automated inverted microscope, equipped with a 4× lens. The individual images from a culture are stitched together to a large image file by proprietary microscope software (Cellomics Array Scan VTI, Thermo Fisher) to allow a full overview of the ROI and its surrounding area (Fig. 2).

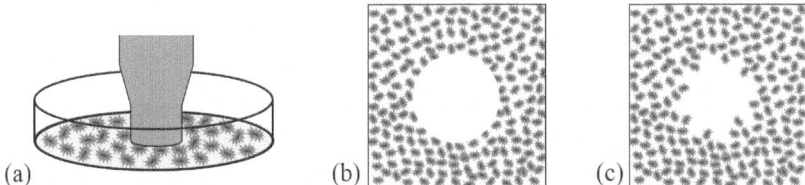

(a)   (b)   (c)

Fig. 1. Principle of the "non invasive" migration assay of NC (MINC): (a) insert stoppers and seed cells onto cell culture plate (side view), (b) remove stoppers to create detection zone (top view), (c) allow cells to migrate into detection zone (top view).

2.2   Image data

Each acquired composite image of a culture dish consists of two color channels: a blue-fluorescent channel indicating nuclei (stained with H-33342) and a green-fluorescent channel indicating the total cell area (cytoplasmic stain through use of calcein-AM).

2.3   Estimation of ROI

The initial step to quantify cell migration is to detect the circular ROI. Due to the aforementioned difficulties to manually determine the coordinates of the stopper before acquiring cell images, an automated image processing method to estimate the ROI in a cell image is required. To estimate the circle, we select the green channel to avoid noise observed in the blue channel.

The segmentation of the central region (i.e. the area that is not populated by cells) is performed in polar coordinates, where the horizontal axis corresponds to the angle axis, and the vertical axis corresponds to the radius axis, respectively. As an example, the cell image (Fig. 3a) is first transformed to polar coordinates using the center of the whole image as the pole (Fig. 3b). Usage of the polar image improves the segmentation result over pure smoothing and thresholding the cartesian image [2]. After applying morphological operations, i.e. dilation and flood-fill operations, a binary mask is generated (Fig. 3c). It is transformed back to Cartesian coordinates and only the segment with the largest area is selected (dark region in Fig. 3d). The initial estimate of the origin of the circle is computed as the center of gravity of this segment, and the estimated ROI is outlined (Fig. 3e).

However, the initial estimate may not be reasonable for some cell images in which the cells are not evenly distributed. A "hole" is observed in these images, as shown at the bottom-right corner in Fig. 3a. Looking back at the segmentation result in Polar coordinates (Fig. 3c), the protruding part of the dark region is connected to the upper margin, corresponding to the "hole" in Cartesian coordinates. Ideally, the dark region will be a rectangle if its counterpart in Cartesian coordinats is a regular circle and the origin of the circle is set as the pole for Cartesian-to-Polar coordinates transformation.

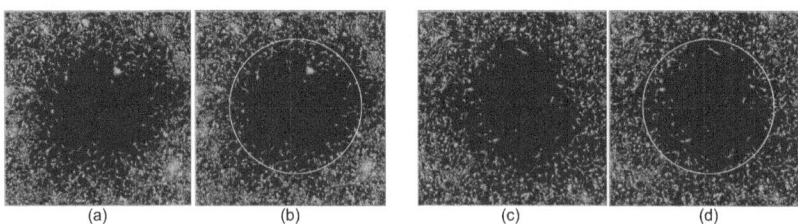

Fig. 2. Examples of dual channel microscopy images (a,c) used for identification of the ROI (b,d).

Based on this observation, the optimal estimation of the origin (x_{opt}, y_{opt}) is a coordinate that, if it is set as the pole, the dark region in the polar image approximates a rectangle. To measure how well the dark region in the polar image approximates a rectangle, the variance of the y-coordinate value of its upper outline is computed. The smaller the variance, the more the dark region approximates a rectangle. (x_{opt}, y_{opt}) is searched within a window around the initial estimate, and the one with the smallest variance is found and kept as the optimized result (Fig. 3f).

2.4   Cell segmentation and quantitative analysis

Once the ROI is determined, segmentation of individual cells is applied in this region. We use several KNIME (The Konstanz Information Miner [3]) nodes including Voronoi segmentation [4] for cell segmentation.

There are numerous segmentation algorithms for cell segmentation. The Voronoi-based algorithm is used in this paper due to its robustness to noise. Based on a metric defined in the image plane and based on seed points, seed-to-pixel distances are calculated and each pixel is assigned to the closest seed under that metric [4]. The nuclei images are segmented using the local maxima of each segment as the seed, and the cytoplasm images are segmented using the nuclei of each cell as the seed.

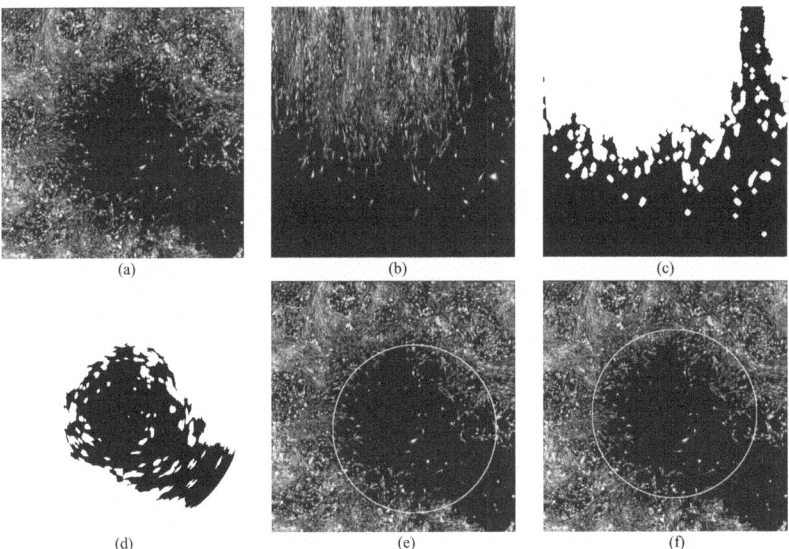

Fig. 3. An example image (green channel) with unevenly distributed cells (a) and its polar image (b). Segmentation result with morphological operations (c) and the largest segment transformed to Cartesian coordinates (d). Initial estimation of ROI (e). Optimized estimation (f).

The number of cells within the ROI is calculated based on the Voronoi segmentation result. As there are outliers in both channels (noise in blue channel and cell debris in green channel), the cytoplasm image and nuclei image are converted to binary images using global threshoding, and are then multiplied with each other to exclude the aforementioned outliers. The multiplication results in an image with noise and cell debris excluded, and the number of cells is calculated based on this image.

3   Results and discussion

The proposed image processing framework was applied to 68 microscopy images of human NC cells, including both untreated cells (28 images) and cell populations treated with five chemicals (C1-C5), for each of which eight images were obtained.

In order to evaluate the performance of the proposed algorithm to estimate the location of the ROI, the origin of the circle was manually located by three human raters. Each human rater manually positioned a circle on the cell image using computer painting tools. The means and standard deviations of the Euclidean distance between the origins of circles of human raters vs. the results of the proposed algorithm (green), and between human raters only (black), are illustrated in Fig. 4a, on all six experimental groups of cell images. The mean and standard deviation of the Euclidean distance averaged across all cell images is 18.8 ± 12.6 pixels for human raters vs. the proposed approach (mean $\pm$ std deviation), and 19.5 ± 12.2 pixels between different human raters. The results show that the estimation by the proposed approach is comparably accurate as human raters, which proves the efficacy of the proposed algorithm in estimating the ROI. The algorithm is also compared to the result of circle detection based

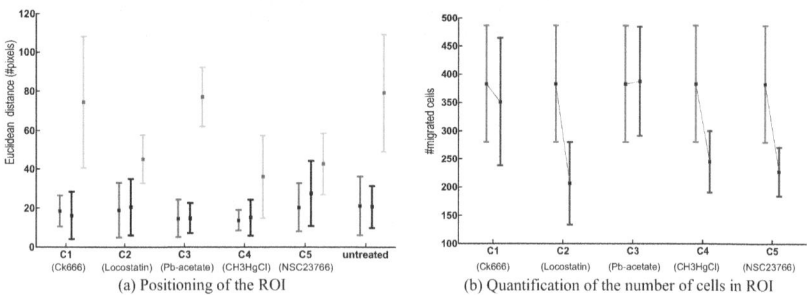

(a) Positioning of the ROI   (b) Quantification of the number of cells in ROI

Fig. 4. Results for cell populations treated with five different chemicals (C1-C5). (a) Means and standard deviations of the Euclidean distance between the origins of circles of human raters vs. the results of the proposed algorithm (green), the origins of circles of human raters vs. a standard circular Hough transformation (pink), and between human raters only (black). (b) Means and standard deviations of numbers of untreated cells (red) and cells treated with different chemicals, respectively (blue).

on the standard circular Hough transformation (Fig. 4a, pink). It can be clearly seen that the proposed circle detection outperforms the standard circular Hough transformation, which has a much higher estimation error (64.8 ± 30.6). Some example results of the estimated ROI are provided in Fig. 2.

In a next step, the accuracy of the cell counts was examined by biologists. For this purpose, the human raters manually counted the number of cells and observed the automated segmentation results of the proposed algorithm to determine the false-positives. The percentage of false-positives was within the range of 1.56% to 9.76%. The results show that the segmentation algorithm tends to oversegment the cells, but according to the biologists this percentage of false-positives is acceptable and in the range of the manual counting variation. A small trend towards oversegmentation is well acceptable to the biologists as they care more about the relative change of the number of cells after treatment with different chemicals.

Fianlly, the cell counts are used in order to assess the effect of chemicals on cell migration. For this purpose, the means and standard deviations of numbers of untreated cells and cells treated with five chemicals are shown in red and blue, respectively (Fig. 4b). For example, the number of cells decreases significantly after treatment with Locostatin (C2), which indicates that this chemical affects cell migration. In contrast, the cell number does not change significantly after treatment with Pb-acetate (C3), which indicates that C3 is not likely to inhibit cell migration.

4   Conclusion

An automated image processing framework for cell migration analysis is proposed in this paper. The main contribution is an approach to estimate the location of the ROI, followed by segmentation of individual cells within the ROI. In order to evaluate the approach, the ROI estimation and cell segmentation are examined by biologists. The results of the proposed image processing approach proved to be comparable to human raters, which verifies that the automatic image processing framework is a useful tool to quantify cell migration.

References

1. Zimmer B, Lee G, Balmer NV, et al. Evaluation of developmental toxicants and signaling pathways in a functional test based on the migration of human neural crest cells. Environ Health Perspect. 2012;120(8):1116–22.
2. Riess T, Dietz C, Tomas M, et al. Automated Image Processing for the Analysis of DNA Repair Dynamics. In: Proc. 3rd International Conference on Bioinformatics, Biocomputational Systems and Biotechnologies (BioTechno); 2011. p. 31–6.
3. Berthold MR, Cebron N, Dill F, et al. KNIME: The Konstanz Information Miner. In: Proc. Data Analysis, Machine Learning and Applications; 2008. p. 319–26.
4. Jones TR, Carpenter AE, Golland P. Voronoi-Based Segmentation of Cells on Image Manifolds. In: Proc. Computer Vision for Biomedical Image Applications (CVBIA); 2005. p. 535–43.

Impact of Segmentation in Quantitative Computed Tomography
A Simulation Study

Bastian Gerner, Dominique Töpfer, Oleg Museyko, Klaus Engelke

Institute of Medical Physics (IMP), University of Erlangen-Nuremberg, Germany
bastian.gerner@imp.uni-erlangen.de

Abstract. Due to limited spatial resolution of CT scanners, cortices with submillimeter thickness are substantially blurred, which leads to problems when estimating their extent and intensity. In the present work, we used three different algorithms to determine cortical thickness, cortical bone mineral density and cortical bone mineral content and investigated their ability to detect a change of these three parameters.

1 Introduction

Cortical bone is an important component of bone strength and therefore the quantification of cortical bone thickness and bone mineral density (BMD) at the hip, spine and forearm is of major interest in the field of osteoporosis. However, if the cortical thickness is smaller than 1 mm, the limited spatial resolution of whole body clinical CT scanners causes partial volume artifacts and as a consequence, cortical thickness may be over- and cortical BMD underestimated in quantitative computed tomography (QCT) [1].

The consequences of spatial blurring have been extensively studied in Literature. Prevrhal et al. proposed a method based on local adaptive 50 % thresholds, which is a fast method but leads to an overestimation of cortical thickness for thin cortices [2]. Other methods based on thresholding also suffer from inaccuracies when thin bone cortices are observed [3]. Recent publications use optimization techniques to overcome these problems. In this context, the method proposed by Treece et al. must be named as a prime example [4].

These results show that the accuracy with which the cortical thickness and density can be determined depends on the segmentation method. Here, we investigated the effects of three different segmentation techniques on simulated changes in cortical BMD and thickness.

2 Materials and methods

2.1 Simulation of image acquisition

After an initial segmentation, which can be performed by using the volume growing method, the bone surface is triangulated. For each vertex, a linear

H.-P. Meinzer et al. (Hrsg.), *Bildverarbeitung für die Medizin 2013*, Informatik aktuell, DOI: 10.1007/978-3-642-36480-8_29, © Springer-Verlag Berlin Heidelberg 2013

bone profile BMD (x) is obtained by measuring the BMD values along a line p perpendicular to the outer bone surface (Fig. 1).

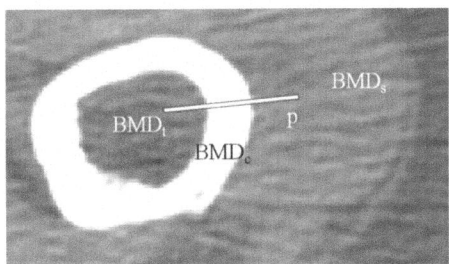

Fig. 1. Acquisition of a linear bone profile. BMD_t represents trabecular bone, BMD_c cortical bone and BMD_s soft tissue.

BMD (x) can be modeled as a sum of step functions of varying width and height and can be described as

$$\text{BMD}(x) = \text{BMD}_t + (\text{BMD}_c - \text{BMD}_t)\, H(x - x_1) \\ + (\text{BMD}_s - \text{BMD}_c)\, H(x - x_2) \tag{1}$$

Here, BMD_t represents trabecular bone, BMD_c cortical bone and BMD_s soft tissue. $H(x)$ is the Heaviside Function while x_1 and x_2 determine the position of the inner and outer bone surfaces. Therefore, the true cortical thickness is $t_c = x_2 - x_1$.

1 was convoluted with a Gaussian function $g(x; \sigma, \mu = 0)$ approximating the point spread function of the CT scanner. The full width at half maximum (FWHM) was assumed to be the scanner resolution. Therefore, the blurred profile $\text{BMD}_b(x)$, simulating the density distribution within a reconstructed CT image, can be calculated by

$$\text{BMD}_b(x) = \int_{-\infty}^{+\infty} \text{BMD}(t)\, g(x - t)\, dt \tag{2}$$

Fig. 2 shows the results of 2 for two different t_c and BMD_c values.

2.2 Estimation of cortical thickness and BMD

To calculate cortical thickness, we used three different algorithms: a global threshold (GT) and two local adaptive thresholds, one based on 50 % thresholds (AT), and the second one inverting 2 using an optimization method based on Levenberg-Marquardt algorithm (OM).

GT uses global threshold values to separate soft tissue, cortical and trabecular bone. In our study, we used $400\,\text{mg/cm}^3$ to segment cortical bone from soft tissue and $150\,\text{mg/cm}^3$ to differentiate cortical and trabecular bone.

AT calculates threshold values, which are locally adjusted for each profile perpendicular to the bone surface. The positions of the outer and inner bone surface x_1 and x_2 are determined by calculating 50 % threshold values for each side of the cortex [2].

OM is based on a method described in [4]. Here, 2 is fitted to each profile and the parameters $\mathrm{BMD_t}$, $\mathrm{BMD_s}$, x_1, x_2 and σ are determined using the Levenberg-Marquardt method. $\mathrm{BMD_c}$, the cortical bone density, is measured in a location where $t_c \gg$ FWHM and therefore cortical intensity is not affected by partial volume artifacts.

To estimate cortical density $\mathrm{BMD_e}$ at the location of interest, where usually $t_c <$ FWHM, we integrated the density distribution between the edges x_1 and x_2 and divided the result by t_e [2]

$$\mathrm{BMD_e} = \frac{1}{t_e} \int_{x_1}^{x_2} \mathrm{BMD_b}(x)\,\mathrm{d}x \tag{3}$$

By multiplying $\mathrm{BMD_e}$ and t_e, the cortical bone mass (the so called cortical bone mineral content $\mathrm{BMC_e}$) can be calculated.

2.3 Simulation parameters

In our study, we simulated a change of true cortical thickness t_c and true cortical $\mathrm{BMD_c}$, which can be caused by ageing, disease or treatment. We simulated a longitudinal 2.5 %, 5.0 % and 7.5 % increase of $\mathrm{BMD_c}$ and a longitudinal 5 %, 10 % and 20 % increase of t_c for different initial cortical thickness values. For each profile, we estimated the changes Δt_e, $\Delta\mathrm{BMD_e}$ and $\Delta\mathrm{BMC_e}$ using the methods described in 2.2 and compared the results with the simulated true values.

Baseline $\mathrm{BMD_c}$ was assumed to be $1400\,\mathrm{mg/cm^3}$. The remaining parameters were set to $\mathrm{BMD_t} = 75\,\mathrm{mg/cm^3}$, $\mathrm{BMD_s} = 0\,\mathrm{mg/cm^3}$, FWHM $= 0.5\,\mathrm{mm}$ and kept constant during the simulation process.

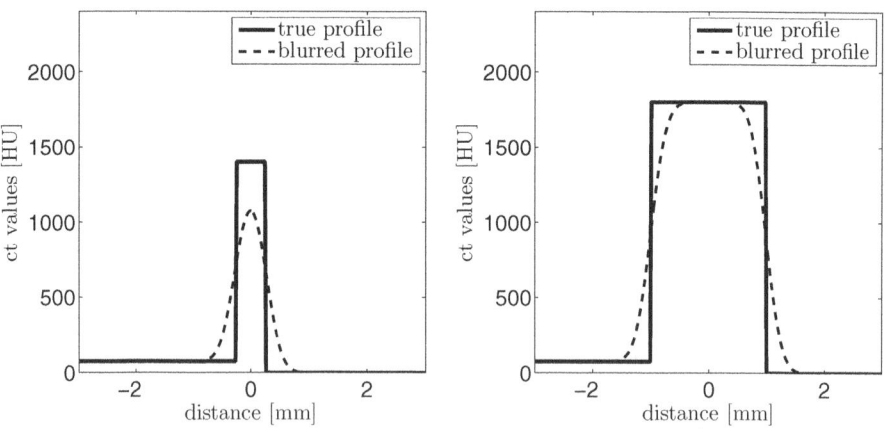

Fig. 2. True and blurred profiles (left: $t_c = 0.5\,\mathrm{mm}$, $\mathrm{BMD_c} = 1400\,\mathrm{HU}$; right: $t_c = 2.0\,\mathrm{mm}$, $\mathrm{BMD_c} = 1800\,\mathrm{HU}$; FWHM $= 0.5\,\mathrm{mm}$).

3   Results

3.1   Variation of cortical thickness

The effects of an assumed longitudinal 5%, 10% and 20% cortical thickness increase on measured changes (cortical Δt_e, ΔBMD_e and ΔBMC_e) are illustrated in Fig. 3 as a function of t_c/FWHM.

With AT, an increase of cortical thickness is underestimated for thin cortices, but this method provides a good accuracy for $t_c > 2\,\text{FWHM}$, whereas GT leads to an underestimation of Δt_c even for $t_c = 4\,\text{FWHM}$. OM showed the best results

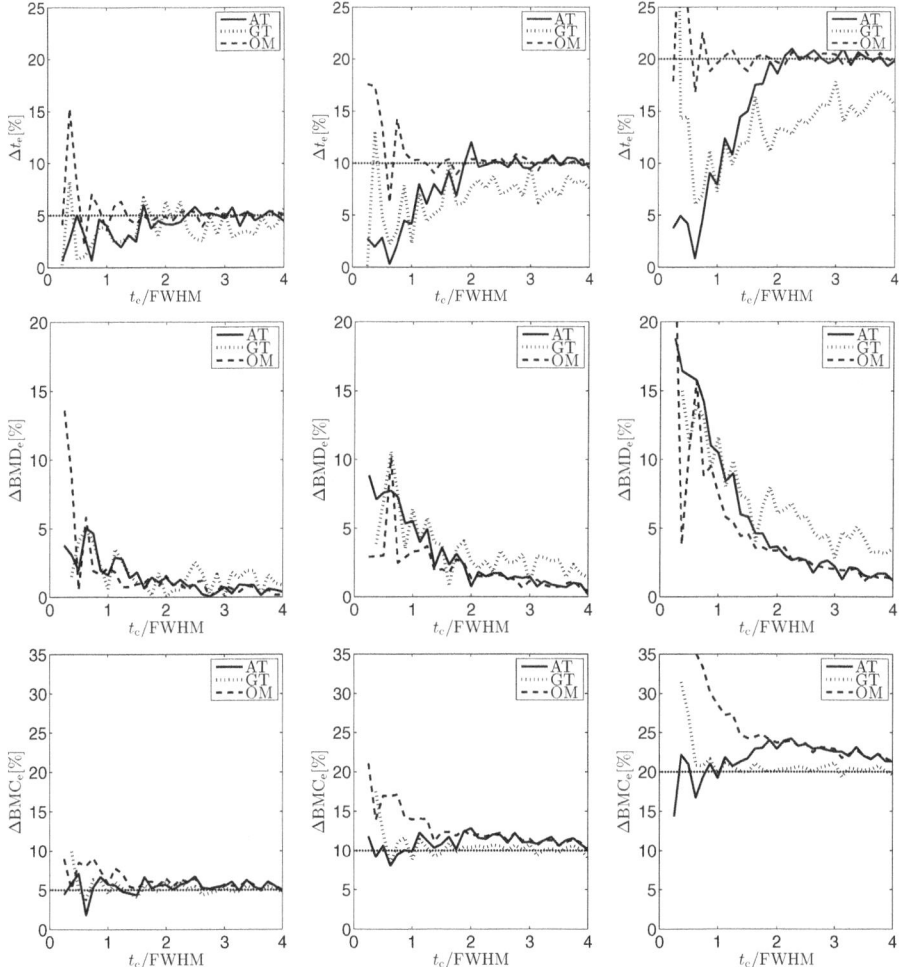

Fig. 3. Results for cortical Δt_e (first row), ΔBMD_e (second row) and ΔBMC_e (third row). Results are shown for an assumed 5% (first column), 10% (second column) and 20% (third column) increase of true cortical thickness t_c.

in particular in the range $0.5\,\mathrm{FWHM} < t_\mathrm{c} < 2\,\mathrm{FWHM}$. For even smaller t_c, OM was severely impacted by noise. For all three segmentation techniques, the assumed increase in cortical thickness resulted in an artificial increase of cortical BMD, which was larger for thinner cortices. For $t_\mathrm{c} > 1.5\,\mathrm{FWHM}$, GT showed larger errors in estimating $\Delta\mathrm{BMD_e}$. With respect to $\Delta\mathrm{BMC_e}$, GT resulted in the lowest errors. OM largely overestimated $\Delta\mathrm{BMC_c}$ for $t_\mathrm{c} < 1\,\mathrm{FWHM}$.

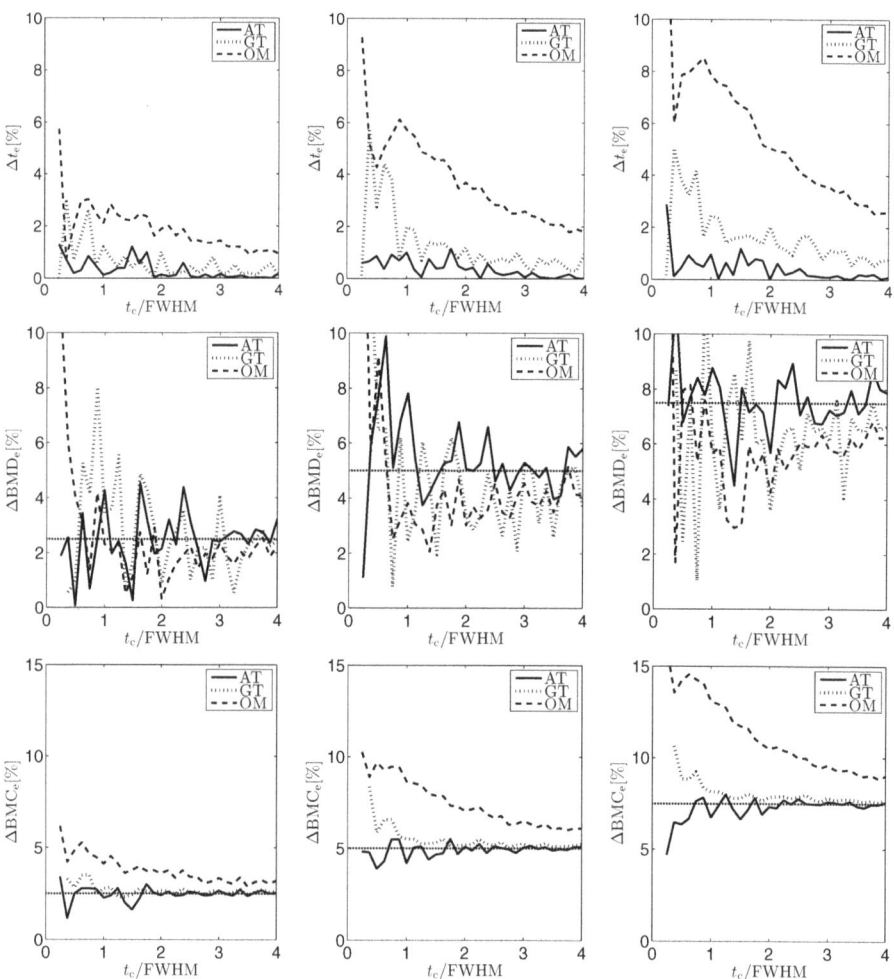

Fig. 4. Results for cortical Δt_e (first row), $\Delta\mathrm{BMD_e}$ (second row) and $\Delta\mathrm{BMC_e}$ (third row). Results are shown for an assumed 2.5 % (first column), 5 % (second column) and 7.5 % (third column) increase of true cortical $\mathrm{BMD_c}$.

3.2   Variation of cortical BMD

The effects of an assumed longitudinal 2.5%, 5% and 7.5% cortical BMD increase on measured changes (cortical ΔBMD_e, Δt_e and ΔBMC_e) are illustrated in Fig. 4 as a function of $t_c/FWHM$.

With GT, the simulated increase in BMD_c resulted in an increase of Δt_e, which was larger for thinner cortices, and an underestimation of ΔBMD_c even for $t_c = 4\,FWHM$. OM showed much larger errors for cortical thickness, BMD and BMC. However, it must be remembered that BMD_c used in 2 was set to $1400\,mg/cm^3$ and was not adapted to the simulated BMD_c change. Furthermore, it can be questioned whether a 5 % change at the location of interest also occurs in the region where the true value is determined. The use of AT showed small changes in Δt_e and a slight underestimation of ΔBMD_c for $t_c < FWHM$. For $t_c < 2\,FWHM$, GT overestimated the change in cortical BMD and showed small errors in ΔBMC_e for $t_c < FWHM$.

4   Discussion

With the use of global segmentation thresholds, a longitudinal change in cortical BMD is underestimated while cortical thickness falsely increases. An increase of t_c is underestimated and an artificial increase in BMD_c can be detected. It may be more accurate to determine BMD_c changes instead.

With local 50 % thresholds, results for Δt_e, ΔBMD_e and ΔBMC_e are accurate at least as long as $t_c > FWHM$, as far as increases in cortical BMD are concerned. A change of cortical thickness can be satisfyingly detected for $t_c > 2\,FWHM$, while cortical BMD falsely increases.

While OM showed good results in estimating changes in cortical thickness, a falsely assumed value for cortical BMD leads to errors when detecting an increase in cortex intensity.

These results must still be verified in more advanced simulations, e. g. considering different noise levels or periosteal apposition.

References

1. Adams JE. Quantitative computed tomography. Eur J Radiol. 2009;71(3):415–24.
2. Prevrhal S, Engelke K, Kalender WA. Accuracy limits for the determination of cortical width and density: the influence of object size and CT imaging parameters. Phys Med Biol. 1999;44(3):751.
3. Hangartner TN. Thresholding technique for accurate analysis of density and geometry in QCT, pQCT and microCT images. J Musculoskelet Neuronal Interact. 2007;7(1):9–16.
4. Treece GM, Gee AH, Mayhew PM, et al. High resolution cortical bone thickness measurement from clinical CT data. Med Image Anal. 2010;14(3):276–90.

Bone Age Assessment Using Support Vector Machine Regression

Daniel Haak, Hendrik Simon, Jing Yu, Markus Harmsen, Thomas M. Deserno

Department of Medical Informatics, RWTH Aachen University
dhaak@mi.rwth-aachen.de

Abstract. Bone age assessment on hand radiographs is a costly and time consuming task in radiology. Recently, an automatic approach combining content-based image retrieval and support vector machines (SVM) has been developed. In this paper, we we apply support vector regression (SVR) as a novel method, yielding a gain in performance. Our methods are designed to cope with the age range 0-18 years as compared to the age range 2-17 of the commercial product BoneXpert. On a standard data set from University of South Carolina, our approaches reach a root-mean-square error of 0.95 and 0.80 years for SVM and SVR, respectively. This is slightly below the performance of the commercial product using an active shape approach.

1 Introduction

Bone age assessment (BAA) is a frequently and time consuming method for growth disturbances determination in the human body. Usually this task is done manually by radiologists on hand radiographs, requiring domain knowledge and experience [1, 2]. Previous work on BAA [3, 4, 5] presented first approaches in automation of this process with content-based image retrieval (CBIR) methods. In [4, 5] new results have been published by combining a support vector machine (SVM) for classification and cross-correlation similarity to a prototype image as feature vector. Although this is a promising method the SVM needs to be extended by multiclass adaption for BAA. The age is discretized in 30 classes and the prediction is calculated by one-against-one voting.

In this work, we apply with support vector regression (SVR) [6, 7, 8] a regression model as a novel approach that naturally supports multiclass problems.

2 Materials and methods

Fig. 1 illustrates the processing pipeline of our approach. At first, the epiphysal centers are located on the radiographs. Then eROIs are extracted, and rotated into a reference position. Cross correlation features are extracted. Classification is done by SVM and SVR.

H.-P. Meinzer et al. (Hrsg.), *Bildverarbeitung für die Medizin 2013*, Informatik aktuell, DOI: 10.1007/978-3-642-36480-8_30, © Springer-Verlag Berlin Heidelberg 2013

2.1   Evaluation data

The standard data available for research is the USC hand atlas that is composed of 1,097 images from different age classes, gender and ethnics [9]. In previous work an automatic approach for eROI extraction, presented by Fischer et al. [10], has been used. However, the automatic method can suffer from artefact, e.g. noise and misplacement, in the images. This leads to errors in feature extraction and affects the classication performance. To avoid those errors, here a semi-automatic approach for eROI extraction is used, where eROI location is performed manually. To be comparable to [4, 5], the USC data has been reprocessed. In total, 14 available epiphyseal regions are used dismissing the five regions close to the wrist. Fig. 2 shows the epiphysal centers and their corresponding region numbers. eROIs are extracted and normalized with respect to vertical alignment (rotation). Based on 512×512 pixel images, an eROI is of size 60×50. Hence, our experiments are based on 29,050 eROIs.

In [11], 15 images have been removed from USC data. This data is denoted USC-15.

2.2   SVM and SVR

Prototypes for each class are determined and the cross-correlation function (CCF) is used for feature extraction to represent similarities between the images [4, 5]. The resulting feature vectors include the gender of the patient and CCF values for each class and epiphyseal region. Data management is performed using the Image Retrieval in Medical Applications (IRMA) framework (http://irma-project.org).

To cope with the high number of classes, the one-against-one approach is used as multi-class extension for SVM. Contrarly, the SVR inherently handles

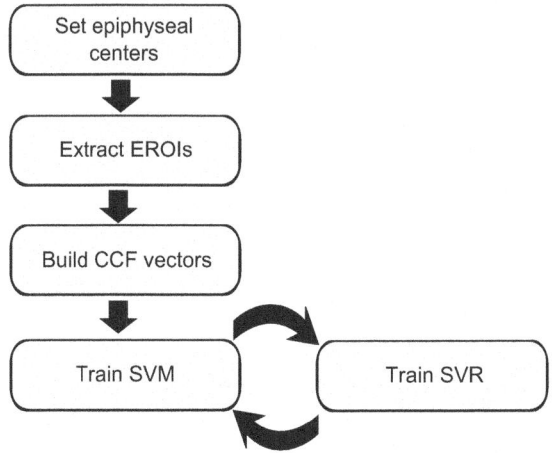

Fig. 1. Integration of SVR into the processing pipeline.

multi-class prediction. Given a training data set $\{(x_1, y_1), (x_2, y_2), ..., (x_n, y_n)\}$ of size n with corresponding target values, SVR tries to approximate a target function $f(x)$. This function has maximum deviation of ϵ from target values y_i in the training data. The parameter ϵ is critical and needs to be chosen carefully. A too high ϵ might result in an arbitrarily bad approximation of the target value function, where a too small ϵ leads to overfitting. Optimizing the approximation with respect to a ϵ-intensive loss function results in a hyperplane regression model. The ϵ-intensive loss function penalizes data points with higher deviation than ϵ.

Like in SVM, this hyperplane is only affected by the support vectors, which are those data points having a loss greater than 0 or lying directly on the ϵ-border. The main difference to SVM is that the resulting hyperplane function produces a continuous output, which can be interpreted as a soft class assignment. Unlike SVM, the regression function is already multi-class capable, since it approximates the target values, i.e. the class labels. For our method we use the SVR library coming with libSVM, which is also used by [4, 5]. Further, the ν-SVR method is used, since it indirectly controls ϵ via a parameter ν. This new parameter trades off ϵ against the model complexity and individual error tolerances of the training data, also known as slack variables [7]. Since the regression function is trained on the class labels, the output represents a class and needs to be discretized, which is done by a mapping to discrete values. In this first approach, the mapping is done by simple truncation of the SVR output.

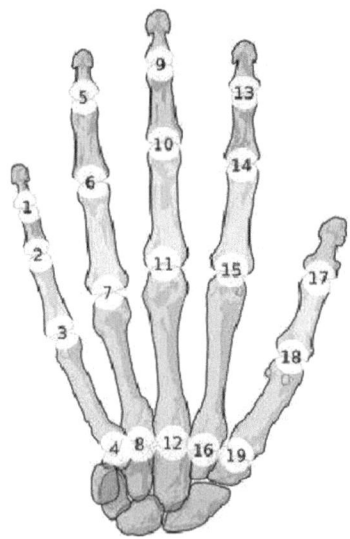

Fig. 2. EROIs and corresponding region numbers.

Table 1. SVM & SVR optimal parameters and regions.

Method	C	γ	ν	Regions
SVM	2048	0.0078125	0.5	2,6,11,13,15,18
SVR	128	0.003125	0.5	6,7,9,10,11,13,14,15,18

2.3 Evaluation

To produce comparable results SVM experiments done by [4, 5] were repeated with reprocessed USC images. SVM and SVR were evaluated using five-fold cross-validation. Class prototypes were chosen randomly from both datasets, but fixed for all experiments. Optimal parameters for SVM and SVR were determined using grid search and grid regression, respectively. The optimal subsets of regions for SVM and SVR were analyzed by calculating experiments on each possible subset of the 14 regions. The determined parameters and best regions for both methods are shown in Tab. 1.

For all experiments, the mean error (ME) was computed

$$\text{ME} = \frac{1}{n} \cdot \sum_{i=1}^{n} \left| r_{\text{est}}^i - r_{\text{rad}}^i \right| \tag{1}$$

where n denotes the size of the dataset, r_{est} and r_{rad} denote the estimated age and the radiologist reading respectively.

3 Results

The recomputation of the experiments done by [4, 5] with semi-automatic feature extraction can be found in Tab. 2, where the same data set and SVM parameters were used here. Although we used a different processing pipeline, resulting in different EROIs, the results are very similiar. So we can conclude that the semi-automatic approach shows the same performance as the automatic method. For all other experiments on the USC atlas, new optimal parameters and subsets were used, resulting in slightly deviating results.

Comparing SVR to SVM (Tab. 3) it turns out that the mean error decreases from 0.832 to 0.768 by 7% for the age range 0-18 years and drops even more significantly from 0.798 to 0.692 by 13% in the age range 2-17 years. Comparing with BoneXpert the RMS error decreases from 0.95 to 0.80 by 15%. The percentage of correctly classified hands is reduced from 35.42% to 32.52% (Tab. 4),

Age range (years)	USC atlas	USC atlas (new EROIs)
$0-18$	0.832	0.835
$2-17$	0.826	0.819

Table 2. Mean classification error in years, using the setup of [4, 5].

Table 3. Mean error and standard deviation in years. RMS denotes the root mean squared error.

Dataset	Age range (years)	SVM	SVR	BoneXpert [11]
USC	0 – 18	0.832 ± 0.775	0.768 ± 0.657	–
	2 – 17	0.798 ± 0.658	0.692 ± 0.572	–
USC-15	2 – 17	0.950 (RMS)	0.799 (RMS)	0.61 (RMS)

but the overall class distance is significantly lower. Most hands have a class distance of at most two, which indicates an error of approximately one year.

4   Discussion

USC data has been re-processed, resulting in new training data. The performance of SVM comparing the old and new USC dataset is stable and yields negligibly different results. So the semi-automatic and automatic approach show the same performance. A reason for this might be that the standard USC data set with carfeully selected images only sparsely contains radiographs with artefacts. Probably this image set is not optimal for showing improvement by manual eROI center location. Further experiments with additional BAA image sets including noisy images from daily routine can result in further knowledge. Anyway the SVM produces stable results and seems to be robust against small shifts in the data.

With SVR a novel method was introduced and evaluated on USC data. It turned out that this approach yields significantly better results than SVM, especially on the age range 2-17 years, but still does not yet reach the performance of BoneXpert. A smarter class mapping from SVR output could even further decrease the error rate. Another idea is the interpretation of BAA as natural regression problem, avoiding detour over (artificial) age classes. Here, the SVR can directly work on data with age readings as labels and can predict the age without classification.

The fixed random prototype selection also offers potential for improvement. Generation of prototypes by mean values or optimizied selection of prototype images can yield in better results.

Class distance	0	1	2	3	4	5	6	7	8	9	10	≥ 11
SVM hits(%)	35.42	42.33	14.35	5.18	1.27	0.54	0.54	0.18	0.00	0.00	0.00	0.18
	$\leftarrow 92.1 \rightarrow$						$\leftarrow 7.9 \rightarrow$					
SVR hits(%)	32.52	46.23	15.53	3.36	1.09	0.73	0.09	0.27	0.09	0.00	0.00	0.09
	$\leftarrow 94.28 \rightarrow$						$\leftarrow 5.72 \rightarrow$					

Table 4. Class distances of SVM & SVR in the range of $0 - 18$ years on the USC data.

Furthermore, the best region selection can be optimized. An option is training several SVM classifiers working on different region sets. Preprocessing of data can then be used to assign each image to the most applicable classifier. Anyway, comprehensive evaluation of hand radiograph data has shown that BAA prediction in computer-aided diagnostics (CAD) offers promising results for further investigations. In special, the suitability of this methods in practical routine should be evaluated.

References

1. Greulich WW, Pyle SI. Radiographic atlas of skeletal development of the hand and wrist. Am J Med Sci. 1959;238(3):393.
2. Tanner J, Healy M, Goldstein H, et al. Assessment of skeletal maturity and prediction of adult height (TW3). WB Saunders, London. 2001.
3. Martin M, Martin-Fernandez M, Alberola-Lopez C. Automatic Bone Age Assessment: A Registration Approach. Proc SPIE. 2003;5032:1765–76.
4. Harmsen M, Fischer B, Schramm H, et al. Support vector machine classification using correlation prototypes for bone age assessment. Proc BVM. 2012; p. 434–9.
5. Harmsen M, Fischer B, Schramm H, et al. Support vector machine classification based on correlation prototypes applied to bone age assessment. IEEE Trans Inf Technol Biomed. 2012;PP(99):1.
6. Basak D, Pal S, Patranabis DC. Support vector regression. Neural Inform Process Lett Rev. 2007;11(10):203–24.
7. Schölkopf B, Smola AJ, Williamson RC, et al. New support vector algorithms. Neural Comput. 2000;12(5):1207–45.
8. Schölkopf B, Burges CJC, Smola AJ. Advances in kernel methods: support vector learning. MIT Press; 1998.
9. Gertych A, Zhang A, Sayre J, et al. Bone age assessment of children using a digital hand atlas. Comput Med Imaging Graph. 2007;31(4-5):322.
10. Fischer B, Brosig A, Welter P, et al. Content-based image retrieval applied to bone age assessment. Proc SPIE. 2010;7624:762412.
11. Thodberg HH, Sävendahl L. Validation and reference values of automated bone age determination for four ethnicities. Acad Radiol. 2010;17(11):1425–32.

Using the Monogenic Signal for Cell-Background Classification in Bright-Field Microscope Images

Firas Mualla[1], Simon Schöll[1,2,3], Björn Sommerfeldt[4], Joachim Hornegger[1,3]

[1]Pattern Recognition Lab, Friedrich-Alexander University Erlangen-Nuremberg
[2]ASTRUM IT GmbH, Erlangen
[3]SAOT Graduate School in Advanced Optical Technologies
[4]Institute of Bioprocess Engineering, Friedrich-Alexander University
Erlangen-Nuremberg
firas.mualla@cs.fau.de

Abstract. Some cell detection approaches which deal with bright-field microscope images utilize defocussing to increase the image contrast. The latter is related to the physical light phase through the transport of intensity equation (TIE). Recently, it was shown that it is possible to approximate the solution of the TIE using a modified monogenic signal framework. We show empirically that using the local phase of the previous monogenic signal in place of the defocused image improves the cell-background classification rate. The evaluation was performed on L929 adherent cell line with more than 1000 manually labeled cells. The improvement was 6.8% using a random forest classifier and 10% using a support vector machine classifier with a radial basis function kernel.

1 Introduction

Detecting cells in microscope images is a crucial step in the cell image analysis. Several approaches in different image modalities tackle the problem as a classification problem. A fixed-size square patch is sampled at each pixel and used to train a cell-background classifier. The features can be either the patches themselves as in [1] or the patches after applying traditional feature extraction schemes as in [2, 3, 4].

It is known that bright-field microscopy delivers insufficient contrast at focus especially for the adherent cells [5, 6]. More contrast can be obtained by defocussing the microscope [5]. Moreover, in quantitative phase microscopy (QPM) approaches, the physical light phase can be reconstructed computationally from the amplitude information in order to get both more contrast and more object details.

A QPM approach in [7] suggests approximating the TIE (section 2.1) solution in the monogenic signal (section 2.2) domain. In fact, the obtained results approximate the local phase and the local energy of the physical light phase.

It is expected that the defocused image delivers higher discrimination between the background and the cells compared to the at-focus image. In this paper, we show that using the previously mentioned local phase instead of the

H.-P. Meinzer et al. (Hrsg.), *Bildverarbeitung für die Medizin 2013*, Informatik aktuell,
DOI: 10.1007/978-3-642-36480-8_31, © Springer-Verlag Berlin Heidelberg 2013

defocused image yields even higher discrimination power for the cell-background classification problem. Section 2.3 discusses the details of the used classifier models and features.

The experiments were performed on bright-field images of an unstained adherent L929 cell culture. Section 2.4 clarifies the acquisition and the labeling details. Section 3 shows the results of these experiments which are further discussed and summarized in section 4.

2   Materials and methods

2.1   Transport of intensity equation

As mentioned in the introduction, defocussing a bright-field microscope yields more contrast in the acquired images. In fact, there is a relation between this contrast and the physical phase of light. The transport of intensity equation TIE [8] models this relation

$$\frac{2\pi}{\lambda}\frac{\partial I}{\partial z} = -\nabla . I \nabla \phi \qquad (1)$$

Where λ is the wavelength of light, I is the intensity image at the defocus distance z, and ϕ is the physical phase of light.

2.2   Monogenic signal

The monogenic signal is a 2D generalization of the analytic signal [9]. Like its 1D counterpart, it is computed in practice by convolving the signal with a band-pass quadrature filter yielding the local phase and local energy of the input.

In [7], a link between the physical phase and the local phase was established using the monogenic signal. According to [7], it is possible to use the monogenic signal framework to approximate the solution of equation (1) under two conditions: First, the derivative image, i.e. the left side of equation (1), is used as an input instead of the image itself. Second, a low-pass filter is used in the monogenic signal framework instead of the band-pass filter.

2.3   Learning

We want to investigate the discriminative power of the local phase as defined in section 2.2 compared to the defocused images in the cell-background separation problem. Obviously, it is possible to measure the discriminative power difference by learning a classifier for each of them and then comparing the test errors.

As a classifier model, we use the support vector machine (SVM) and the random forest (RF). The kernel of the SVM was set to the radial basis function (RBF) kernel. The cost parameter and the RBF γ parameter were set to the default parameters in LibSVM. The trees number in the RF and the number of the randomly selected variables at each node were set following [10] to 500 and $N/5$, respectively. N is the feature number.

The feature vectors are 5×5 patches. Therefore, the number of features is 25. We did not conduct a thorough analysis of the effect of the patch size. However, cell areas in our data are considerably larger than the chosen patch area.

The data was z-scored for the SVM, while it was used without normalization for the RF.

Cutting patches at each pixel is computationally expensive. Therefore, only P patches are randomly sampled from each image. P was set to 100.

2.4   Materials

The evaluation was performed on L929 adherent cells. The images were acquired with an inverted Nikon Eclipse TE2000U microscope using Nikon USB camera. The used microscope objective has a numerical aperture of 0.45, a working distance of 7.4 mm, and 20x magnification. Image resolution is 1280×960 pixels with 0.49 μm/pixel.

The acquired data consists of five pairs of images. Each pair consists of an image at focus (Fig. 1(a)) and another positively defocused image (Fig. 1(b)) of the same scene at distance $+30$ μm. The total number of cells is 1078. All of them were labeled by two bioprocess engineering experts. This was done by manually delineating the borders of the cells in the defocused images.

The software SePhaCe [6] was used to generate the local phase (Fig. 1(c)) and the local energy (Fig. 1(d)) images for each image pair.

3   Results

One of the five at-focus images was used to train both the SVM and the RF, then the learned models were applied on the other at-focus images. This was repeated for each at-focus image and the mean test error was computed. The previous experiment was repeated 10 times with one mean test error obtained from each repetition. The mean and the standard deviation of all these mean test errors are shown in the first column of table 1.

The same was done on the positively defocused images and the results are shown in the second column of the table.

The third and the fourth columns show the results when the same process applied on the local phase and the local energy, respectively.

The results show that the defocused image contains more discriminative power than the at-focus image, while the local phase contains more discriminative power than the defocused image.

4   Conclusion and discussion

We have empirically showed that the pixel wise cell-background classification yields considerably better results when the local phase as obtained in [7] is used

Table 1. Comparing the discriminative power of the at-focus, the defocused, and the monogenic output using classification test errors.

	At-focus	Defocused	Phase	Energy
RBF SVM	39.9%±3.6%	32.8%±2.5%	22.8%±1.7%	33.6%±3.4%
RF	45.0%±3.3%	32.0%±2.6%	25.2%±1.1%	37.6%±2.4%

instead of the defocused image. Nevertheless, the defocused image still delivers better results compared to the at-focus image.

More than 1000 manually labeled adherent cells were used in the evaluation. This relatively large number of cells supports the soundness of the paper statement.

One might criticize the evaluation as being done using one defocus distance, i.e. the distance of 30 μm described in section 2.4. Actually, the very short distances do not deliver sufficient contrast. On the other hand, very long distances smash out the image information due to the excessive blurring by the point spread function of the optical system. Therefore, there is an optimal distance which maximizes the contrast. During the image acquisition, we tried to pick out this optimal distance experimentally. However, this was judged subjectively.

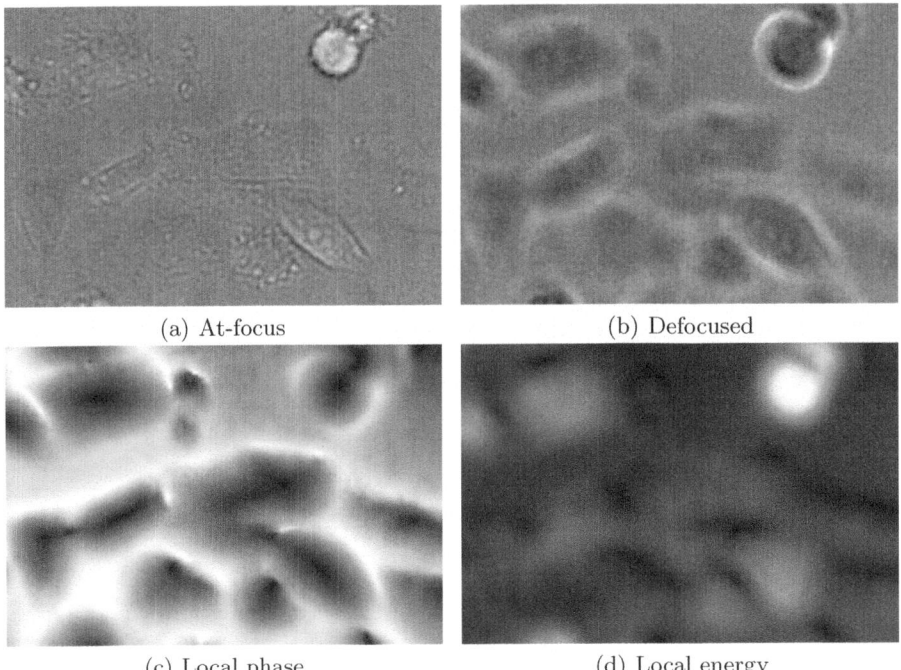

(a) At-focus (b) Defocused

(c) Local phase (d) Local energy

Fig. 1. Examples cut from evaluation images. The histograms of all four cuts were linearly stretched for the clarity.

We are currently developing methods to choose this distance objectively. In fact, other factors should be considered for the defocus distance selection because it is used to estimate a derivative image. Further research will tackle this issue.

Acknowledgement. The authors would like to thank the Bavarian Research Foundation BFS for funding the project COSIR under contract number AZ-917-10.

References

1. Jesper Sjöström P, Frydel BR, Wahlberg LU. Artificial neural network-aided image analysis system for cell counting. Cytometry. 1999;36(1):18–26.
2. Nattkemper TW, Ritter H, Schubert W. Extracting patterns of lymphocyte fluorescence from digital microscope images. Intell Data Anal Med Pharmacol. 1999;99:79–88.
3. Long X, Cleveland WL, Yao YL. A new preprocessing approach for cell recognition. IEEE Trans Inf Technol Biomed. 2005;9(3):407–12.
4. Long X, Cleveland WL, Yao YL. Automatic detection of unstained viable cells in bright field images using a support vector machine with an improved training procedure. Comput Biol Med. 2006;36(4):339–62.
5. Agero U, Monken CH, Ropert C, et al. Cell surface fluctuations studied with defocussing microscopy. Phys Rev E. 2003;67(5):051904.
6. Ali R, Gooding M, Szilágyi T, et al. Automatic segmentation of adherent biological cell boundaries and nuclei from bright-field microscopy images. Mach Vis Appl. 2012;23(4):607–621.
7. Ali R, Szilagyi T, Gooding M, et al. On the use of low-pass filters for image processing with inverse Laplacian models. J Math Imaging Vis. 2010; p. 1–10.
8. Teague MR. Deterministic phase retrieval: a Green's function solution. J Opt Soc Am. 1983;73(11):1434–41.
9. Felsberg M, Sommer G. The monogenic signal. IEEE Trans Signal Process. 2001;49(12):3136–44.
10. Khoshgoftaar TM, Golawala M, Van Hulse J. An empirical study of learning from imbalanced data using random forest. Proc IEEE Int Conf Tool Artif Intell. 2007; p. 310–7.

Bildgebende Charakterisierung und Quantifizierung der Vaskulogenese bei Arthritis

Svitlana Gayetskyy[1], Oleg Museyko[1], Andreas Hess[3], Georg Schett[2], Klaus Engelke[1]

[1]Institut für Medizinische Physik, FAU Erlangen-Nürnberg
[2]Innere Medizin 3, Universitätsklinikum Erlangen
[3]Lehrstuhl für Pharmakologie und Toxikologie, FAU Erlangen-Nürnberg
svitlana.gayetskyy@imp.uni-erlangen.de

Kurzfassung. Angiogenese ist ein wesentlicher pathophysiologischer Prozess bei chronischen Entzündungsreaktionen, insbesondere bei Arthritis, der das Fortschreiten und den Verlauf der Krankheit beeinflusst. Bei der Suche nach möglichen Arthritistherapien sind die therapeutischen Ansätze gegen Angiogenese von großem Interesse. Um die Änderungen der Knochendurchblutung bei Mäusen mit rheumatoider Arthritis (RA) zu quantifizieren, wurde ein mehrstufiges Segmentierungsverfahren entwickelt. Dabei wurden die Blutgefäße im Bereich des entzündetes Kniegelenks segmentiert und anschließend quantitative 3D histomorphometrische Parameter berechnet. Zwei Gruppen von Mäuse (RA und WT) wurden in-vitro untersucht und die Ergebnisse miteinander verglichen.

1 Einleitung

Arthritis ist eine entzündliche Gelenkerkrankung, die durch Vermehrung der Gelenkflüssigkeit charakterisiert werden kann und zum Gelenkknorpel- und Knochenabbau führt [1]. Angiogenese bezeichnet die Gefäßneubildung, die zusammen mit der Entzündung das Fortschreiten und den Verlauf der Krankheit beeinflusst. Angiogenese entsteht in der Gelenkflüssigkeit, um die wachsende Gelenkkapsel zu versorgen. Das Eindringen der Blutgefäße in den Knorpel wird durch die Abtragung der Knorpelmatrix begleitet. Angiogenese und Entzündung interagieren miteinander. Die Entzündungsfaktoren werden durch die neugebildeten Gefäße transportiert, um die Ausbreitung der Entzündung zu unterstützen. Bei der Suche nach möglichen Arthritistherapien sind die therapeutischen Ansätze gegen Angiogenese von großem Interesse. Aufgrund arthroskopischer Beobachtungen an menschlichen Gelenken und durch histologische Untersuchungen an Tiermodellen mit Arthritis ist eine erhöhte Vaskularisierung des Entzündungsgewebes bei Arthritis bekannt [2, 3].

Die Segmentierung der Gefäße im Kniegelenk ist schwierig, da die Absorptionswerte von Kontrastmittel und Knochens sich oft nicht unterscheiden. Die Verwendung eines einfachen Schwellwert-basierten Verfahren ist daher i.a. nicht möglich. Aus diesem Grund werden die Knochen häufig dekalzifiziert. Die Fähigkeit, Blutgefäße zu segmentieren, ohne die Gelenke vorher zu dekalzifizieren,

H.-P. Meinzer et al. (Hrsg.), *Bildverarbeitung für die Medizin 2013*, Informatik aktuell,
DOI: 10.1007/978-3-642-36480-8_32, © Springer-Verlag Berlin Heidelberg 2013

würde die Segmentierung und Analyse von Knochen und von Gefäßen in einem Datensatz ermöglichen.

2 Material und Methoden

Für die Untersuchung der Knochenvaskularisierung wurden 7 Mäuse mit rheumatoider Arthritis (RA) sowie 7 Wildtype-Mäuse (WT) verwendet. Für die Darstellung des Gefäßnetzes wurden beide Gruppen mit bleihaltigem Kontrastmittel Microfil MV-122 über die Aorta perfundiert und 24-Stunden im Kühlraum zwecks Aushärtens der Gefäße aufbewahrt. Anschließend wurden die Kniegelenke mit umgebendem Weichteilgewebe entnommen und mit hochauflösender 3D μCT (70 kV und 140 μA) untersucht. Die 3D-Volumina wurden mit einer isotropen Voxelgröße von 15 μm rekonstruiert. Die Segmentierung der Gefäße erfolgte in mehreren Schritten.

2.1 Initiale Segmentierung der Gefäße

Um eine Gefäßsegmentierung zu ermöglichen, sollten zunächst die einzelnen Knochen segmentiert werden. Die Segmentierung des Knochens wird allerdings durch die in der Nähe der periostealen Oberfläche verlaufenden größeren (0,6 mm) Gefäße (Abb. 1a) erschwert. Daher ist zunächst eine initiale Gefäßsegmentierung notwendig. Ein Histogramm wurde für das komplette Kniegelenk erstellt und daraus wurden zwei Schwellen abhängig von den maximalen Intensitätswert berechnet (Abb. 2a). Alle Voxel, deren Intensitätswerte sich innerhalb dieser zwei Schwellen befinden, wurden als „Gefäßvoxel"bezeichnet. Anschließend wurde ein Opening mit einer Kernelgröße von 5 und einem sphärischen Strukturelement durchgeführt. Die nahe am Knochen liegenden Gefäße konnten so separiert und aus der Region, die für die Segmentierung des Knochens benutzt wird, ausgeschlossen werden.

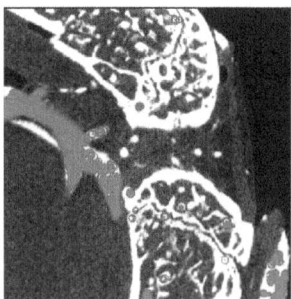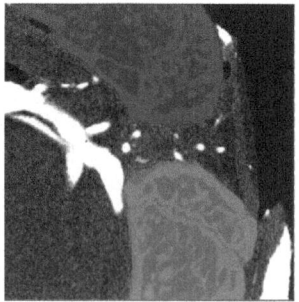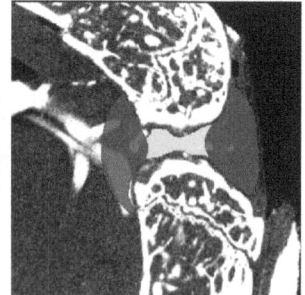

Abb. 1. Ergebnisse der ersten Segmentierungsschritte. Links: Initiale Gefäßsegmentierung (blau); mitte: Segmentierte Knochen (rot: Tibia, blau: Femur); rechts: VOIs (weiß: KGS, lila: KGS-VOI).

2.2 Segmentierung der Knochen

Die Knochensegmentierung erfolgt in zwei Schritten [4]: 1) Volume-Growing-Verfahren (Setzen des Saatpunktes durch Operator) und 2) kombinierte morphologische Operationen (Dilatation, Holefilling, Erosion). Bei Bedarf besteht die Möglichkeit, das Ergebnis (Abb. 1b) manuell zu korrigieren. Mit diesem Verfahren werden alle Knochen wie Tibia, Fibula, Femur, Patella usw. segmentiert.

2.3 Segmentierung des Weichteilgewebes

Bei der Perfusion des Kontrastmittels in die Aorta, fließt oft ein Teil des Kontrastmittels aus dem Herz heraus und gelangt an die Außenseite der Haut. Bei der Gefäßsegmentierung würden diese Bereiche aufgrund der gleichen Intensitätswerte ebenfalls als Gefäße identifiziert. Aus diesem Grund wird zuerst derjenige Bereich segmentiert, der Luft und Kontrastmittel an der Haut ausschließt. Hierzu wird die initiale Gefäßsegmentierung (Segmenterung des Kontrastmittels an der Haut und großer Gefäße) und ein Schwellwert für Weichteilgewebe (aus dem Histogramm in Abb. 2a) verwendet. Das globale Volume-Growing-Verfahren erfasst das zusammenhängende Volumen unter Ausschluss der initialen Gefäße. Anschließend werden durch das Ausschließen der großen Gefäße entstandenen Löcher, die innerhalb der VOIs liegen, gefüllt (Abb. 1c).

2.4 Segmentierung des Kniegelenkspaltes (KGS)

Zum Vergleich der Vaskularisierung in den beiden Gruppen wird ein Anatomie orientiertes Volume of Interest (VOI) benötigt, das in allen Mäusen möglichst gleich positioniert ist. Aus diesem Grund wurde der Kniegelenkspalt (KGS) segmentiert. Zur Segmentierung des KGS wurde auf das Segmentierungsergebnis der Tibia und des Femurs ein Closing mit einem großen Kernel angewendet. Hiervon wurde die initiale Segmentierung substrahiert und mit einem Volume-Growing nach der größten zusammenhängenden Region gesucht. Im Schwerpunkt des

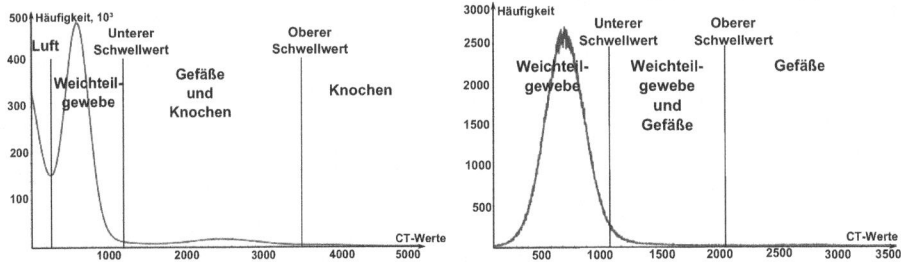

Abb. 2. Histogramme in unterschiedlichen VOIs, die für die Schwellwertberechnungen verwendet wurden. Links: komplettes Kniegelenk mit 3 Peaks (Luft, Weichteilgewebe und Knochen bzw. Gefäße); rechts: KGS-VOI mit einem Peak für Weichteilgewebe und Gefäße ohne einen klaren Peak.

KGS wurde eine Kugel von der Größe der maximalen Ausdehnung des KGS erzeugt und als VOI verwendet (Abb. 1c).

2.5 Segmentierung der Gefäße

Für die Segmentierung der Gefäße wurde ein lokal adaptives Verfahren mit Homogenitätskriterium verwendet. Aus dem Histogramm der KGS-VOI (Abb. 2b) wurden mit (1) zwei Schwellen berechnet

$$T_{\text{low}} = \text{HistoPeak} + 2 \cdot \sigma$$
$$T_{\text{high}} = 0,65 \cdot \text{HistoMax}$$

(1)

Die Klassifikation des Voxels erfolgte in zwei Stufen. Zuerst wurde sein Intensitätswert mit den Schwellen aus (2) verglichen.

$$f(I_{xyz}) = \begin{cases} \text{if } I_{xyz} < T_{\text{low}}, & \text{Softtissue} \\ \text{if } I_{xyz} \geq T_{\text{high}}, & \text{Vessel} \\ \text{sonst}, & \text{local adaptive segmentation} \end{cases}$$

(2)

Falls eine Entscheidung nicht möglich war (Intensitätswert des Voxels befindet sich im Bereich zwischen den beiden Schwellen), wurde ein lokal adaptives Verfahren verwendet. Für die Klassifikation jedes Voxels wurden Mittelwert μ und Variationskoeffizient σ der Intensitätswerte in der 26-Nachbarschaft der zu untersuchenden Voxel ermittelt. τ ist ein vom Rauschen abhängiger Parameter und wird als $\tau = \frac{\sigma}{\text{HistoPeak}}$ berechnet. Die Einteilung wurde dann mittels (3) getroffen.

$$f(\mu_{xyz}, \sigma_{xyz}) = \begin{cases} \text{if } \frac{\sigma}{\mu} < \tau, & \text{Vessel} \\ \text{sonst}, & \text{Softtissue} \end{cases}$$

(3)

Das Ergebnis der Segmentierung der Gefäße innerhalb der großen VOI ist in Abb. 3a dargestellt und innerhalb der KGS-VOI in Abb. 3b.

2.6 Berechnung der quantitativen Parameter

Zur Quantifizierung der Knochenvaskularisierung wurden mehrere histomorphologische Parameter verwendet: relatives Gefäßvolumen (VV/TV), Gefäßdicke ($V.Th$), Gefäßanzal pro mm ($V.N$) und Gefäßabstand ($V.Sp$) [4]. Die Gefäßoberfläche ($V.S$) wurde mittels Marching-Cubes-Verfahren berechnet. Außerdem wurde die Anzahl der zusammenhängenden Gefäßbaumstücke ($V.N^*/TV$) durch das Volume-Growing-Verfahren bestimmt. Zur Untersuchung der Homogenität der Gefäßverteilung im Bereich des GS wurden drei VOIs (VOI_1, VOI_2 und VOI_3) unterschiedlicher Größe verwendet (Abb. 4).

3   Ergebnisse

In der RA-Gruppe war TV (Kugelvolumen minus Volumen des Knochens innerhalb der Kugel) aufgrund der Knochenerosion in allen drei VOIs signifikant erhöht (Tab. 1). Bei RA-Mäusen waren das relative Gefäßvolumen (VV/TV) und Gefäßdicke ($V.Th$) niedriger aber nicht immer signifikant (z.B. für VV/TV in VOI_2 $3, 7 \pm 1, 5$ für RA-Gruppe und $7, 2 \pm 4, 3$ für WT-Gruppe). Weiterhin waren in der RA-Gruppe unabhängig von der Kugelgröße $V.Sp$ signifikant niedriger und $V.N$ signifikant höher als in der WT-Gruppe. Ein weiterer signifikanter Parameter war die erhöhte Anzahl der zusammenhängenden Gefäßsegmente pro mm^3 in der RA-Gruppe.

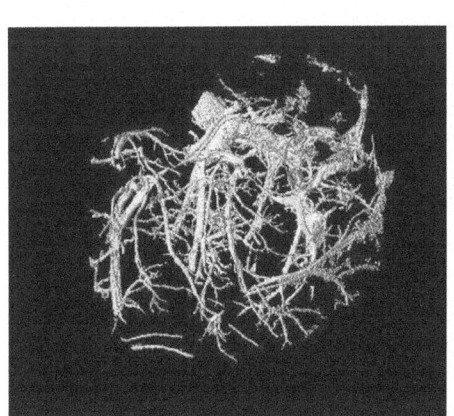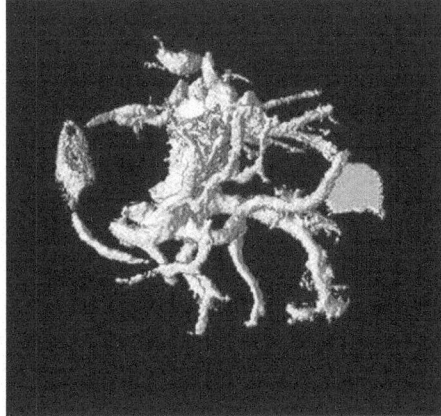

Abb. 3. 3D Volume Rendering der segmentierten Gefäßen. Links: große VOI, KGS-VOI als Kreis dargestellt; rechts: KGS-VOI.

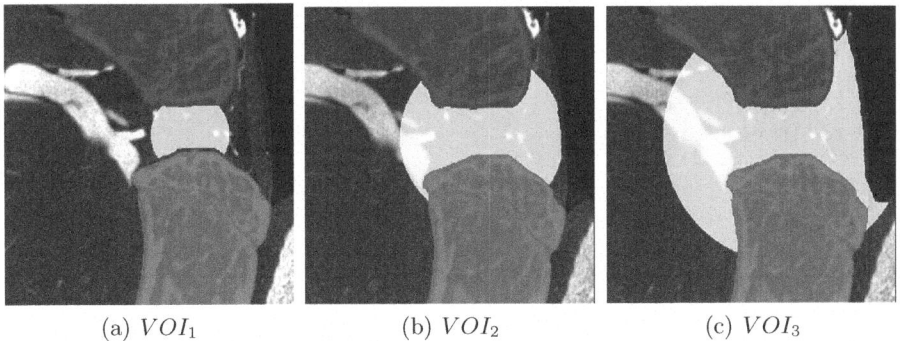

(a) VOI_1 (b) VOI_2 (c) VOI_3

Abb. 4. Unterschiedliche VOIs bei der Variation der Kugelgröße.

Tabelle 1. Vergleich der berechneten Parameter in den beiden Gruppen: Totales Volumen (TV), Relatives Gefäßvolumen (VV/TV), Gefäßdicke ($V.Th$), Gefäßabstand ($V.Sp$), Gefäßanzahl pro mm ($V.N$) sowie Anzahl der zusammenhängenden Gefäßbaumstücke ($V.N^*/TV$) für drei Kugel-VOIs (VOI_1, VOI_2, VOI_3). † : $p < 0,001$; ⋆ : $0,001 \leq p < 0,01$; * : $0,01 \leq p < 0,05$.

	VOI_1		VOI_2		VOI_3	
	RA	WT	RA	WT	RA	WT
$TV\,[\mathrm{mm^3}]$	$1,2 \pm 0,4^\star$	$0,7 \pm 0,2$	$8,8 \pm 3,4^\star$	$5,1 \pm 2,3$	$33 \pm 11,4^\star$	22 ± 8
$VV/TV\,[\%]$	$2,1 \pm 1,5$	$3,7 \pm 4,4$	$3,7 \pm 1,5^*$	$7,2 \pm 4,3$	$3,2 \pm 1,2$	$3,6 \pm 2$
$V.Th\,[\mu m]$	$4,3 \pm 1,2^*$	$7,6 \pm 4,3$	16 ± 11	$20 \pm 8,5$	$18,8 \pm 8,8$	$23,4 \pm 3,3$
$V.Sp\,[\mathrm{mm}]$	$0,4 \pm 0,1^*$	$0,6 \pm 0,2$	$0,6 \pm 0,1^*$	$0,8 \pm 0,2$	$0,9 \pm 0,15^*$	$1,1 \pm 0,2$
$V.N\,[\frac{1}{\mathrm{mm}}]$	$2,4 \pm 0,5^\star$	$1,8 \pm 0,7$	$1,6 \pm 0,2^*$	$1,4 \pm 0,3$	$1,1 \pm 0,2^*$	$1,0 \pm 0,2$
$V.N^*\,[\frac{1}{\mathrm{mm}}]$	$298 \pm 225^*$	104 ± 190	$26 \pm 10^\dagger$	$13 \pm 5,4$	$7 \pm 2,5^\dagger$	3 ± 1

4 Diskussion

Aus histologischen Untersuchungen ist bei RA die durch Stenosen erhöhte Fehlfunktion von Blutgefäßen bekannt [2]. Aufgrund begrenzten μCT-Auflösung stellt sich eine Gefäßverengung wegen der damit verbundenen Partialvolumenartefakte im rekonstruierten Volumen oft als Gefäßunterbrechungen dar. Dies kann die erhöhte Anzahl der Gefäßsegmente pro Volumen in der RA Gruppe erklären. Aus unseren Ergebnissen könnte auch gefolgert werden, dass in der RA-Gruppe der Gefäßabstand geringer ist und es mehr Gefäße pro Volumeneinheit geben könnte. Außerdem ist die Größe des KGS bei den RA-Mäusen signifikant erhöht, was bereits ein klares Zeichen für ein fortgeschrittenes Krankeitsstadium wäre. Der nächste Schritt ist die Untersuchung von Mäusen, bei denen der Fortschritt der Krankheit noch nicht das Stadium der Schwellung und erhöhten Knochenerosion erreicht hat. Außerdem fehlt noch die Information über den Aufbau des Gefäßbaums und ob die Änderungen in ihm auch als Parameter bei der Krankheitsdiagnostik verwendbar sind.

Literaturverzeichnis

1. Kennedy A, Ng CT, Biniecka M, et al. Angiogenesis and blood vessel stability in inflammatory arthritis. Arthritis & Rheumatism. 2010;62(3):717–21.
2. Raatz Y, Ibrahim S, Feldmann M, et al. Gene expression profiling and functional analysis of angiogenic markers in murine collagen-induced arthritis. Arthritis & Reasearch Therapy. 2012;14(4):R169.
3. Zhao Q, Shen X, Zhang W, et al. Mice with increased angiogenesis and osteogenesis due tu conditional activation of HIF pathway in osteoblasts are protected from ovariectomy induced bone loss. Bone. 2012;50(3):763–70.
4. Lu J. Advanced methods for the quantification of trabecular bone structure and density in micro computed tomography images. PhD Thesis, Friedrich-Alexander-University of Erlangen; 2010.

Towards Fully Automated Tracking of Carotid and Vertebral Arteries in CT Angiography

Igor Pener, Michael Schmidt, Horst Karl Hahn

Fraunhofer Institute for Medical Image Computing MEVIS, Bremen, Germany
igor.pener@mevis.fraunhofer.de

Abstract. This paper presents an approach towards fully automated vessel tracking and segmentation in computed tomographic (CT) images. The proposed algorithm operates in 3D and is fast enough for interactive usage once preprocessing has been done. This approach focuses on vessel segmentation in the neck region, particularly the carotid arteries. Especially, potential apoplectic stroke patients can benefit from this approach due to the automatic visualization of the carotid arteries.

1 Introduction

Vessel segmentation in CT angiography (CTA) images has been addressed by several authors and a review of existing methods was published by Lesage et al. [1]. Artery tracking in CTA of the head and neck region has been acknowledged as a particularly difficult problem due to the frequent bone-vessel contacts and possibly due to the presence of plaques [2]. At the same time, the unhindered 3D visualization of carotid and vertebral arteries is of major importance for diagnosis and decision support for stroke patients. Not only can patients benefit from a specific therapy, but also can the chance of a stroke be assessed from preventive explorations.

Currently, software solutions exist which require the user to interactively construct vessel trees by setting seed points inside a 3D image. These semi-automatic approaches are comparatively stable, but require training from the user in order to efficiently and correctly segment the vessel structure. Alternatively, various algorithms were developed in order to be able to extract the centerlines [3] with the perspective to dilate them in the next step [4]. Furthermore, existing software based on tracking multiple hypothetical vessel trajectories in combination with Dijkstra's algorithm are already able to produce very accurate centerlines [5]. However, problems occur at regions where the vessel winds around bone structures or calcification heavily blocks the vessel. This specifically applies to the carotid and the vertebral arteries.

The initial motivation of this project was to develop a fully automated algorithm to accurately segment the carotid arteries. In this paper, all preprocessing steps, the core algorithm, and its validation will be described.

H.-P. Meinzer et al. (Hrsg.), *Bildverarbeitung für die Medizin 2013*, Informatik aktuell,
DOI: 10.1007/978-3-642-36480-8_33, © Springer-Verlag Berlin Heidelberg 2013

2   Materials and methods

This section presents the underlying segmentation and 3D tracking algorithm which we refer to as the *Sphere-Shift* algorithm. Furthermore, we want to introduce and explain all significant preprocessing steps and the seed point generation.

2.1   Preprocessing

Prior to generating the marker seed points, fast morphological and filter operations were utilized. In particular, noise was reduced by an opening and homogeneity was increased by self-dual reconstruction [6] with a white marker with black borders. The kernel size of the structuring element used for the opening can be modified appropriately depending on the degree of noise in the image. In order to reduce the number of segmented objects used for the seed point generation, the image is modified according to Equation (1) prior to applying the self-dual reconstruction, where t_l and t_u are the lower and upper threshold respectively (in this case $t_l = 100$ GV and $t_u = 700$ GV, where GV is the unit for gray scale intensity)

$$f(x; t_l, t_u) = \begin{cases} x & x \in [t_l, t_u] \\ 0 & \text{otherwise} \end{cases} \tag{1}$$

After reconstruction, a binary threshold $t = 1$ GV was applied, i.e. all positive values are kept. As a last preprocessing step, an image labeling algorithm [6] was applied in order to assign unique values to the individual connected components in each slice.

2.2   Seed point generation

We propose a method to identify points with a high chance to lie inside a vessel using the object based image analysis framework (OBIA) by Homeyer et al. [7]. The classification process is based on four object properties and works on each 2D slice individually. At first, all objects which have a bounding box greater than 50×50 pixel are dismissed. Secondly, rather homogeneous objects are selected, i.e. whose median value lies between $100 - 400$ GV. The next selection is based on the object size, which has to lie between $55 - 350$ pixels. In the further step, only objects with a circularity between values $0.98 - 1.02$ are kept. In parallel, a selection of objects with size between $95 - 250$ pixels and a circularity between $0.99 - 1.01$ is assumed to be the *true* vessels. From all previously found objects only those are kept whose median value lies with some threshold around the average median value of the true vessel objects. Lastly, a further selection of objects with a standard deviation of less than 100 GV is kept as the resulting seed points. After the seed point generation, a list of positions as well as the radii of the seed points was passed on to the final tracking step. An illustration of detailed object selections is shown in Fig. 1.

2.3   3D vessel tracking

The main concept of the algorithm was to create a virtual sphere which can recursively update its position and diameter. It consists of two shells (inner and outer) and a core where the two shells are each one voxel thick and the core diameter is not smaller than five voxels. Having two shells allows the sphere to either shrink or grow. In particular, the sphere grows when the mean value of all voxels inside the outer shell is within some threshold with respect to the mean inside the core. Similarly, it must shrink when the mean value inside the inner shell is outside some threshold with respect to the core's mean. By default, the sphere is constructed such that only the core and the inner shell lie completely inside the vessel. The core itself is used for position and direction determination in each step. Starting with a precomputed or default direction, weighted mean values for all voxels lying inside the core, the inner, and the outer shell are computed according to Eq. (2), respectively, where f is the input image, μ is the previously computed mean for the core voxels, and n is some weighting constant (in our case $n = 20$)

$$v = \exp\left(-\left(\frac{f(v) - \mu}{n}\right)^2\right) \tag{2}$$

Furthermore, the center of mass is determined for all voxels inside the core in a similar procedure as above. Consequently, voxels outside this range are disregarded and the computed center of mass forms the center of a second sphere, which we call the prototype sphere for simplicity. This process is recursively executed until the center of mass is stable. Since the center of mass is rounded to integers, the recursive process will terminate. Once the prototype sphere is

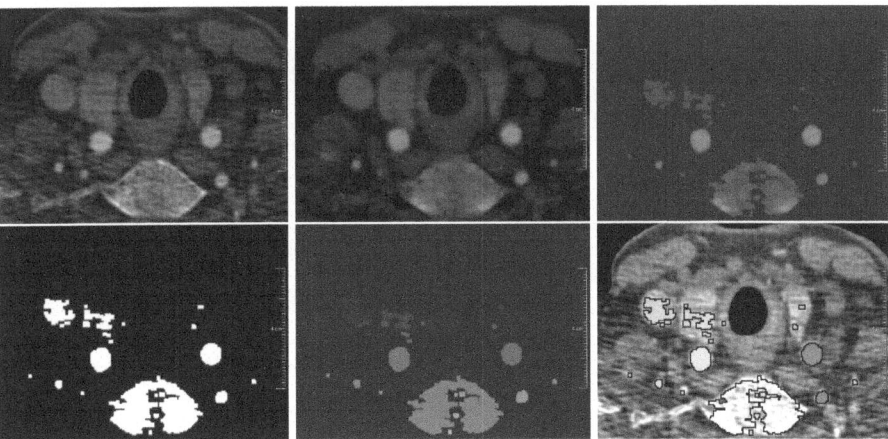

Fig. 1. OBIA selection process for the seed point search. The first row shows the original image (left), the result after an opening (middle), and the output image after reconstruction (right). The lower row illustrates the image after thresholding (left), labeling (middle), and finally after the classification in OBIA (right).

stabilized, its radius is adapted using the mean value information inside the inner and outer shell (Fig. 2). Here, we formed the constraint that the radius always either changes by ±1 voxel or stays constant. This assumption is based on the fact that vessels are rather smooth and cannot change their diameter abruptly. At the end of every iteration step, the prototype sphere becomes fixed and the voxels it contains as well as the center position are added to a set respectively.

Continuing this concept for each seed point, the algorithm places two spheres with opposite directions at the center of the seed point. By restricting the direction change, it is assured that no prototype sphere can change its direction abruptly and as such models the flow of a vessel. The simplest method is to restrict the angle $\phi = \arccos(\frac{v_0 \cdot v_1}{|v_0||v_1|})$ to some legitimate value, e.g. 45° or 90°. Besides the exceedance of this limit, further terminating conditions are collisions of two or more moving spheres, image border hits, as well as a sphere diameter value smaller than five voxels.

3 Results

In the following section, the evaluation of the general algorithmic complexity and its performance on the carotid and vertebral artery segmentation will be addressed. In order to validate the performance, the ratio between the output mask of the program and the manually drawn centerlines was computed. The Sphere-Shift algorithm has a time complexity of $O(n \log n)$ for each sphere, where n is the number of traversed voxels. The spacial complexity is $O(n)$ since the container to store all traversed voxels is a set from the Standard Template

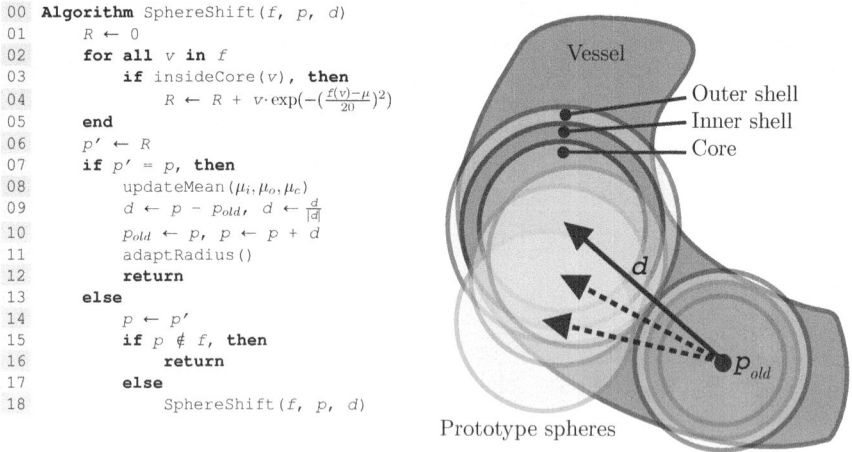

```
00  Algorithm SphereShift(f, p, d)
01      R ← 0
02      for all v in f
03          if insideCore(v), then
04              R ← R + v·exp(-(f(v)-μ/20)²)
05      end
06      p' ← R
07      if p' = p, then
08          updateMean(μi, μo, μc)
09          d ← p - pold, d ← d/|d|
10          pold ← p, p ← p + d
11          adaptRadius()
12          return
13      else
14          p ← p'
15          if p ∉ f, then
16              return
17          else
18              SphereShift(f, p, d)
```

Fig. 2. Pseudocode of the algorithm, where f is the input image, p is the position and d the direction vector, R is the center of mass, and μ_x is the mean for the inner and outer shell, and the core (left). Sphere stabilization after three iterations (right).

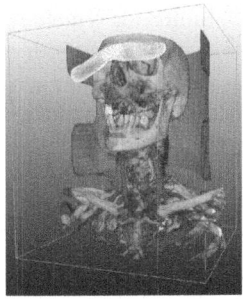 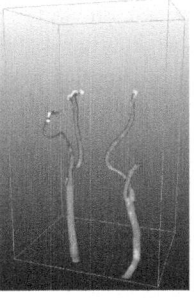 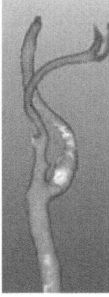

Fig. 3. Original image (left), the obtained segmentation of the carotid arteries (middle), and a close-up on the obtained result (right).

Table 1. Average processing time (left). Segmentation validation based on the type I error ε_α and type II error ε_β where subscript c refers to carotid and v to vertebral artery (right). The values are given as relative errors from 0 to 1.

Operation	Time (sec)
Opening	$\approx 120 - 140$
Self-dual reconstruction	$\approx 30 - 50$
Labeling image regions	$\approx 10 - 30$
Seedpoint generation	$\approx 60 - 110$
Gauss smoothing	$\approx 20 - 30$
Sphere-Shift	$\approx 5 - 10$

N$^{\underline{o}}$	$\varepsilon_{\alpha,c}$	$\varepsilon_{\beta,c}$	$\varepsilon_{\alpha,v}$	$\varepsilon_{\beta,v}$
1	0.158	0.124	0.813	0.000
2	0.219	0.023	0.922	0.212
3	0.232	0.026	1.000	0.000
4	0.331	0.149	0.591	0.052
5	0.326	0.537	0.610	0.322
6	0.127	0.105	0.390	0.351
7	0.368	0.073	0.919	0.147

Library (STL). On average, for an image containing 20 mio. voxels it requires between $300 - 600$ milliseconds per sphere. Considering an average amount of 50 spheres per image, the algorithm runs between 15 and 30 seconds in the worst case (assuming that every sphere traverses the whole image). However, in practice the computation time is generally around 5 seconds. Despite these fast executions, the preprocessing takes between 4 and 6 minutes in the most accurate settings. Table 1 illustrates the time spent in the different processing steps as well as the type I (false negatives) and type II (false positives) error for seven unknown data sets. The exact validation formulae for the type I error ε_α and type II error ε_β are listed in Eq. 3, where c is the true centerline, M is the segmented vessel mask, and c_M is the mask's centerline

$$\varepsilon_\alpha = 1 - \frac{|c \cap M|}{|c|}, \qquad \varepsilon_\beta = 1 - \frac{|c \cap M|}{|c_M|} \qquad (3)$$

Fig. 3 illustrates a fully automatic segmentation of the left and right carotid.

4 Discussion and conclusion

To our best knowledge, we are the first to address a fully automated segmentation method dedicated to the carotid and vertebral arteries in routine clinical CTA data. The current implementation was based on naive 3D buffering which is comparatively slow for images of a size between 20 and 200 mio. voxels. In order to reduce the computation time, the sphere's direction vector can be scaled such that each sphere performs a larger step in every iteration. Additionally, a better seed point generation by considering the neighbor relations using OBIA could be a significant, additional improvement. It would detect and remove potential outliers and hence reduce the number of falsely placed spheres. Consequently, ε_β and ε_α would both decrease. Lastly, the algorithm needs to be trained on more data sets to find a heuristic which reduces the break-out into regions outside the vessel. In particular vertebral arteries, once having a small diameter, are prone to such breaks, since the ratio between the shell mean and the core mean is no longer robust.

Despite its simplicity, the results are promising and encourage a further refinement of our approach and evaluation on an extended set of test data. The algorithm is an alternative to the current preprocessing strategies as it automatically segments a significant part of the desired arteries. Furthermore, it is fast enough for interactive usage and can be even used to remove falsely segmented regions in future work. Lastly, it can be used as a preprocessing step for more accurate semi-automatic segmentation tools.

References

1. Lesage D, Angelini ED, Bloch I, et al. A review of 3D vessel lumen segmentation techniques: models, features and extraction schemes. Med Image Anal. 2009;13(6):819–45.
2. Schaap M, Manniesing R, Smal I, et al. Bayesian tracking of tubular structures and its application to carotid arteries in CTA. Med Image Comput Comput Assist Interv. 2007;10(2):562–70.
3. Mohan V, Sundaramoorthi G, Stillman A, et al. Vessel segmentation with automatic centerline extraction using tubular tree segmentation. Proc MICCAI Workshop CI2BM. 2009.
4. Kirbas C, Quek F. A review of vessel extraction techniques and algorithms. ACM Comput Surv. 2004;36(2):81–121.
5. Friman O, Kühnel C, Hindennach M, et al. Multiple hypothesis template tracking of small 3D vessel structures. Med Image Anal. 2010;14(2):160–71.
6. Soille P. Morphological Image Analysis. Principles and Applications. Berlin Heidelberg: Springer; 2004.
7. Homeyer A, Schwier M, Hahn HK. A generic concept for object-based image analysis. Proc VISAPP. 2010;2:530–3.

Qualitative Evaluation of Feature Lines on Anatomical Surfaces

Kai Lawonn, Rocco Gasteiger, Bernhard Preim

Otto-von-Guericke University Magdeburg
lawonn@isg.cs.uni-magdeburg.de

Abstract. This paper deals with the application of feature lines on patient-specific anatomical surfaces used for treatment planning. We introduce the most commonly used feature line methods and evaluate them qualitatively. The evaluation is conducted by physicians and medical researchers to assess shape interpretation and visual impression of these methods compared to surface shading. We utilize several anatomical models, which were derived from clinical image data. Furthermore, we identify the limitations of this kind of illustrative visualization and discuss requirements for their application.

1 Introduction

In medicine, illustrations are primarily known from anatomical atlases where they are used for illustrating anatomical structures and treatment procedures. Only essential information of the object are depicted and unnecessary information are omitted to avoid visual clutter. Moreover, illustrative visualization has a high potential in medical applications such as surgery planning [1] and intraoperative visualizations [2]. They are useful to present integrated or contextual information, e.g., from pre- and intraoperative image data or multimodal diagnostic data. In this paper, we focus on illustrative surface visualizations of anatomical structures rather than on illustrative volume visualizations. The surfaces are derived from clinical image data and binary segmentation masks. In general, surface data are visualized with common surface shading. For integrated visualizations, however, this can cause occlusions or increased visual complexity. Sparse representations like feature lines depict only certain surface features like concave and convex regions. Studies have shown that existing feature line techniques are highly valued as scientific illustrations based on artificial surface data [3]. Inspired by these techniques illustrative visualization methods like point and line renderings have been adapted for medical applications [4]. Tietjen et al. [1] employ silhouettes and feature lines to depict anatomical context structures and object boundaries in surgery and therapy planning visualizations. Another example of line rendering is hatching, which is used by Ritter et al. [2] for vascular structures to emphasize shape and thus to support depth perception. Among these techniques we focus on feature lines and their application and

H.-P. Meinzer et al. (Hrsg.), *Bildverarbeitung für die Medizin 2013*, Informatik aktuell,
DOI: 10.1007/978-3-642-36480-8_34, © Springer-Verlag Berlin Heidelberg 2013

usability on patient-specific surfaces which are not well investigated. For artificial surfaces several studies have shown that current approaches can effectively depict shape and even match the effectiveness of hand drawings [3].

Existing feature line techniques can be categorized in image-based and object-based approaches. Image-based techniques operate entirely on RGB or gray value input images of the scene and extract feature lines with convolution kernels [5]. However, the resulting lines are represented as pixel with limited control over the final rendering style, e.g., line thickness and dotted lines. Object-based methods use the surface model as input. Furthermore, additional information like camera and light position as well as curvature information are used to detect features.

The extracted lines are represented as explicit 3D lines and arbitrary rendering styles can be applied. Our evaluation is based on four object-based methods for the automatic generation of feature lines: ridges and valleys [6], suggestive contours [7], apparent ridges [8], and photic extremum lines [9]. We give an overview about the underlying approach in Section 2.

The contribution of this paper is to investigate the application of modern and powerful feature line methods on patient-specific anatomical surfaces. In contrast to artificial data sets, on which these methods are currently applied, the anatomical surfaces exhibit surface noise and artifacts (e.g., staircases). We want to evaluate the application and usability of these feature lines techniques in terms of shape depiction and visual impression. In particular, we perform a qualitative evaluation conducted by two physicians and one medical researcher to assess how much the medical experts can derive advantages from feature line drawings compared to surface shading.

2   Materials and method

In this section we briefly explain the four feature line methods, we want to evaluate.

2.1   Ridges and valleys

Ridges and valleys (RV) [6] are defined as the loci of points at which the principle curvatures assumes an extremum in the principle direction

$$D_{e_1} k_1 = 0,$$

where k_1 is the principle curvature and e_1 is the associated principle curvature direction. Additionally, we have: $D_{e_1} D_{e_1} k_1 < 0$, for ridges and $D_{e_1} D_{e_1} k_1 > 0$, for valleys. Here $D_{e_1} k_1$ means the derivative of k_1 in the direction of e_1. Furthermore, ridge and valley lines are drawn if the magnitude of the maximum principal curvature exceeds a user-defined threshold. As ridges and valleys are view-independent they can not capture salient features in smooth regions and require additionally object contours.

2.2 Suggestive contours

Suggestive contours (SC) [7] are view-dependent and of second order. These lines are defined as the set of minima of $n \cdot v$ in the direction of w, where n is the unit surface normal, v is the view vector, and w is the projection of the view vector on the tangent plane. Precisely

$$D_w(n \cdot v) = 0, \text{ and } D_w D_w(n \cdot v) > 0$$

Furthermore, lines are drawn if the derivative magnitude is larger than a user-defined threshold. However, objects without concave regions have no suggestive contours.

2.3 Apparent ridges

Apparent ridges (AR) [8] extend the definition of ridges by using the maximum view-dependent curvature q_1 and its corresponding view-dependent principle curvature direction t_1. Formally, these lines are defined as a set of points satisfying $D_{t_1} q_1 = 0$. The maximum is identified with the orientation of the view-dependent principle curvature directions. To reduce lines they used a threshold based on q. Since q depends on the projection to the view screen it follows that features turned away from the viewer have a much higher curvature than feature regions facing the viewer.

2.4 Photic extremum lines

A photic extremum line (PEL) [9] is of third order and view- as well as light-dependent. These feature lines are defined as the set of points where the variation of illumination in its gradient direction is a local maximum

$$D_w \|\nabla f\| = 0, \text{ and } D_w D_w \|\nabla f\| < 0$$

with $f = n \cdot v$ as the headlight illumination function and $w = \frac{\nabla f}{\|\nabla f\|}$ as the unit gradient of f. Additionally, the light-dependency can be used to improve the line drawing result. They check if $\int \|f\| ds$ exceeds a user-defined threshold to filter out noisy lines.

2.5 Evaluation

We performed a qualitative evaluation of the four feature line techniques to assess their capabilities in capturing important surface features compared with surface shading. The evaluation is conducted with two physicians and one medical researcher who are familiar with medical visualizations. Three representative surface models are chosen: a cerebral aneurysm, a trachea seen from an endoscopic view, and a liver. All surface models are derived from clinical image data and binary segmentation masks. Thus, they exhibit surface noise and other artifacts like staircases. Since all four feature line methods are based on higher order derivatives, they are sensitive to noise and the underlying tessellation. To ensure a reliable comparison between the different methods and to reduce these artifacts, we smooth each surface model with a low pass filter according to the recommendations in Bade et al. [10]. Furthermore, we ensure an equal and appropriate degree of tessellation among the surface models. Finally, we employed the original feature line implementations provided by the corresponding authors.

The evaluation itself was conducted in two parts. In the first part, each participant was shown the shaded surface models, which could be explored interactively to gain an impression of important surface features. For each surface model one out of four feature line methods was overlayed successively. For each method, the participants were asked to adjust the corresponding threshold (recall Sec. 2) until the resulting feature lines capture as much as possible surface features compared to the shaded representation. Thereby, a tradeoff between inherent feature lines and false-positive feature lines resulting from surface artifacts should be considered. During the evaluation the participants were also able to hide the shaded surface model. At the end of each adjustment the final threshold was recorded. The second part consists of a visual comparison and a qualitative assessment between the feature line methods. Based on the recorded threshold the participants should assess which method is more appropriate to capture surface features and which limitations they observed.

3   Result

In Figure 1 the three shaded surface models are shown. For each model the underlying rows represent the feature line representation with one of the four techniques. Thereby, the result of the best-choice for the given technique is rated by the participants. For the aneurysm model, participant #1 (P#1) observed that the generated lines by RV and SC are not sufficient to gain a 3d impression. For AR and PEL the resulting lines are reasonable but some lines are distracting. Finally, P#1 preferred the PEL method. P#2 and P#3 rated the result of the SC method as their favored technique. For RV, AR, and PEL P#2 stated that most of the generated lines are not meaningful or distracting but depicts parts of the bifurcation well. Additionally, P#3 mentioned that AR produces lines on small vessel parts which lead to the impression that the vessel is very wrinkly.

The inner view of the trachea has two main features: the elongated structure and the bifurcation. P#1 stated that RV gives no satisfactory impression on the 3d structure. Apart from that, SC, AR, and PEL depict the elongated structures but fail to enhance the bifurcation. Although, PEL produces more unnecessary lines which are distracting, P#1 preferred the result of the PEL method. P#2 and P#3 preferred the SC method because it conveys the elongated structure as well as the tracheal cartilage. Furthermore, the resulting lines depict also the bifurcation appropriately. Both participants noted that they could not figured out the bifurcation when using the RV, AR, or PEL method.

The liver model failed for the illustration since too many distracting lines are generated. This is probably due to the fact that the liver shape has few

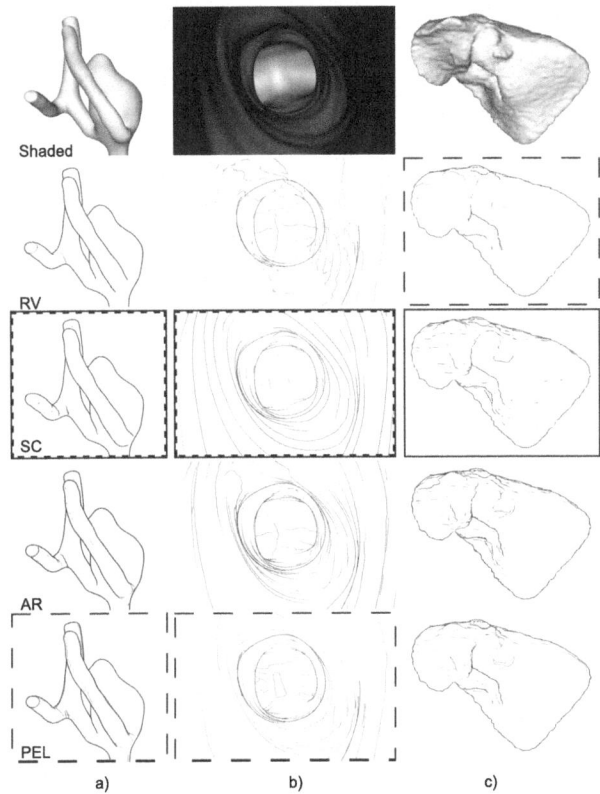

Fig. 1. Application of the four feature line techniques applied on: (a) a cerebral aneurysm, (b) an inner view of a trachea, and (c) a liver surface. The resulting images are obtained by best-choice adjustments of the domain experts. Favored results of the experts are depicted with corresponding borders. The dashed line border stands for the best-choice by P#1, e.g. (a) and PEL. The dashed points represent the choice by P#2, e.g. (a) and SC. The line border depicts the favored result by P#3, e.g. (b) and SC.

prominent surface features and the lines emphasize artifacts from image acquisition and surface generation instead of real anatomical features. Thus, without the shaded underlying model the participants were not able not recognize the model as a liver. From an illustrative point of view, P#1 chose the RV method as his favored. P#2 did not favored a particular technique and noted that it is necessary to rotate the model in order to gain an impression of the model. Finally, P#3 chose SC as the favored method but noticed that the differences between the feature line methods are not significant when using the liver model.

4   Discussion

The results of our evaluation can be summarized in two conclusions. First, reasonable depictions of patient-specific surface models with current feature line methods are obtained only if the models exhibit a smooth and regularly tessellated surface. Due to the high order derivations of the methods they are sensitive in terms of surface noise and artifacts. Advanced smoothing and remeshing algorithms are necessary to reduce these artifacts but preserve important anatomical surface shape and features. Thereby, the user has to find a tradeoff between surface shape and plausible resulting feature lines. However, for some cases it seems that current feature line methods are not able to detect important features of the underlying model. Additional surface shading and exploring the model by interactively changing the camera are needed. Furthermore, the evaluation shows a subjective rating in terms of choosing a preferred method. It seems that the SC method tends to be the most expressive technique. The second conclusion considers the application of feature line visualizations. Since they are able to provide a sparse representation of the underlying model they can be used for context-aware medical illustrations in which the model should not be in the focus but serve as anatomical context.

References

1. Tietjen C, Isenberg T, Preim B. Illustrative Rendering-Techniken für die medizinische Ausbildung und Therapieplanung. Proc BVM. 2005; p. 282–6.
2. Ritter F, Hansen C, Preim B, et al. Real-time illustration of vascular structures for surgery. IEEE Trans Vis. 2006;12:877–84.
3. Isenberg T, Neumann P, Carpendale S, et al. Non-photorealistic rendering in context: an observational study. In: Proc ACM 4th Int Symp Non-Photorealistic Animation and Rendering; 2006. p. 115–26.
4. Preim B, Tietjen C. Illustrative rendering for intervention planning: methods, applications, experiences. Proc Eurographics Workshop. 2006.
5. Nadernejad E, Sharifzadeh S, Hassanpour H. Edge detection techniques: evaluations and comparisons. Appl Math Sci. 2008;2(31):1507–20.
6. Interrante V, Fuchs H, Pizer S. Enhancing transparent skin surfaces with ridge and valley lines. Proc Vis. 1995; p. 52.
7. DeCarlo D, Finkelstein A, Rusinkiewicz S, et al. Suggestive contours for conveying shape. ACM Trans Graph. 2003;22(3):848–55.
8. Tilke J, Frédo D, Edward A. Apparent ridges for line drawing. Proc ACM SIGGRAPH. 2007.
9. Xie X, He Y, Tian F, et al. An effective illustrative visualization framework based on photic extremum lines (PELs). IEEE Transactions on Visualization and Computer Graphics. 2007;13:1328–35.
10. Bade R, Haase J, Preim B. Comparison of fundamental mesh smoothing algorithms for medical surface models. In: Simulation und Visualisierung. SCS-Verlag; 2006. p. 289–304.

Bestimmung der Lage der Papilla Duodeni Major im Bild eines Duodenoskops

Duygu Özmen

Institut für Informatik, Heinrich-Heine-Universität Düsseldorf
duygu.oezmen@hhu.de

Kurzfassung. Mit Hilfe eines am Universitätsklinikum Tübingen erstellten Phantoms des Gastrointestinaltrakts lassen sich ERCP-Eingriffe realitätsnah trainieren. Es wird ein Verfahren vorgestellt, mit dem die Papilla duodeni major im Bild eines Duodenoskops detektiert wird und beurteilt werden kann, ob ihre Lage für die Kanülierung geeignet ist.

1 Einleitung

Bei der endoskopisch retrograden Cholangiopankreatikographie (ERCP) handelt es sich um eine Methode zur direkten röntgenologischen Darstellung von Gallenwegen, Gallenblase und Ausführungsgang der Bauchspeicheldrüse. Hierbei werden Beschwerden am Pankreas (Bauchspeicheldrüse), am Ductus Prankreatikus (Hauptbauchspeicheldrüsengang) und am Ductus Choledochus (Hauptgallengang) diagnostiziert und therapiert. Diese Beschwerden sind unter anderem Tumore, Steine, Ablagerungen oder Verengungen.

Bei der ERCP wird dem Patienten ein Seitenblickendoskop, das Duodenoskop, oral eingeführt. Dieses wird durch den Ösophagus (Speiseröhre) in den Magen und von dort durch den Pylorus in das Duodenum navigiert, wo schließlich die Papilla duodeni major aufgesucht wird. Dort angekommen wird das Endoskop so eingestellt, dass es die Papille frontal ansieht.

Der nächste Schritt besteht nun im Eindringen in die Papille. Da dies mit dem Duodenoskop selbst aufgrund seines Durchmessers nicht erreicht werden kann, besitzt es einen Arbeitskanal. Durch diesen werden kleinere Instrumente, wie zum Beispiel ein Papillotom, hindurchgeleitet.

Seit einigen Jahren darf die ERCP nur noch zu interventionellen Zwecken durchgeführt werden. Für diagnostische Zwecke ist die ERCP zu risikoreich und kann durch die MRCP (Magnetresonanz-Cholangiopankreatikographie) ersetzt werden. Deshalb gibt es zur Zeit keine vertretbaren Trainingsmöglichkeiten am Patienten. Rein virtuelles Training am Computer findet bei Experten keine Akzeptanz. Aus diesem Dilemma weist das Tübinger Phantom einen Ausweg [1, 2]. Es besteht aus anatomisch getreuen Organnachbildungen mit gewebeähnlichen Eigenschaften. Daran lassen sich alle relevanten diagnostischen und operativen Eingriffe mit üblichen Instrumenten üben. Das Training wird mit Sensorik überwacht. Gegenstand dieser Arbeit ist die Überprüfung der korrekten Lage der Papille für ihre Kanülierung.

H.-P. Meinzer et al. (Hrsg.), *Bildverarbeitung für die Medizin 2013*, Informatik aktuell,
DOI: 10.1007/978-3-642-36480-8_35, © Springer-Verlag Berlin Heidelberg 2013

2   Material und Methoden

Die drei Beispiele für Duodenoskopbilder in Abb. 1 geben einen Überblick über die zugrunde liegende Situation.

2.1   Detektion von Papille und Papilleneingang

Bei den üblichen Duodenoskopen erscheint das Papillotom „von 5 Uhr" im Bild und muss zwischen „10 und 12 Uhr" in die Papille eindringen, um in den Gallengang zu gelangen. Die Papille sollte also ein wenig links vom Zentrum positioniert werden. Der Gallengang sollte in Richtung „11 Uhr" verlaufen. Da er orthogonal zu der Darmfalte ist, auf der die Papille liegt, kann man an der Richtung der Darmfalte beurteilen, ob sich der Papillenwinkel für die Kanülierung eignet. Die Darmfalte lässt sich nicht immer verlässlich detektieren, deshalb gibt es im Phantom eine grüne Leuchtdiode (Abb. 2), die die Richtung des Gallenganges angibt. Sie lässt sich bei Bedarf einschalten und ist leicht detektierbar.

Zur Beurteilung der Papillenposition im Duodenoskopbild muss die Papille also zunächst detektiert werden. Die Papille zeichnet sich durch ihre starke rötliche Färbung aus (Abb. 1). Daher kann man ausgehend von den HSV-Werten der Pixel durch eine empirisch ermittelte Schwelle für den H-Wert eine erste grobe

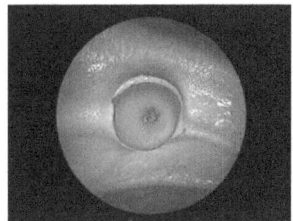 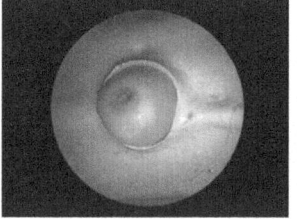 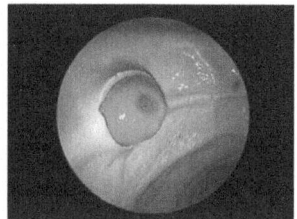

Abb. 1. Beispielbilder für verschiedene Papillenlagen.

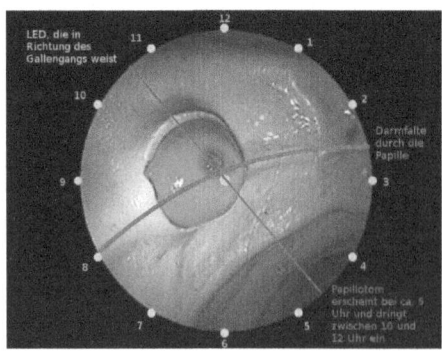 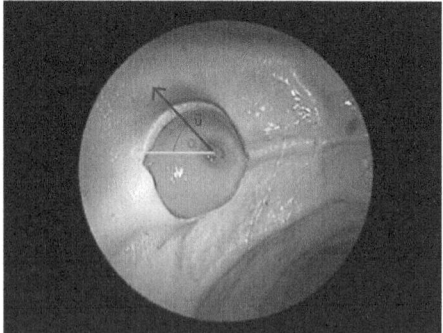

(a) Optimale Papillenlage   (b) Optimaler Papillenwinkel

Abb. 2. Optimale Papillenpositionierung und Winkel α.

Segmentierung der Papille erhalten (Abb. 3). Durch morphologische Operationen wie Minimums- und Maximumsoperatoren werden Binärisierungfehler wie mehrfacher Zusammenhang oder Lücken beseitigt.

Die Detektion des Papilleneingangs gelingt mit dieser Methode nicht. Die nähere Betrachtung des Papilleneingangs und der unmittelbaren Umgebung zeigt eine homogene Helligkeitsverteilung in der Umgebung und eine starke Streuung dieser innerhalb des Eingangs (Abb. 4).

Zur Segmentierung des Eingangs wird daher die Varianz σ_V der V-Werte der Pixel innerhalb der Papille herangezogen. Dazu wird für jedes Pixel p in einer Umgebung $U(p)$ die Varianz $\sigma_V = E(V^2) - E(V)^2$ berechnet. Dabei ist $E(V) = \frac{1}{|U|} * \sum_{q \in U} V(q)$ der Erwartungswert der V-Werte. Anschließend wird eine wiederum empirisch ermittelte feste Varianzschwelle zum Binärisieren gewählt. Das Resultat zeigt sich in Abb. 5.

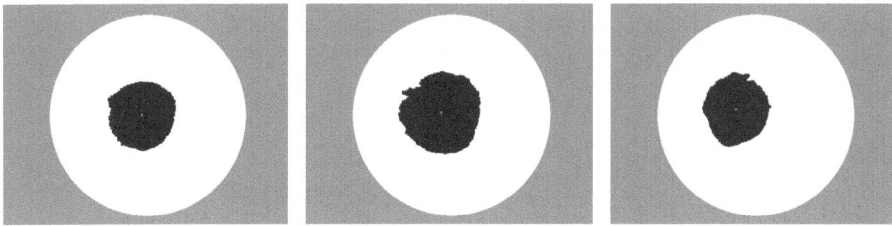

Abb. 3. Segmentierungsergebnisse der Papillen in den Bildern aus Abb. 1.

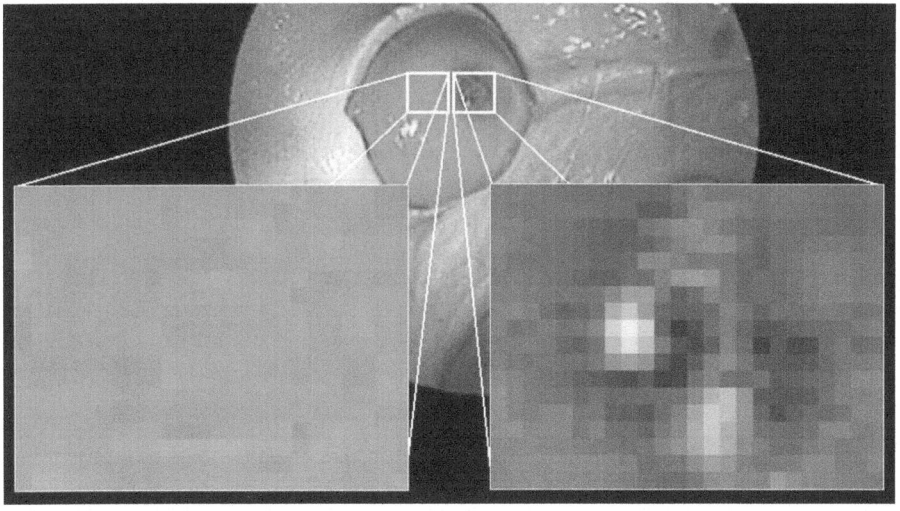

Abb. 4. Detailansicht des Papilleneingangs.

Abb. 5. Segmentierungsergebnisse der Papilleneingänge in den Bildern aus Abb. 1.

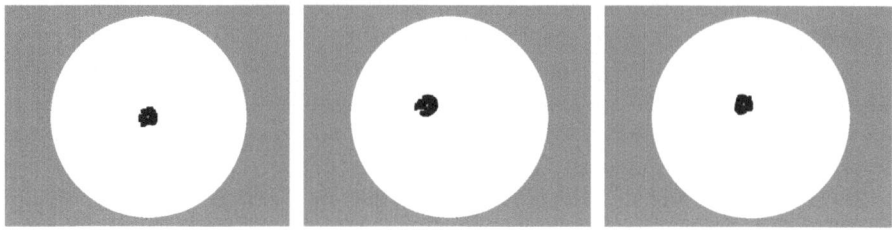

2.2   Kriterien zur Beurteilung der Detektion

Abb. 2 zeigt eine nach Expertenmeinung optimale Papillenpositionierung. Um die Güte der Papillenposition zu beurteilen, wird der Papillenschwerpunkt in dem zu bewertenden Bild mit dem in Abb. 2 verglichen. Um unterschiedliche Bildgrößen auszugleichen, wird eine Normierung vorgenommen. Der auf 0 bis 1 normierte Abstand δ der Papillenschwerpunkte wird als Maß für die Güte der Papillenlage verwendet (Tab. 1).

Tabelle 1. Güte der Papillenlage.

Lage	Bewertung
$0,00 < \delta < 0,15$	sehr gut
$0,15 < \delta < 0,30$	gut
$0,30 < \delta < 0,45$	schlecht
$0,45 < \delta < 1,00$	sehr schlecht

Eine optimale Winkellage der Papille liegt genau dann vor, wenn das Papillotom bei 4-5 Uhr im Bild erscheint und zwischen 10 und 12 Uhr in die Papille eindringt. Dies ist genau dann der Fall, wenn der Vektor $\vec{u}$ vom Schwerpunkt des Papilleneingangs zum Schwerpunkt der grünen LED, die in Gallengangrichtung weist, mit der Horizontalen $\vec{v}$ einen Winkel α von ungefähr 60° aufspannt (Tab. 2).

Tabelle 2. Güte des Papillenwinkels.

Winkel	Bewertung
$55° < \alpha < 75°$	sehr gut
$30° < \alpha < 55°$	gut
$75° < \alpha < 80°$	gut
$\alpha < 30°$ oder $\alpha > 80°$	schlecht

Tabelle 3. Evaluation.

Bild	Menschliche Bewertung	Bewertung des Programms
01	Position: Gut	Position: Gut
	Winkel: Sehr gut	Winkel: Sehr gut
02	Position: Gut	Position: Gut
	Winkel: Schlecht	Winkel: Schlecht
03	Position: Schlecht	Position: Schlecht
	Winkel: Sehr gut	Winkel: Sehr gut
04	Position: Sehr schlecht	Position: Sehr schlecht
	Winkel: –	Winkel: –
05	Position: Schlecht	Position: Sehr schlecht
	Winkel: –	Winkel: –
06	Position: Sehr gut	Position: Gut
	Winkel: Sehr gut	Winkel: Sehr gut
07	Position: Schlecht	Position: Sehr schlecht
	Winkel: Sehr gut	Winkel: –
08	Position: Sehr schlecht	Position: Sehr schlecht
	Winkel: Sehr gut	Winkel: –
09	Position: Schlecht	Position: Schlecht
	Winkel: Gut	Winkel: Sehr gut
10	Position: Gut	Position: Gut
	Winkel: Sehr gut	Winkel: Sehr gut
11	Position: Sehr schlecht	Position: Sehr schlecht
	Winkel: –	Winkel: –
12	Position: Sehr schlecht	Position: Sehr schlecht
	Winkel: –	Winkel: –

3 Ergebnisse

Zur Verifikation der korrekten Funktionsweise des Programms standen zwölf Papillenbilder zur Verfügung. Tabelle 3 zeigt für jedes der zwölf Bilder eine Gegenüberstellung der Bewertung des hier vorgestellten Verfahrens und der eines Experten. In den Fällen, in denen die Papillenposition mit „sehr schlecht" bewertet wird, erfolgt keine Bewertung des Winkels durch das Programm.

4 Diskussion

Es gibt nur wenige Abweichungen der Bewertung des Programms von der des Experten. Diese Abweichungen rühren daher, dass das Programm die Bewertung anhand von festen Schwellwerten trifft. Ein Mensch jedoch bewertet die Position nicht anhand fester Schwellwerte, sondern nach Intuition und Erfahrung.

Zwar ändert sich die Grundtendenz nicht, doch die Bewertung im Detail ist Er-messenssache und daher nicht immer reproduzierbar. Solange die Unterschiede zwischen Programm und Mensch jedoch nur im Detail liegen und die Grund-tendenzen, also gut/sehr gut bzw. schlecht/sehr schlecht, übereinstimmen, sind diese Abweichungen nicht von praktischer Bedeutung für die Einsetzbarkeit des Verfahrens im Tübinger Phantomprojekt.

Literaturverzeichnis

1. Grund KE, Ingenpaß R, Durst F, et al. Neuartiges Hands-on-Phantom für das realistische Training der gesamten diagnostischen und therapeutischen ERCP. Endo Heute. 2012;25:1–4.
2. Grund KE, Ingenpaß R, Schweizer U, et al. Neues ERCP-Trainingsmodell für alle diagnostischen und therapeutischen Eingriffe. 23 Kongress der Südwestdeutschen Gesellschaft für Gastroenerologie. 2012.

Object-Based Boundary Properties

Teodora Chitiboi[1,2], Andre Homeyer[1], Lars Linsen[2], Horst Hahn[1,2]

[1]Fraunhofer MEVIS
[2]Jacobs University Bremen
teodora.chitiboi@mevis.fraunhofer.de

Abstract. While object-based image analysis specializes in using region features for object detection, it lacks the possibility to use border strength and local geometry, common in edge detection. We propose to enhance common object-based image representation with boundary features that measure strength and continuity. Using these we formulate strategies for merging regions in a partitioned image to identify potentially regular shapes. To illustrate the capacity of this approach, we apply the proposed concepts to CT bone segmentation.

1 Introduction

Object-based image analysis (OBIA) has emerged as a powerful solution to the shortcomings of pixel-based analysis, giving the possibility to encode context information in an image representation. Formally defined for the first time by Hay and Castilla [1] in the context of Geo-imaging, OBIA has become popular through the Definiens software [2] and later made its way to medical image analysis in applications based on the framework proposed by Homeyer et al. [3]. In OBIA the nuclear semantical structures used to analyze images are not individual pixels but pixel regions called objects. Determined by an initial image partition, the objects are described by a set of properties regarding their appearance and relative position.

However, one of the pitfalls of OBIA approaches is that they rely mostly on region features and do not make use of edge information such as strength and local geometry. But one fundamental criterion that humans rely on to find meaningful structures that have been over-segmented is how the boundaries of small fragments fit together. For example, in Fig. 1(a) we recognize the triangular shape because the boundaries group together in three prominent lines. Moreover, in human perception object boundaries which are not justified by a significant local gradient perpendicular to the edge direction are automatically pruned. In edge detection these ideas correspond to contour grouping and salient edges.

Few other OBIA approaches [4, 5] combine region and boundary features using supervised learning to obtain general purpose segmentation solutions. However the feature extractors considered do not account for noisy boundaries when computing boundary continuity and rank edge strength only according to the

H.-P. Meinzer et al. (Hrsg.), *Bildverarbeitung für die Medizin 2013*, Informatik aktuell,
DOI: 10.1007/978-3-642-36480-8_36, © Springer-Verlag Berlin Heidelberg 2013

absolute gradient rather than check if the gradient direction reinforces border saliency.

In this work we extend the object-based image representation [3] with additional border information for encoding strength and local boundary geometry. In the given examples we apply an OBIA approach by starting with a highly over-segmented image using the watershed algorithm that preserves local details. Then we successively merge pairs of adjacent objects in greedy fashion, using the boundary criteria on which we elaborate in Section 2, until we obtain the final segmentation.

2   Measuring continuity and strength

2.1   Border continuity in an image partition

Given an image partition in the OBIA sense, such as in Fig. 1(a), we perceive a set of objects as belonging to the same structure if their boundaries flow continuously in a straight line or a smooth curve. This idea is seconded by the Gestalt law of *good continuation*.

Considering the simple setting in Fig. 2, we want to know if the two neighboring objects have a continuous boundary and may be part of the same structure. Specifically, we want to compute the boundary curvature at their junction nodes.

For this we need to robustly estimate the direction of the adjacent boundary segments. The main challenge here is to find the right scale to approximate the boundary directions. The reason why digitally straight segment algorithms find high curvature values that do not correspond to the actual shape is because they consider only the pixel scale where any local changes in boundary curvature are exacerbated because of discretization.

We would like to adapt to the general trend perceived in the boundary direction without completely losing grip on local continuity information. This is

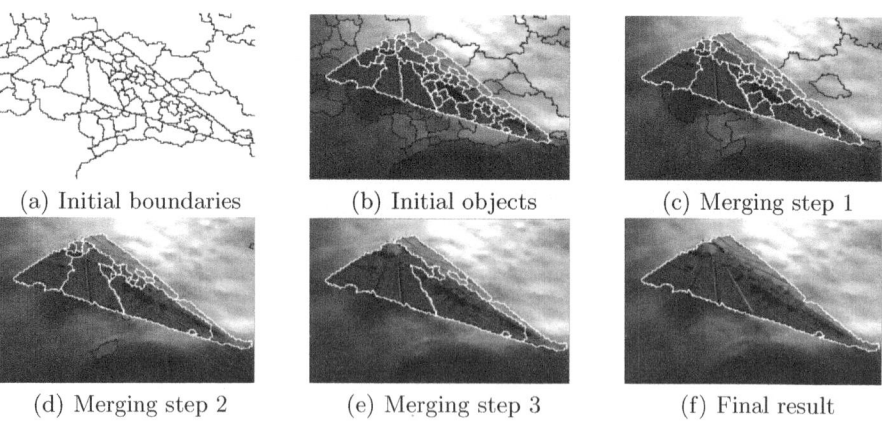

(a) Initial boundaries   (b) Initial objects   (c) Merging step 1

(d) Merging step 2   (e) Merging step 3   (f) Final result

Fig. 1. Segmenting regular shape using boundary strength and continuity.

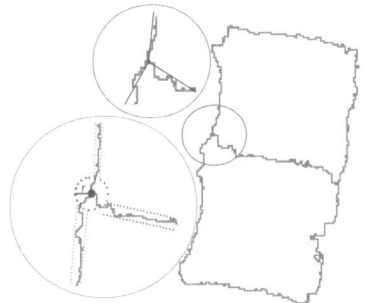

Fig. 2. Measuring continuity is challenging on a pixel scale (upper-left bubble). To find the right scale to estimate border direction we first compute the blurred segments. Pixels close to junction point are skipped. We then define the local curvature as the angle between pairs of adjacent borders.

possible with Debled-Rennesson's concept of blurred segments [6], further optimized by Roussillon et al. [7]. Extending the digitally straight segments, blurred segments can cope with noise and irregularities, preserving only the general direction of a digitized curve.

The blurred segment represents a minimum width band that encloses a corresponding boundary segment, described by a thickness ω. Roussillon's algorithm starts with a seed point (and a given direction) and adds consecutive points on the boundary until the width reaches a maximum given value. By computing the blurred segments for all border segments meeting at a junction point we obtain a local, noise-robust estimation of their direction. Using this information we can then compute the curvature as the angle formed by pairs of boundary segments. Finally, by choosing the pair with the least curvature we can determine the most likely adjacent objects to be part of a larger image structure.

However, one problem we face is that boundaries are especially noisy in the close vicinity of the junction point because edge descriptors are generally poorly defined at corners. One solution for this is to skip pixels on a radius r from the junction when constructing blurred segments, as shown in Fig. 2. As a consequence, the blurred segments become thinner and the approximation of the overall boundary direction is more precise.

2.2 Border strength as significance measure

Boundary strength is another powerful tool that helps distinguish whether neighboring objects should be merged to the same structure. In case of a strong line edge (when the boundary is brighter or darker that both opposite regions) or a step edge (when one region is brighter than the other), without further information the two objects will be perceived as distinct.

However, the usual edge detectors, such as Sobel, do not offer enough information for OBIA because once an image is partitioned, the only edges considered are corresponding to object boundaries. Moreover, for each boundary we want to measure the strength of the relevant gradient perpendicular to its direction, which reinforces gradient saliency. This feature can be computed on the same image used by the segmentation algorithm for the initial OBIA partition (either the original to detect line edges or the gradient image for step edges).

One way to do this is to consider for each point $\boldsymbol{b}$ on the border a pair of points from the two opposite objects obtained by a step in the normal direction $\boldsymbol{n}$ with a small step size d. Let $\boldsymbol{b_1} = \boldsymbol{b} + d\boldsymbol{n}$ and $\boldsymbol{b_2} = \boldsymbol{b} - d\boldsymbol{n}$ be the respective points, where the border and normal directions were estimated by principal component analysis. Their corresponding intensity values are obtained through bilinear interpolation. Then for each pixel center $\boldsymbol{b}$ on a boundary B in image I, we can define a boundary strength indicator

$$\text{Strength}(\boldsymbol{b}) = \frac{1}{2} \cdot (|I(\boldsymbol{b}) - I(\boldsymbol{b} + d\boldsymbol{n})| + |I(\boldsymbol{b}) - I(\boldsymbol{b} - d\boldsymbol{n})|) \cdot (\max(I) - \min(I))^{-1} \quad (1)$$

The value is scaled to the size of the intensity value range of the original image. Then the values of all individual sampled positions can be aggregated to obtain a significance measure for the entire boundary segment using one of the methods existing in literature: based on the maximum value used by Canny [8] edge detector, minimum used to rank watersheds, or using the average like Harris [9] (depicted in bottom-right picture of Fig. 3).

3   Results

In this section we explore the idea of reconstructing fragmented regular structures using only boundary information. In the first small example we would like to segment the triangular structure (Star Destroyer) in Fig. 1. After computing the image gradient and applying a morphological closing, we use the watershed algorithm to obtain an initial image partition (Fig. 1 top-left). Our task is to merge the objects that belong to the destroyer without including objects from the background.

We can achieve this by iteratively merging pairs of adjacent objects with border strength $< 15\%$ and continuity $> 170°$ for at least one pair of adjacent border segments, in Fig. 1(c), 1(d). However, some objects are too small to offer border continuity information, so in order to reduce granularity, in Fig. 1(e)

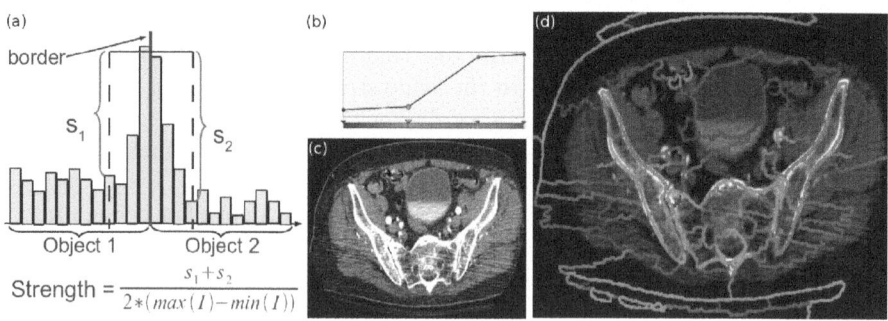

Fig. 3. Algorithm for computing boundary strength in 1D (a). Blue-red color map (b). Original CT image (c). Watershed lines colored by their average strength (d).

the strength threshold is decreased to 8%. Finally, some borders inside the structure have a higher intensity than the borders separating the shape from the background. Therefore, as image regions become bigger, only the border continuity remains a criterion for merging neighboring regions (Fig. 1(f)). So, by alternating strength- and continuity-based merging where the strength threshold decreases we obtain the final result.

As a second example we choose the task of reconstructing the boundaries of over-segmented hip bones in axial CT image slices. The segmentation strategy is based on the assumption that the outer layer surrounding the bone is composed of compact, dense tissue which forms a high intensity boundary. Using the watershed algorithm directly on the image, the high-intensity cortical bone layer separates the bone from the surrounding tissue by a high local maximum. However, because of noise, image artifacts or pathological conditions the boundary is sometimes discontinuous. In order to prevent leaking, the image is over-segmented and the bones are divided into smaller irregular fragments. Our goal is to reconstruct the fragmented hip bones using, as previously, only boundary information.

Because the structures we are looking for have a regular, smooth shape, we can use boundary continuation to merge regions where the blurred segments form an angle $> 160°$ for both junction points. However, in Fig. 4(b) we can see that some surrounding regions which are accidentally aligned because of linear artifacts were also merged. This can be avoided by using an empirically determined threshold for the average boundary strength. In case this threshold is exceeded, the neighboring objects are probably separated by a high intensity bones shell and they are not merged (Fig. 4(c)).

4   Conclusion and future work

Boundary continuity and strength are essential perceptual cues to determine which objects belong together. In this work, we have shown how to compute features that describe both properties in a partitioned image. Using border information, one can define merging criteria for pairs of neighboring objects to reconstruct larger, significant image structures. We have tested this idea on regular shapes (artificial and anatomical) where the thresholds for boundary strength

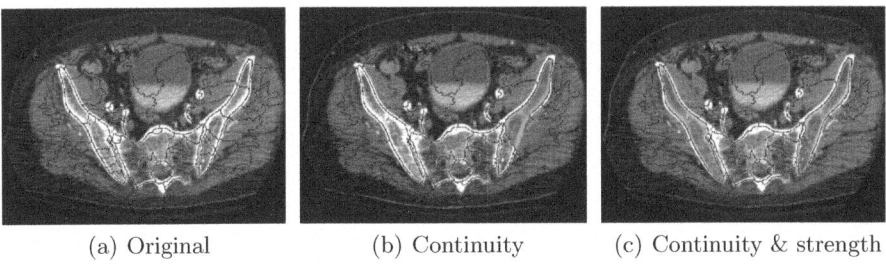

| (a) Original | (b) Continuity | (c) Continuity & strength |

Fig. 4. Reconstruct fragmented hip bones in CT image.

and continuity and the maximum width of blurred segments were chosen empirically. These very promising early experiments provide the basis to integrate the features in a more comprehensive image segmentation scheme, where the parameters are learned from a training dataset.

Furthermore, another interesting problem appears when combining region-based and edge-based features which traditionally belong to separate segmentation strategies. We know from perception psychology that region and border characteristics, such as color and shape, are complementary in recognition tasks [10]. But it was not established exactly how the two are distilled by our perception and what causes one or the other to have a higher relevance. One future possibility would be to combine the merging strategy based on region similarity and minimum basin depth used in hierarchical watersheds with border strength and continuity used in OBIA.

In the future we will continue to investigate the application of boundary features in the context of OBIA to problems where traditional pixel, edge, or region based approaches tend to fail.

References

1. Hay GJ, Castilla G. Object-based image analysis: strengths, weaknesses, opportunities and threats (SWOT). Proc OBIA. 2006 July.
2. Definiens eCognition Developer XD 1.0 Reference Book. Definiens AG; 2008.
3. Homeyer A, Schwier M, Hahn HK. A generic concept for object-based image analysis. VISAPP. 2010; p. 530–33.
4. Luo J, Guo C. Perceptual grouping of segmented regions in color images. Pattern Recognit. 2003;36(12):2781–92.
5. Ren X, Malik J; IEEE. Learning a classification model for segmentation. Proc IEEE Int Conf Comput Vis. 2003; p. 10–7.
6. Debled-Rennesson I, Feschet F, Rouyer-Degli J. Optimal blurred segments decomposition of noisy shapes in linear time. Comput Graph. 2006;30(1).
7. Roussillon T, Tougne L, Sivignon I. Computation of binary objects sides number using discrete geometry, application to automatic pebbles shape analysis. Proc CIAP. 2007; p. 763–8.
8. Canny J. A computational approach to edge detection. IEEE Trans Pattern Anal Mach Intell. 1986;8(6):679–98.
9. Haris K, Efstratiadis S, Maglaveras N. Hierarchical image segmentation based on contour dynamics. Proc ICIP. 2001; p. 7–10.
10. Smid H, Jakob A, Heinze H. The organization of multidimensional selection on the basis of color and shape: An event-related brain potential study. Atten Percept Psychophys. 1997;59:693–713.

Merkmalsverfolgung für die Panoramaendoskopie

Sebastian Nowack[1], Thomas Wittenberg[1], Dietrich Paulus[2], Tobias Bergen[1]

[1]Abteilung Bildverarbeitung und Medizintechnik, Fraunhofer Institut für Integrierte Schaltungen IIS, Erlangen
[2]Institut für Computervisualistik, Universität Koblenz-Landau
nowacksn@iis.fraunhofer.de

Kurzfassung. Zur Sichtfelderweiterung in der diagnostischen und interventionellen Endoskopie eignet sich die sogenannte Panoramaendoskopie. Zur Erstellung endoskopischer Panoramen ist es essentiell Korrespondenzen zwischen sukzessiv aufgenommenen Endoskopiebildern zu erstellen. Für die Merkmalsverfolgung existieren bekannte Ansätze wie KLT, SIFT oder SURF. Diese Trackingverfahren, sowie der neue ORB-Algorithmus, werden in diesem Beitrag auf ihre Eignung für die Endoskopie untersucht. Zur Bewertung der verschiedenen Verfahren wurde eine halbautomatische Evaluierungsmethode entwickelt. Darüber hinaus wird ein neuer Hybrid-Algorithmus vorgestellt, der sich besonders für die Verfolgung von Merkmalspunkten in endoskopischem Bildmaterial der Zystoskopie eignet. Die Ergebnisse des neuen Algorithmus wurden evaluiert und mit den bekannten Ansätzen verglichen.

1 Einleitung

Die Verfolgung von Merkmalspunkten in endoskopischen Bildsequenzen stellt elementare Informationen zur Verfügung, auf deren Basis sich unterschiedliche Anwendungen im Bereich der diagnostischen und therapeutischen Endoskopie realisieren lassen. So können Ergebnisse der Merkmalsverfolgung zur Erweiterung des Blickfelds mittels Image Stitching [1] für die Panoramaendoskopie oder für die Erstellung von 3D-Rekonstruktionen aus endoskopischen Bildern genutzt werden.

Im Bereich der Merkmalsverfolgung stellen die Algorithmen KLT [2], SIFT [3] und SURF [4] etablierte Verfahren dar. Diese werden, ebenso wie der jüngst vorgestellte ORB-Algorithmus (Oriented FAST and Rotated BRIEF) [5], in diesem Beitrag auf ihre Eignung für die Endoskopie untersucht[1]. Dazu wurde eine Methode entwickelt, mit der es möglich ist, eine Aussage darüber zu treffen, wie präzise und zuverlässig diese Algorithmen Merkmalspunkte auf endoskopischem Bildmaterial verfolgen. In der Literatur wird zwischen pixel- und merkmalsbasierten Trackingansätzen unterschieden. Masson et al. [6] untersuchen beispielsweise pixelbasierte Ansätze, indem kleine Bereiche auf der Geweboberfläche von

---

[1] Für KLT, SIFT, SURF und ORB wurden die Implementierungen aus OpenCV 2.4.1 verwendet.

H.-P. Meinzer et al. (Hrsg.), *Bildverarbeitung für die Medizin 2013*, Informatik aktuell, DOI: 10.1007/978-3-642-36480-8_37, © Springer-Verlag Berlin Heidelberg 2013

Schweinemägen durch Koagulation markiert werden, wodurch die Grundwahrheit festgelegt wird. Luó et al. [7] untersuchen merkmalsbasierte Ansätze auf ihre Verwendbarkeit in der Bronchoskopie. Zur Evaluierung der Tracker werden die Ergebnisse der Punktverfolgung genutzt, um mittels Epipolargeometrie die Kamerabewegung zwischen den Bildern zu berechnen. Mit diesen Informationen wird ein synthetisches Bild mit Hilfe eines Volume Rendering basierend auf 3D-CT-Daten erstellt. Stimmen das echte Bild und das synthetische Bild überein, so gelten die Punkte als korrekt verfolgt. Im Gegensatz zu den direkten Ansätzen, bei denen besonders markante Punkte als Grundwahrheit gewählt werden können, gestaltet sich diese Festlegung bei merkmalsbasierten Ansätzen als schwierig. So ist es in Endoskopiebildern in der Regel nicht möglich die neuen Positionen pixelgenau in einem Folgebild festzulegen. Wurde ein Merkmal in einem für das menschliche Auge weitestgehend homogenen Bereich extrahiert, so wird diese Problematik noch deutlich erhöht.

2 Material und Methoden

Die Algorithmen KLT, SIFT, SURF und ORB wurden auf ihre Eignung für die Panoramaendoskopie untersucht. Dafür wurden je zwei Videosequenzen der Zystoskopie und Koloskopie ausgewählt, die im Rahmen einer konventionellen ärztlichen Untersuchung entstanden sind. Abb. 1 zeigt Bilder der verwendeten Datensätze. Die ersten beiden Sequenzen entstammen einer Untersuchung der Blasenwand, wobei der zweite Datensatz starkes Bildrauschen und Kompressionsartefakte aufweist. Die Sequenzen 3 und 4 zeigen koloskopische Untersuchungen der Darmwand und eines Polypen. Das Bildmaterial der Zystoskopie weist fast planare Strukturen und wenige Glanzlichter auf. Im Gegensatz dazu handelt es sich bei den Koloskopieaufnahmen vorwiegend um 3D-Strukturen mit deutlich mehr Glanzlichtern. Jede Sequenz besteht aus 300 Einzelbildern, die für die Trackingvorgänge verwendet wurden. Alle untersuchten Algorithmen verfolgen die extrahierten Merkmalspunkte auf dem gleichen Videomaterial. Um einen Vergleich der Ergebnisse zu ermöglichen, werden die Maße *recall* (r) und *1-precision* (p) verwendet, die in [8] zur Untersuchung von Trackingergebnissen

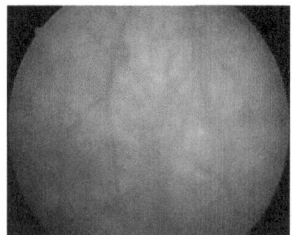 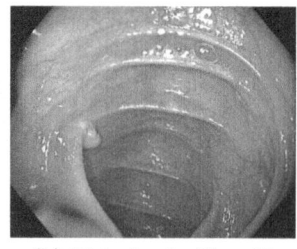 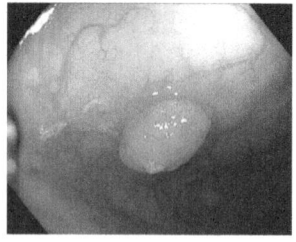

(a) Zystoskopie (Seq. 2)   (b) Koloskopie (Seq. 3)   (c) Koloskopie (Seq. 4)

Abb. 1. Typische Einzelbilder der verwendeten Videosequenzen.

vorgeschlagen werden

$$r = \frac{|C|}{|M|}, p = \frac{|F|}{|C| + |F|} \tag{1}$$

Recall liefert eine Aussage, wie viele korrekte Treffer C im Verhältnis zu allen Korrespondenzen gefunden wurden. Da recall einen Wert abhängig von allen theoretisch ermittelbaren Korrespondenzen M darstellt, liefert dieses Maß keine Aussage darüber, wie präzise der Algorithmus für gefundene Korrespondenzen ist. Hierfür wird das Maß 1-precision verwendet, das angibt wie viele der gefundenen Korrespondenzen korrekt sind. F bezeichnet die Menge der falschen Korrespondenzen. Zur Evaluierung der gefundenen Korrespondenzen wird ein halbautomatisches Verfahren eingesetzt, das die extrahierten Merkmalspunkte der Algorithmen mit Hilfe eines interaktiven Template-Matching-Ansatzes verfolgt. Ist diese Ausgabe augenscheinlich korrekt, wird sie als Grundwahrheit für die weiteren Trackingverfahren verwendet. Andernfalls wird das Ergebnis manuell korrigiert, um eine Grundwahrheit zu erhalten. Um das Template-Matching möglichst effektiv einzusetzen, wird die Größe des Templates für jedes Merkmal individuell bestimmt. Durch die Kombination von automatischer und manueller Vorgehensweise ist gewährleistet, dass eine Grundwahrheit zur Verfügung steht und gleichzeitig der Aufwand der manuellen Bearbeitung reduziert wird.

Die Bewertung der Trackingalgorithmen erfolgt auf Basis des euklidischen Abstandes der Merkmalspunkte zur entsprechenden Grundwahrheit. Sofern die euklidische Distanz unter einem Schwellwert von fünf Pixeln liegt, wird die gefundene Position als korrekte Korrespondenz akzeptiert. Für die weitere Verarbeitung ist es vorteilhaft, wenn das Ergebnis eines Trackingalgorithmus nicht nur eine möglichst hohe Präzision (precision), sondern auch eine hohe Wiederauffindungsrate (recall) aufweist. Recall und 1-precision sind etablierte Maße, um Trackingverfahren zu bewerten. Zusätzlich messen wir die Lebensdauer der Merkmalspunkte nach ihrer Extraktion.

Die in Kapitel 3 beschriebenen Ergebnisse zeigen, dass Merkmale der untersuchten Algorithmen in der Regel nur über wenige Einzelbilder verfolgt werden können, obwohl sie augenscheinlich auch in Folgebildern noch vorhanden sind. Dies führt zu einem geringen recall. Daher wurde ein hybrider Tracking-Algorithmus mit dem Ziel entwickelt, extrahierte Merkmalspunkte über längere Zeiträume zu verfolgen. Dieser Ansatz stellt eine Kombination aus merkmals- und pixelbasierter Methode dar. Zunächst werden mit Hilfe des SIFT Ansatzes Merkmalspunkte extrahiert. In jedem Einzelbild werden mittels Ratio-Test [3] Punktkorrespondenzen gesucht. Für Merkmalspunkte, die nicht gefunden wurden, wird ein Suchbereich um die letzte bekannte Position aufgespannt. Anschließend wird für jedes Pixel im Suchbereich ein SIFT-Deskriptor erstellt. Aus der neu entstandenen Menge von Deskriptoren wird mittels Bruteforce-Matcher [3] der beste Deskriptor ausgewählt. Mit Hilfe des Template-Matching, basierend auf normalisierter Kreuzkorrelation, wird ebenfalls die neue Position des Merkmalspunktes gesucht. Wenn beide Positionen übereinstimmen, gilt der Merkmalspunkt als gefunden.

Tabelle 1. Die Tabelle zeigt die gemittelten Ergebnisse aller Trackingverfahren auf vier verschiedenen Videosequenzen. Die besten Werte jeder Videosequenz sind fett dargestellt.

	Zystoskopie				Koloskopie			
	Datensatz 1		Datensatz 2		Datensatz 3		Datensatz 4	
	r	p	r	p	r	p	r	p
KLT	0,52	0,48	0,33	0,65	0,12	0,88	0,47	0,53
SIFT	0,25	**0,05**	0,16	**0,2**	0,11	0,32	0,16	**0,25**
SURF	0,17	0,21	0,07	0,59	0,1	0,48	0,14	0,4
ext. SURF			0,05	0,48				
ORB	0,09	0,13	0,02	0,62	0,07	**0,2**	0,03	0,34
Hyb. Ansatz	**0,74**	0,22	**0,4**	0,47	**0,64**	0,34	**0,52**	0,41

3 Ergebnisse

Werden nur die Ergebnisse von recall und 1-precision betrachtet (Tab. 1), so fällt auf, dass der KLT-Tracker über alle Videosequenzen den besten recall-Wert aufweist. SIFT erreicht nach dem KLT Tracker in jeder Sequenz den zweithöchsten recall-Wert und fast immer die beste Präzision. SURF schneidet etwas schlechter ab. Lediglich im zweiten Datensatz mit sehr verrauschtem Bildmaterial ist die Präzision von SURF deutlich schlechter als die von SIFT. ORB erreicht mit einer Ausnahme gute Präzisionswerte bei einem sehr geringen recall. In allen Sequenzen erreicht der hybride Ansatz einen höheren recall Wert. Die Präzision bleibt allerdings hinter der von SIFT zurück. Anhand des in Abb. 2a dargestellten „Lebenszeithistogramms" für SIFT ist zu erkennen, dass der größte Teil der Korrespondenzen nach der ersten Korrespondenzbildung nur noch in einem bis drei Folgebildern gefunden wird. Dies trifft ebenfalls auf SURF und ORB zu. Nahezu kein Merkmal „lebt" länger als 20 Einzelbilder. Die Merkmale des hybriden Ansatzes (Abb. 2b) weisen hingegen eine deutlich längere Lebenszeit auf. Als Grundlage für beide Histogramme dienen ausschließlich als korrekt gewertete Korrespondenzen.

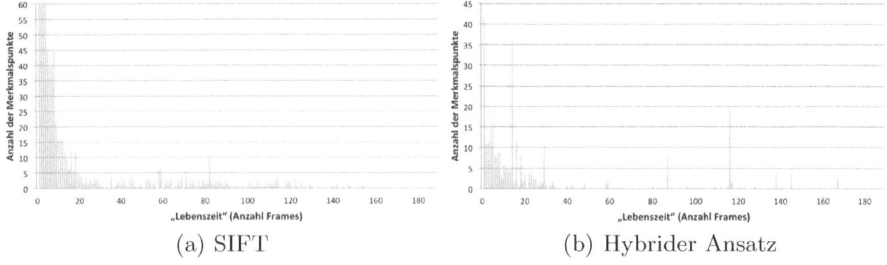

(a) SIFT   (b) Hybrider Ansatz

Abb. 2. Lebenszeithistogramme von SIFT und dem hybriden Ansatz (Datensatz 1).

4 Diskussion

Der KLT-Tracker weist über alle Videosequenzen den höchsten recall-Wert aller getesteten Standardverfahren auf. Die 1-precision-Werte relativieren das bessere Abschneiden gegenüber den anderen drei Algorithmen, da der KLT-Tracker in allen Sequenzen die geringste Präzision aufweist. Dies ist darauf zurückzuführen, dass der KLT-Tracker eine fest vorgegebene Anzahl von Merkmalspunkten auf allen Bildern verfolgt. Daher liegt in der Regel für jeden Merkmalspunkt in jedem Bild ein Trackingergebnis vor, unabhängig davon, ob dieses richtig oder falsch ist. Bei der verwendeten Implementierung werden die Ergebnisse des vorherigen Bildes als Grundlage für die Merkmalsverfolgung im Folgebild genutzt. SIFT, SURF und ORB hingegen bilden nur Korrespondenzen, wenn eine definierte Deskriptorähnlichkeit vorliegt. Daher erreicht der KLT-Tracker trotz schlechter Präzision einen deutlich höheren recall Wert als die anderen Algorithmen. Die schlechte Präzision von KLT lässt sich in erster Linie damit begründen, dass viele Merkmalspunkte nach einiger Zeit anfangen zu driften. Auffällig ist der besonders geringe recall Wert von ORB, der je nach Videosequenz zwischen 0,02 und 0,09 liegt. Dies ist darauf zurückzuführen, dass ORB sehr viele Merkmalspunkte extrahiert, aber nur sehr wenige davon wiederfindet. Aufgrund der nicht mehr gefundenen Korrespondenzen müssen regelmäßig neue Punkte extrahiert werden.

Bei der Präzision schneidet SIFT deutlich besser ab als die restlichen Tracker. Lediglich im dritten Datensatz (Koloskopie) erreicht ORB eine höhere Präzision. Besonders gut ist die Präzision von SIFT auf Bildern der Zystoskopie. Im zweiten Datensatz erreichen die anderen Tracker lediglich einen 1-precision-Wert von etwa 0,6. Dies zeigt, dass sie im Gegensatz zu SIFT deutliche Probleme mit starkem Bildrauschen und Bildartefakten haben, da mehr falsche als richtige Korrespondenzen gebildet wurden. Ein oft genannter Grund für das schlechtere Abschneiden von SURF gegenüber SIFT ist der kleinere 64-dimensionale Merkmalsvektor. Für die zweite Videosequenz wurde daher ein Test mit „extended SURF" (128-dimensionaler Merkmalsvektor) durchgeführt. Allerdings wurden dabei keine signifikant besseren Trackingergebnisse erzielt. Die Ergebnisse des Vergleichs von SURF und extended SURF stützen die These von Luó et al. [7], dass die schlechteren Ergebnisse vor allem durch die geringere Qualität der extrahierten Merkmalspunkte und nicht durch den Deskriptor bedingt ist. ORB liefert für die Präzision bessere Ergebnisse als KLT und SURF. Lediglich in der stark verrauschten zweiten Videosequenz liefert ORB ein schlechtes Ergebnis. Da zur Erstellung des ORB-Deskriptors 256 Pixelvergleiche verwendet werden, führt starkes Bildrauschen hier zu Problemen bei der Korrespondenzbildung. Die verwendeten FAST-Merkmale eignen sich zur Merkmalsextraktion allerdings nur bedingt, da es zu Clusterbildungen in bestimmten Bildbereichen kommt und in anderen Bereichen kaum Merkmale extrahiert werden. Grundsätzlich weisen die Algorithmen SIFT, SURF und ORB das Problem auf, dass Merkmalspunkte nur wenige Einzelbilder nach der Extraktion wiedergefunden werden. Der Hybrid-Ansatz weist zwar eine geringere Präzision als SIFT auf, aber verfolgt dafür Punkte länger als alle getesteten Algorithmen. Besonders auf dem ersten Datensatz wird ein hoher recall-Wert bei guter Präzision erreicht. Abb. 2 zeigt das „Lebenszeithistogramm" für SIFT und den hybriden Ansatz für die erste Sequenz. Da die Merkmalspunkte des Hybrid-Ansatzes deutlich länger verfolgt werden können, weisen sie eine deutlich längere „Lebenszeit" auf als die Punkte von SIFT. Die Präzisionswerte für die Datensätze zwei bis vier bleiben deutlich hinter denen des ersten Datensatzes zurück. Hier zeigt sich, dass sich diese Methode nur bedingt für Sequenzen eignet, die deutliche 3D-Strukturen oder starkes Bildrauschen aufweisen.

5 Fazit

Im Rahmen dieses Beitrags wurden die Algorithmen SIFT, SURF, KLT und ORB auf ihre Eignung für die Panoramaendoskopie untersucht. SIFT liefert die besten Trackingergebnisse, kann aber Merkmalspunkte nur über wenige Einzelbilder verfolgen. Dies führt zu häufiger Extraktion neuer Merkmalspunkte. Im Zuge der Evaluierung der verschiedenen Ansätze wurde auch der ORB-Algorithmus untersucht, dessen Deskriptor vielversprechende Ergebnisse für die Merkmalsverfolgung in der Panoramaendoskopie liefert. Darüber hinaus wurde ein neuer Hybrid-Algorithmus vorgestellt, der einen merkmalsbasierten mit einem pixelbasierten Ansatz verbindet, um Merkmalspunkte in endoskopischen Daten länger verfolgen zu können. Dieser zeigt besonders im Bereich der Zystoskopie überzeugende Ergebnisse, da die Verfolgung von Merkmalspunkten deutlich länger als mit den untersuchten Ansätzen gelingt und gleichzeitig eine gute Präzision erreicht wird.

Literaturverzeichnis

1. Bergen T, Ruthotto S, Münzenmayer C, et al. Feature-based real-time endoscopic mosaicking. Proc Int Symp Image Signal Process Anal. 2009; p. 695–700.
2. Tomasi C, Kanade T. Detection and tracking of point features. Carnegie Mellon University; 1991.
3. Lowe DG. Distinctive image features from scale-invariant keypoints. Int J Comput Vis. 2004;60(2):91–110.
4. Bay H, Ess A, Tuytelaars T, et al. Speeded-up robust features (SURF). Comput Vis Image Underst. 2008;110(3):346–59.
5. Rublee E, Rabaud V, Konolige K, et al. ORB: An efficient alternative to SIFT or SURF. Proc IEEE Int Conf Comput Vis. 2011; p. 2564–71.
6. Masson N, Nageotte F, Zanne P, et al. Comparison of visual tracking algorithms on in vivo sequences for robot-assisted flexible endoscopic surgery. Proc IEEE Int Conf Eng in Med and Biol Soc. 2009; p. 5571–6.
7. Luó X, Feuerstein M, Reichl T, et al. An application driven comparison of several feature extraction algorithms in bronchoscope tracking during navigated bronchoscopy. Proc MIAR. 2010; p. 475–84.
8. Mikolajczyk K, Schmid C. A performance evaluation of local descriptors. IEEE Trans Pattern Anal Mach Intell. 2005;27(10):1615–30.

Konturverfeinerung über Fourierdeskriptoren

David Friedrich[1], Adrián Luna Cobos[1], Stefan Biesterfeld[2], Alfred Böcking[2],
Dietrich Meyer-Ebrecht[1]

[1]Lehrstuhl für Bildverarbeitung, RWTH Aachen
[2]Funktionsbereich Cytopathologie, H.-H. Universität Düsseldorf
david.friedrich@lfb.rwth-aachen.de

Kurzfassung. Algorithmen zur Konturverfeinerung können die Produktivität im klinischen Workflow steigern, indem sie hochbezahlten medizinischen Experten die manuelle Korrektur schlechter oder grober Segmentierungen ersparen. In dieser Veröffentlichung beschreiben wir ein Verfahren zur Konturverfeinerung basierend auf Fourierdeskriptoren. Eine Quasi-Newtonmethode optimiert dafür die Fourierdeskriptoren derart dass die zugehörige Kontur maximal bezüglich einer Gütefunktion wird. Der Suchraum für die Optimierung wird durch eine Beschränkung auf die Fourierdeskriptoren mit niedrigen Frequenzen verkleinert. Das vorgestellte Verfahren wird mit etablierten Verfahren zur Konturverfeinerung, den parametrischen und geometrischen Aktiven Konturen verglichen. Auf einem Testset von 197 mikroskopischen Aufnahmen von Zellkernen konnte die Methode eine initiale Schwellwertsegmentierung von einer Hausdorff-Distanz von $2.63\,\mu$m auf $1.78\,\mu$m verbessern. Dabei wurden durchschnittlich 3.37 Sekunden für die Verfeinerung benötigt. Bezüglich der Segmentierungsqualität liegt die Methode dabei im Bereich der etablierten Verfahren, mit $1.66\,\mu$m für die parametrischen und $1.97\,\mu$m für die geometrischen Aktiven Konturen.

1 Einleitung

Die DNA Bildzytometrie ist ein nicht-invasives Verfahren zur Krebsfrüherkennung anhand von Zellabstrichen, die Krebs bis zu zweieinhalb Jahre früher als herkömmliche Methoden erkennen kann [1]. Die Diagnose basiert hierbei auf der DNA-Verteilung morphologisch auffälliger Zellkerne. Zellmaterial wird zum Beispiel durch Bürstenabstriche der Mundhöhle gewonnen, auf einen Mikroskop-Objektträger aufgebracht und proportional zum DNA-Gehalt angefärbt. Ein Mikroskop und eine digitale Kamera messen anschließend den DNA-Gehalt der Zellen anhand der Schwächung des Weißlichtes. In Zellen mit hohem DNA-Gehalt ist diese Schwächung aufgrund der verwendeten Färbetechnik und des Lambert-Beerschen Gesetzes stärker. Für eine DNA Bildzytometrie-Messung wird der Objektträger systematisch abgefahren und geeignete Zellkerne durch einen Mausklick im Livebild hinzugefügt. Für die anschließende Messung des DNA-Gehaltes durch das System ist eine präzise Segmentierung der Zellkerne unerlässlich. Diese Segmentierung muss in Echtzeit verfügbar sein, deshalb

H.-P. Meinzer et al. (Hrsg), *Bildverarbeitung für die Medizin 2013*, Informatik aktuell,
DOI: 10.1007/978-3-642-36480-8_38, © Springer-Verlag Berlin Heidelberg 2013

wird ein schneller Schwellwert-Algorithmus verwendet [2]. Liefert dieser Algorithmus keine zufriedenstellende Segmentierung, so muss die Kontur zurzeit manuell nachgezeichnet werden.

Um dem Pathologen diesen zeitaufwändigen Schritt zu ersparen, präsentieren wir in dieser Veröffentlichung einen Algorithmus zur Konturverfeinerung basierend auf Fourierdeskriptoren. Fourierdeskriptoren werden zur Glättung von Konturen oder zur Unterscheidung von Konturen eingesetzt [3, 4]. Sie erlauben eine ein-eindeutige Beschreibung von Konturen aus zweidimensionalen Bildern, in dem man aufeinander folgende 2D-Koordinaten der Konturpixel als N-Tupel komplexer Zahlen auffasst und anschließend eine Fourier-Transformation durchführt. Da sich bei glatten Objekten die meiste Information in den niedrigen Fourierkoeffizienten befindet, lässt sich eine glatte Kontur bei geringem Informationsverlust mit weniger Freiheitsgraden darstellen, indem man die Rekonstruktion der Kontur auf Fourierkoeffizienten aus niedrigen Frequenzen beschränkt. Ein Optimierungsalgorithmus sucht dann in diesem Suchraum mit kleinerer Dimension diejenige Kontur, welche maximal bezüglich einer Gütefunktion wird.

2   Material und Methoden

2.1   Bildgebung und verwendete Materialien

Objektträger mit Zellmaterial von 11 Patienten wurden systematisch abgescannt und alle darauf befindlichen Objekte segmentiert. Zur Bildaufnahme diente ein Motic BA600 Mikroskop (40x Vergrößerung, NA=0.65) mit einer MotiCam 285c (RGB Kamera, 1360x1024 Pixel Auflösung). Ein Pixel im Bild entspricht dabei 0.18 μm auf dem Objektträger. Die Objekte in den Bilddaten wurden durch ein Schwellwertverfahren im HSV-Raum mit anschließender morphologischer Nachbearbeitung segmentiert [2]. Für klinisch relevante Objekte mit unzureichender Segmentierung wurde eine manuelle Referenzsegmentierung entlang der wahren Kontur erstellt, wobei auch lokal starke Krümmungen berücksichtigt wurden. Die Daten wurden in ein Trainingset von 191 Zellkernen und ein Testset von 197 Zellkernen von 5 bzw. 6 Patienten aufgeteilt. Die Berechnungen wurden auf einem Core i5 PC mit vier 2.8 GHz-Kernen durchgeführt.

2.2   Gütefunktion

Um die Güte einer Kontur zu bewerten und anschließend iterativ zu verbessern, wird zunächst eine skalare Gütefunktion erstellt. Die Konturverfeinerung über Fourierdeskriptoren und die parametrischen Aktiven Konturen werten die Gütefunktion entlang der Kontur aus und benötigen deshalb eine hohe Güte entlang der richtigen Kontur und niedrige Werte sonst (kantenbasierte Kostenfunktion). Die geometrischen Aktiven Konturen werten die Kostenfunktion im von der Kontur umschlossenen Bereich aus, benötigen also hohe Werte im kompletten zu segmentierenden Gebiet (regionenbasierte Kostenfunktion).

Zunächst wird das RGB-Bild in ein Grauwertbild umgewandelt. Um eine möglichst hohe Diskriminanz zwischen Zellkern und Hintergrund zu erreichen, wird derjenige Kanal ausgewählt, in dem das Weißlicht am Stärksten geschwächt wird. Zur Ermittlung des Farbkanals mit der größten Schwächung dienen die Bildwerte im Inneren der initialen Kontur. Durch die unterschiedliche Packungsdichte der DNA befinden sich auch Kanten im inneren des Objektes. Um diese zu entfernen, werden ein Medianfilter oder anisotrope Diffusion (Perona-Malik Filter) angewandt. Für den Diffusionsfilter wird dabei der Diffusionskoeffizient

$$g(\|\nabla I\|) = \frac{1}{1 + \left(\frac{\|\nabla I\|}{K}\right)^2} \tag{1}$$

verwendet. Für die Konturverfeinerung über Fourierdeskriptoren und die geometrischen Aktiven Konturen werden die Konturen durch einen Gradientenfilter (Betrag des Gradienten nach numerischer Ableitung) hervorgehoben. Abb. 2.2 zeigt exemplarisch zwei Kostenfunktionen.

2.3 Methoden zur Konturverfeinerung

Das Ergebnis der Schwellwert-Segmentierung im HSV-Raum [2] dient als Initialisierung für Methoden zur Konturverfeinerung.

Für die Konturverfeinerung über Fourierdeskriptoren wird die initiale Kontur dabei als N-Tupel aufeinander folgender Koordinaten $((x_1, y_1), \ldots, (x_N, y_N))$ beschrieben. Dabei variiert die Anzahl der Konturpunkte N von Objekt zu Objekt. Durch ein gleichmäßiges Sampling an N_f Punkten wird sichergestellt, dass für jedes Objekt die Anzahl an Konturpunkten gleich und der Abstand zwischen zwei Punkten auf der Kontur konstant ist. Über die Transformation $c_m = x_m + iy_m$, wird die abgetastete Kontur bijektiv nach $\mathbb{C}^{N_f}$ abgebildet. Durch eine diskrete Fouriertransformation erhält man die Fourierdeskriptoren $a_{-\frac{N_f}{2}+1}, \ldots, a_0, \ldots, a_{\frac{N_f}{2}}$. Die Rekonstruktion einer Kontur C_k aus $a_{-k}, \ldots, a_k$, $|k| \leq L$ und $a_k = 0$ für $|k| > L$ liefert dann eine geglättete Version der Kontur [3].

Durch die erreichte Dimensionsreduktion wird der Suchraum für eine iterative Optimierung reduziert. Ein Iterationsschritt berechnet dabei zu einem Set von Fourierdeskriptoren die Güte durch

1. Rekonstruktion einer Kontur C_k aus den Fourierdeskriptoren $a_{-k}, \ldots, a_k$.

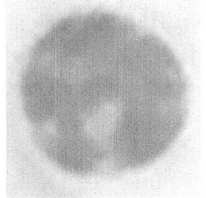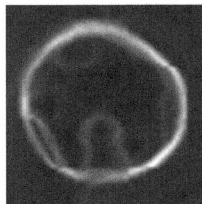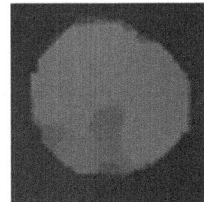

Abb. 1. Beispiel einer Feulgen gefärbten Zelle (links). Kantenbasierte Gütefunktion, berechnet durch Medianfilterung und Gradientenfilter (Mitte). Regionenbasierte Gütefunktion, berechnet durch Anisotrope Diffusion, kein Gradientenfilter (rechts).

Tabelle 1. Optimierung auf dem Trainingset. Zu jeder Methode ist der beste Filter und die optimierten Parameter angegeben, sowie die zugehörige Hausdorff-Distanz.

Algorithmus	Bester Filter und Parameter	Hausdorff-Distanz (μm)
Initiale Segmentierung		2.18
Fourierdeskriptoren	Median, L=3	1.27
Snakes	Median, $\sigma = 2, \alpha = 0.8, \beta = 0.6$	1.40
Chan Vese	Aniso. Diff., $\mu = -100$	1.54

2. Diskrete Berechnung des Linienintegrals über die Gütefunktion durch die Trapezregel und lineare Interpolation der Gütefunktion.
3. Normalisierung der Güte mittels Division durch die Länge der Kontur.

Die Fourierdeskriptoren werden dann durch eine Quasi-Newton Methode [5] auf maximale Güte hin optimiert. Die Normalisierung des Integrals (Punkt 3.) ist nötig, um unnötige Umwege der Kontur oder das mehrfache Durchlaufen der Kontur zu verhindern.

Die vorgestellte Methode wird mit parametrischen Aktiven Konturen (Snakes mit Gradient Vector Flow) [6, 7] und geometrischen Aktiven Konturen (Verfahren von Chan-Vese) [8] verglichen.

2.4 Evaluierung und Optimierung

Um die Gütefunktion zu evaluieren, wurde das Bild zunächst in zwei Klassen aufgeteilt. Für die kantenbasierte Gütefunktion ist die erste Klasse ein $0.58\,\mu$m breiter Ring um die Kontur des Goldstandards. Für die regionenbasierte Gütefunktion wird die Maske des Goldstandards als die erste Klasse verwendet. Die zweite Klasse ist das Komplement der ersten Klasse. Um die Trennbarkeit zwischen diesen beiden Klassen skalierungsinvariant zu bewerten, wurde das Otsu-Kriterium für die Grauwerte der beiden Klassen berechnet. Die Parameter für die verwendeten Filter wurden durch einen Brute-Force Ansatz ausgewählt. Für den Medianfilter wird die Fensterbreite des Filters und für die anisotrope Diffusion der Gewichtsfaktor K im Diffusionskoeffizienten optimiert.

Die Optimierung der Methoden zur Konturverfeinerung erfolgte ebenfalls durch einen Brute-Force Ansatz auf dem Trainingset. Tab. 1 zeigt die beste Filter- und Parameterkonfiguration mit der zugehörigen Hausdorff-Distanz. Für die Konturverfeinerung über Fourierdeskriptoren ist die Anzahl L der Fourierdeskriptoren zu wählen, hier wurden $L = 1$ bis $L = 20$ getestet. Die Anzahl der Samplingpunkte N_f wurde fest auf 200 gesetzt, um den Rechenaufwand gering zu halten. Parameter für die Snakes sind die Gewichte α und β in der internen Energie und das σ des Ableitungsfilters zur Berechnung des Gradient Vector Flows. Freier Parameter für das Chan-Vese Verfahren ist der Gewichtsterm μ, während die anderen Parameter des Energie-Funktionals auf die von Chan und Vese empfohlenen Parameter gesetzt werden [8]. Neben den Parametern für die entsprechende Konturverfeinerungsmethode wurden für die Berechnung

Tabelle 2. Ergebnisse auf dem Testset.

Algorithmus	Hausdorff-Distanz (um)	Dice	Zeit (sec)
Initiale Segmentierung	2.63	0.887	0.01
Fourierdeskriptoren	1.78	0.885	3.37
Chan Vese	1.97	0.900	2.83
Snakes	1.66	0.894	0.77

der Gütefunktion sowohl der beste Medianfilter als auch der beste anisotrope Diffusionsfilter verwendet.

Als Maße für die Segmentierungsgüte dienen der maximale Abstand zwischen den beiden Konturen (Hausdorff-Distanz) und der Dice Koeffizient für den Überlapp der beiden Masken. Als Kriterium für die Optimierung wurde die Hausdorff-Distanz verwendet.

3 Ergebnisse

Die besten kantenbasierten Gütefunktionen erhält man durch eine Medianfilterung mit einer Fenstergröße von 11 oder anisotrope Diffusion mit $K = 3$, für die regionenbasierte Gütefunktion ein Medianfilter mit Größe 13 oder anisotrope Diffusion mit $K = 5$. Durch Optimierung auf dem Trainingset wurden die Parameter für die Konturverfeinerungsmethoden ermittelt (Tab. 1). Auf diesem Datenset schneidet die Konturverfeinerung über Fourierdeskriptoren am Besten ab, mit einer Verkleinerung der Hausdorff-Distanz von $2.18\,\mu m$ auf $1.27\,\mu m$. Für die Rekonstruktion der Kontur aus den Fourierdeskriptoren werden dabei die Fourierkoeffizienten $a_{-3}, \ldots, a_3$ verwendet. Die beste Performance auf dem Testset lieferten die parametrischen Aktiven Konturen mit einer Hausdorff-Distanz von $1.63\,\mu m$ und einem Dice-Koeffizienten von 0.894. Weiterhin waren die Snakes mit durchschnittlich 0.77 Sekunden pro Objekt auch am Schnellsten (Tab. 2).

4 Diskussion

In dieser Veröffentlichung wurde ein Verfahren zur Konturverfeinerung basierend auf Fourierdeskriptoren vorgestellt, um Pathologen die manuelle Korrektur einer schlechten Segmentierung von Zellkernen in der Krebsfrühdiagnose zu ersparen.

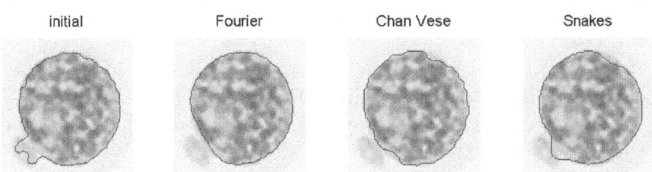

Abb. 2. Beispiel zur Verfeinerung der initial fehlgeschlagenen Segmentierung.

Während dieses Verfahren auf dem Trainingset die besten Ergebnisse lieferte, führte eine Konturverfeinerung durch parametrische Aktive Konturen auf dem Testset zum besten Ergebnis. Die Performance der Fourierdeskriptoren reicht nahe an die etablierten Snakes heran und ist besser als beim Verfahren von Chan Vese. Fourierdeskriptoren eignen sich deshalb gut für die hier vorgestellte Aufgabenstellung, da Zellkerne oft rundlich sind und die verwendeten Basisfunktionen im Fourierraum Kreise mit unterschiedlicher Oszillationsgeschwindigkeit beschreiben. Durch die Beschränkung der Rekonstruktion der Kontur aus wenigen Fourierkoeffizienten wird weiterhin direkt eine geglättete Kontur optimiert, so dass die Ergebnisse visuell oft ansprechend sind (Abb. 2).

Der Trade-off bei der vorgestellten Methode besteht in der Komplexität der darstellbaren Kontur und der Dimension des Suchraums für die Optimierung. Es wurden $L = 1, \ldots, 20$ Fourierdeskriptoren getestet, wobei die durchschnittlich beste Performance mit $L = 3$ Fourierdeskriptoren erreicht wurde. Häufigster Grund für eine unpräzise Segmentierung bei dieser Anzahl von Fourierdeskriptoren ist, dass sie nicht ausreicht um die Kontur komplexerer Zellkerne zu beschreiben. Werden jedoch mehr Fourierdeskriptoren verwendet, werden andere (lokale) Maxima als das der korrekten Kontur gefunden, da die Dimension des Suchraums für die Optimierung größer ist. Als zukünftige Arbeit schlagen wir deshalb einen Multiskalenansatz vor, bei dem zunächst mit wenigen Fourierdeskriptoren eine Kontur auf einem herunter skaliertem Bild gesucht wird. Diese dient dann als Initialisierung für eine weitere Verfeinerung auf dem Bild in Originalgröße mit einer erhöhten Anzahl von Fourierdeskriptoren.

Literaturverzeichnis

1. Remmerbach TW, Meyer-Ebrecht D, Aach T, et al. Towards a multimodal cell analysis of brush biopsies for detection of oral squamous cell carcinoma. Cancer Cytopathol. 2009;117(3):228–35.
2. Würflinger T, Stockhausen J, Meyer-Ebrecht D, et al. Robust automatic coregistration, segmentation, and classification of cell nuclei in multimodal cytopathological microscopic images. Comput Med Imaging Graph. 2004;28:87–98.
3. Jähne B. Practical handbook on image proc for scientific and technical applications. CRC Press; 2004.
4. Zhang D, Lu G. A comparative study of fourier descriptors for shape representation and Retrieval. Proc 5th Asian Conf Comp Vis. 2002; p. 646–51.
5. Broyden CG. The convergence of a class of double-rank minimization algorithms. IMA Journal of Applied Mathematics. 1970;6(1):76–90.
6. Kass M, Witkin A, Terzopoulos D. Snakes: active contour models. Int J Computer Vis. 1988;1:321–31.
7. Chenyang X, Prince JL. Gradient vector flow: a new external force for snakes. Proc IEEE Conf Comp Vis Pattern Recognit. 1997; p. 66–71.
8. Chan TF, Vese LA. Active contours without edges. IEEE Trans Image Process. 2001;VOL. 10, NO. 2:266–77.

Automated Co-Analysis of MALDI and H&E Images of Retinal Tissue for an Improved Spatial MALDI Resolution

Ralf Schönmeyer[1], Günter Schmidt[1], Stephan Meding[2,3], Axel Walch[2], Gerd Binnig[1]

[1]Definiens AG, München [2]Helmholtz Zentrum München, Research Unit Analytical Pathology, Neuherberg [3]University of Adelaide, Adelaide Proteomics Centre, Australia

rschoenmeyer@definiens.com

Abstract. MALDI imaging is a powerful technology to gain proteome information with high mass spectroscopic resolution from tissue slides. As its spatial resolution is lower than that of standard optical microscopy, improving the resolution to allow investigation of cell-sized objects is highly desirable. In this contribution we present an approach to virtually improve MALDI's spatial resolution in cases where the relevant structures have an approximately linear shape and can be transformed into a one-dimensional problem. By applying an automated image analysis to co-registered microscopy data, we can obtain the parameters necessary to support a MALDI-based modeling approach for investigating porcine retinal tissue.

1 Introduction

Matrix-assisted laser desorption/ionization imaging (MALDI) mass spectrometry is an emerging high-throughput label-free molecular analytical technology for spatially-resolved chemical analysis of samples, ranging from biological tissues to polymer films [1, 2]. In the long run it has the potential to deliver dignostic value from unstained tissue samples, which currently in clinical labs are investigated using specific stains [3].

To advance further developments, in this contribution MALDI imaging is used as a substantial part of a multi-modal investigation of mammalian retina that constitutes the basis for a comprehensive systems biology approach. The mammalian retina is chosen because its tissue displays a highly ordered histological and cellular stratification – cells are organized according to function and cross-sections exhibit a well-defined layered structure. The layers of interest, including photoreceptor layer and inner and outer nuclear layer, have a thickness of $\sim 50\,\mu m$ each. MALDI measurements are distributed over the tissue sample with a spatial resolution of $50\,\mu m$. Therefore applied native MALDI data does not allow for more precise observations of the inner structure of layers or their borders.

H.-P. Meinzer et al. (Hrsg.), *Bildverarbeitung für die Medizin 2013*, Informatik aktuell, DOI: 10.1007/978-3-642-36480-8_39, © Springer-Verlag Berlin Heidelberg 2013

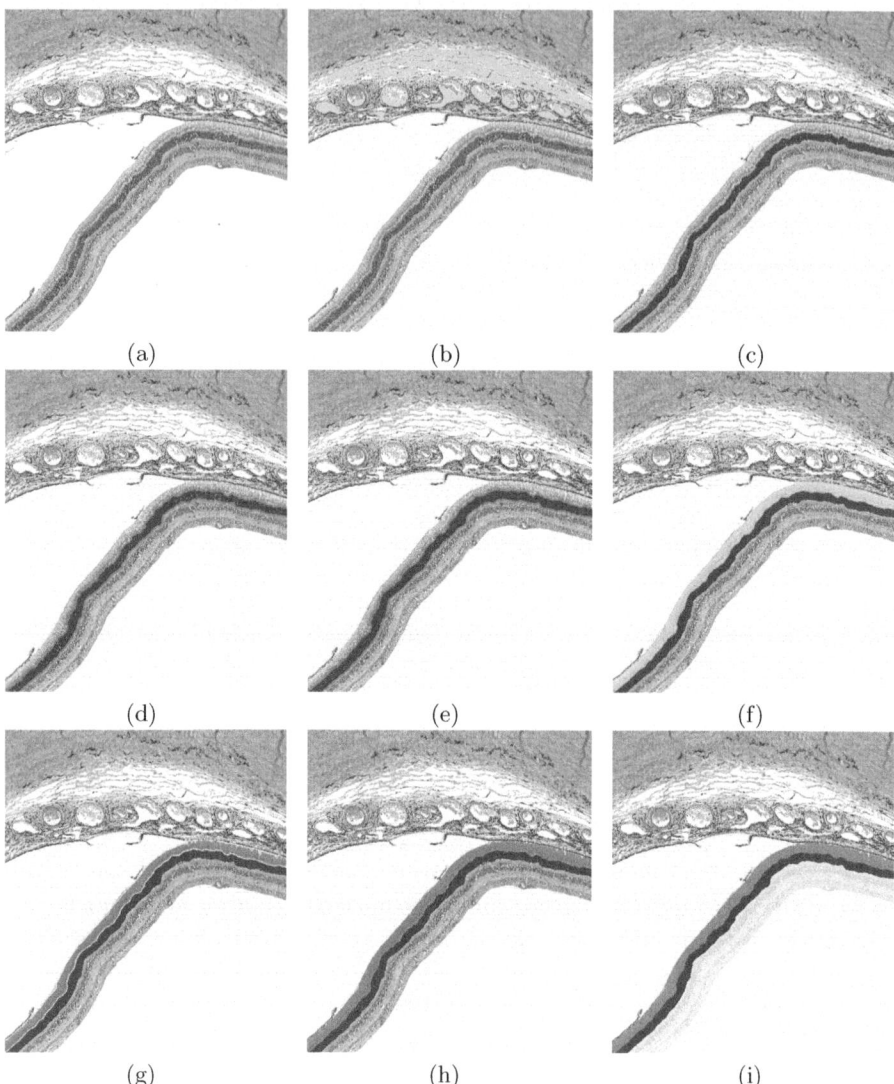

Fig. 1. (a) detail of an input image showing a cross-section from a H&E-stained porcine retina. (b) background (yellow) identification by thresholding and object size constraints. (c) identification of the outer nuclear layer (dark blue) by means of density of pixels within a defined hue and brightness range. (d) coat objects into vicinity of the outer nuclear layer (olive) to (e) smooth its surface by object density in this region. (f) prepare by directed flooding a region (light blue) to find the photoreceptor layer. (g) define layer borders (white) and (h) further form the photoreceptor layer by brightness and surface tension criteria. (i) resulting image includes segmentation of background (yellow), photoreceptor layer (orange), outer nuclear layer (dark blue) and inner layers (white).

Although there are MALDI techniques with higher spatial resolution, they currently do not meet mass spectrometric range and signal-to-noise ratio necessary for comprehensive protein analysis. Standard optical microscopy of tissue samples reaches a resolution below $1\,\mu$m. When slide scans are co-registered to MALDI measurements, we demonstrate that their spatial resolution can be virtually improved. The approach relies on automated image analysis of retinal layers and takes advantage of their structure, which is approximately one-dimensional. The results are used to evaluate spectral channels of MALDI measurements to discriminate between two groups of differently conditioned tissue samples.

2   Materials

Porcine eyes were obtained from a Munich slaughterhouse and transported to the laboratory, where they were cut in half (all in light-free environment). Both halves were Paxgene-fixed and embedded in paraffin – one in darkness and the other following exposure to light. Samples were cut into $4\,\mu$m sections using a microtom. A MALDI imaging protocol ($50\,\mu$m spatial resolution, mass spectrometry with 10k channels covering a range from 2kDa to 25kDa) was then applied, followed by hematoxylin and eosin (H&E) staining. Stained slides were scanned at 40x using a digital slide-scanning system (Mirax Desk, Carl Zeiss MicroImaging, Göttingen, Germany).

3   Methods

A research software prototype has been implemented based on Definiens Cognition Network Technology (CNT) [4, 5]. The software toolbox *Definiens Developer XD* is used to automatically segment and classify retinal layers of interest from H&E-stained slides and transfer resulting information to co-registered MALDI measurements. Registration is assigned by three manually set landmarks in each modality and affine coordinate transformation. On an upper hierarchical image analysis level tissue types – such as inner and outer nuclear layer as well as the photoreceptor layer – are found. Fig. 1 demonstrates the major processing steps which take ~1 minute per slide on a standard PC. On a lower hierarchical analysis level the system is also capable of detecting individual nuclei (data not shown). We use the fact that cross-sections of retinal tissue show a defined sequence of retinal layers. They can be seen as a one-dimensional system where centers of MALDI spots have a certain distance to a reference line – in our case the border line between the outer nuclear layer and the photoreceptor layer. This line and the corresponding distances of all MALDI spots are – as depicted in Fig. 2 (a) – automatically calculated and projected into a one-dimensional system where the reference line represents the origin. It is beneficial if the variation of distances is relatively large, rather than clustered around to a few values. Even for a regular sampling of MALDI spots this is given for the retina due to its moderate curvature. In the one-dimensional system we consider a range from $-50\,\mu$m to $+175\,\mu$m covering the layers of interest. Information from the MALDI mass spectra can then be calculated and plotted on a 2D graph, with the distance of each spectra on the x-axis and the corresponding spectral information on the y-axis. This is performed by data collection and processing with *Definiens Image Miner* software. To demonstrate our approach we have selected a prominent peak from the spectra and averaged the channel values within a small spectral range around it. The result is normalized by the mean of a broader channel range and plotted as the y-value on the 2D graph. The normalization of spectral data is necessary because absolute values of different MALDI measurements vary heavily in magnitude, even when taken from the same type of tissue. Fig. 3 shows such a diagram and it depicts the characteristics from two different sample groups.

4 Results

In total eight available slides were investigated – four light- and four dark-conditioned cases of retinal tissue. Overall, 11,968 MALDI measurements covered the region of interest containing functional retinal layers. These were automatically segmented and classified as described and results were transfered to co-registered MALDI spots. Fig. 2 (b) illustrates the distribution of spot positions and assigned classification results. A visual inspection confirmed the adequate accuracy of the classification results. Regions with non-consistent layer structure – caused by fissures or small wrinkles of the fragile retina tissue samples – were excluded manually from further processing. For the remaining 7,250

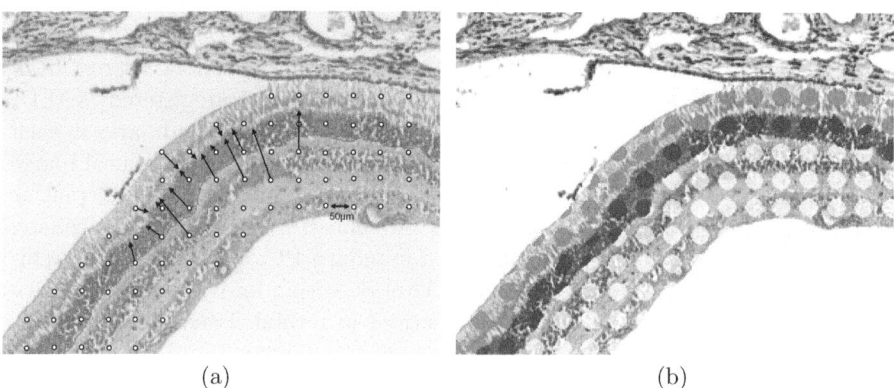

(a)   (b)

Fig. 2. Detail of H&E-stained retinal tissue with co-registered MALDI measurement: (a) yellow points indicate center positions of MALDI measurements and black arrows indicate their distance to the border between photoreceptor and outer nuclear layer (blue line) determined by automated image analysis. (b) for each MALDI spot also classification information in vicinity is linked: photoreceptor layer (orange), outer nuclear layer (blue), inner layers (white), and remaining layers not within region of interest (yellow).

spot positions 1,383 were classified as belonging to the photoreceptor layer, 1,221 to the outer nuclear layer and 4,646 to inner layers.

When the distance of each spot to the border between photoreceptor and outer nuclear layer was measured – the origin of the x-axis – it emerged that, within a range of $10\,\mu m$, 10 to 15 spectra were available. This is enough to resolve a spatial resolution of $\sim5\,\mu m$, which is ten times higher compared to native MALDI measurements. In Fig. 3 values of the selected spectral range for two groups of samples show a difference in characteristics. Plotted values were averaged and based on the available four dark- and four light- conditioned cases.

5 Discussion

In this contribution an automated segmentation and classification of layers from retinal tissue has been implemented to improve spatial resolution of MALDI mea-

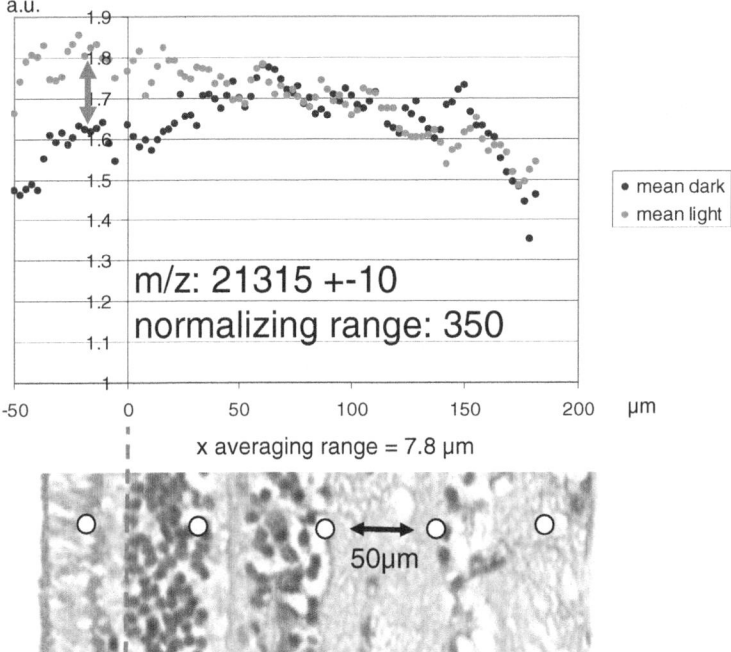

Fig. 3. Plot of two groups of cases (dark- vs. light-conditioned retina): spatial distance of MALDI spots on x-axis and a channel range covering $m/z = 21{,}315\pm10$ of a selected peak from MALDI spectrum on y-axis. Below cross-section of H&E-stained retinal tissue in corresponding scale to illustrate native distance of MALDI spots (yellow). The red dashed vertical line depicts the border between photoreceptor layer and outer nuclear layer as origin of x-axis in diagram. A difference between plots occurs especially in the region of the photoreceptor layer (indicated by red double arrow).

surements. By rapid prototyping with Definiens Cognition Network Technology relevant tissue type and distance parameters are gained. The image analysis works robustly on available tissue slides with sufficient accuracy for further processing. These results make it possible to plot values derived from MALDI spectra against the distance of each spot to a defined baseline. The projection of the spot positions to a one-dimensional system (x-axis) allows for greatly increased spatial resolution compared to original MALDI measurements: a factor of ten. When native MALDI resolution begins to approach those of optical microscopy, then the same methods can be applied to again increase MALDI's virtual resolution. Additionally, using this method MALDI measurements within the same distance to the baseline can be averaged. This helps to improve the signal-to-noise ratio of MALDI spectra compared to single measurements. Two groups of tissue slides (light- and dark-conditioned retina) were investigated for a selected spectral range. The resulting plots show a difference in their course between the two groups – especially in the region of the photoreceptor layer (left of the coordinates x-origin). This gives rise to the assumption that there is a specific mass spectroscopic profile in MALDI measurements across functional layers of retina in response to light and dark conditioning. Our results have inspired further investigations with advanced functional modeling which are currently under preparation and are already supporting assumptions. There, unlike to the data shown here, more than one channel range with a single peak from the MALDI spectrum is taken into account. Also aspects of an unknown convolution kernel from spatial dimensions and structure of MALDI measurements are regarded. Together with other quantitative measurements from image analysis, such as the density of nuclei in distinct nuclear layers, this constitutes valuable input data for an extended MALDI analysis that will help to better understand the retinal function using a comprehensive systems biology – and next-step systems medicine – approach.

Acknowledgement. Parts of the work presented here are funded by the German Federal Ministry for Education and Research (SysTec, grant 0315508).

References

1. Parker C, Smith D, Suckau D, et al. Mass Spectrometry-Based Tissue Imaging. Advanced Imaging in Biology and Medicine. 2009; p. 131–46.
2. Walch A, Rauser S, Deininger SO, et al. MALDI imaging mass spectrometry for direct tissue analysis: a new frontier for molecular histology. Histochem Cell Biol. 2008;130:421–34.
3. Meding S, Balluff B, Elsner M, et al. Tissue-based proteomics reveals FXYD3, S100A11 and GSTM3 as novel markers for regional lymph node metastasis in colon cancer. J Pathol. 2012; p. 10.1002/path.4021.
4. Schäpe A, et al. Fraktal hierarchische, prozeß- und objektbasierte Bildanalyse. Procs BVM. 2003; p. 206–10.
5. Athelogou M, Schönmeyer R, Schmidt G, et al. Bildanalyse in Medizin und Biologie. Medizintechnik – Life Science Engineering. 2008; p. 983–1005.

Fusion von Szintigrafie und CT für die Schilddrüsendiagnostik

Bastian Thiering[1,2], James Nagarajah[2], Hans-Gerd Lipinski[1]

[1]Biomedical Imaging Group, Fachbereich Informatik, Fachhochschule Dortmund
[2]Klinik für Nuklearmedizin, Universitätsklinikum Essen
thiering@biomedical-imaging.de

Kurzfassung. Für die Diagnose und Dignitätsabklärung von Schilddrüsenknoten wird auch heute noch routinemäßig ein Szintigramm verwendet. Um dieses planare, nur gering aufgelöste Bild der Radionuklidaktivität mit der realen Anatomie einer Schilddrüse abzugleichen, wurde ein Bilddatenfusionsverfahren entwickelt, das CT-Bilddaten mit dem Szintigramm verknüpft. Eine räumliche Rekonstruktion der Schilddrüse anhand von CT-Bilddaten wurde erstellt und diese in Richtung der Szintigrafie-Scanebene planar projiziert. Das dadurch erzeugte zweidimensionale Schilddrüsentopogramm wurde hinsichtlich seiner Größe, Lage und Form analysiert und mit der Größe, Lage und Form des Szintigramms mit Hilfe einer Kreuzkorrelation und einem Minimum-Abstandskriterium der Kontur beschreibenden Fourierdeskriptoren (FD) verglichen. Auf diese Weise wurde eine bestmögliche Projektionsrichtung gefunden, die mit der Lage und Form von SD-Topogramm und Szintigramm weitgehend korrelierten, so dass schließlich die aus den CT-Daten abgeleitete Schilddrüsenkontur und die korrespondierenden Szintigrammdaten fusioniert werden konnten.

1 Einleitung

In der Bundesrepublik Deutschland ist die Prävalenz von Schilddrüsenknoten > 1 cm mit etwa 20 % anzusetzen [1]. Die überwiegende Zahl dieser Knoten sind zwar benigne, jedoch kann ein Teil dieser Knoten auch entarten. Mit einer Inzidenz von etwa 3/100 000 gehört zwar das Schilddrüsenkarzinom zu den eher seltenen Tumorerkrankungen, jedoch zu den häufigsten des endokrinen Systems [2]. Nach wie vor führt in der klinischen Routine die klassische Szintigrafie zu relativ zuverlässigen Aussagen über die Entität eines Knotens [3]. Szintigrafisch warme Knoten sind praktisch nicht maligne, kalte jedoch können zu ca. 10 % maligne sein. Da viele Patienten häufig multiple Knoten aufweisen, ist eine genaue Lokalisation des kalten Knotens entscheidend. Leider stellt die konventionelle Szintigrafie lediglich eine zweidimensionale Projektion der Verteilung der Radionuklidaktivität dar. Somit ist ein direkter Vergleich von Szintigramm und Schilddrüsenorgan eingeschränkt. Ein möglicher Ansatz zur Behebung dieses Problems besteht in der Datenfusion von Szintigrafie und Computertomografie, wie sie bereits für andere Organe erfolgreich durchgeführt wurde [4]. Für

H.-P. Meinzer et al. (Hrsg.), *Bildverarbeitung für die Medizin 2013*, Informatik aktuell,
DOI: 10.1007/978-3-642-36480-8_40, © Springer-Verlag Berlin Heidelberg 2013

die Schilddrüse bietet sich eine formbasierte Bildanalyse der aus einem Computertomogramm gewonnenen räumlichen Organ-Rekonstruktion an, wobei die Organlage als ebenes projiziertes Topogramm (Anatomie) mit dem planaren Szintigramm (Funktion) zu verknüpfen ist.

2 Material und Methoden

Mit Hilfe eines konventionellen CT-Gerätes (Siemens Somatom Sensation 16) wurden axiale Bilder aus dem Schilddrüsenareal eines Patienten erzeugt (52 Scans, 512er Bildmatrix, 4,5 mm Schichtdicke). Vom gleichen Patienten wurde ein Szintigramm der Schilddrüse an einer dezidierten Schilddrüsenkamera (Intermedical, MiniCam, 128er Bildmatrix) nach Injektion von ca. 60 MBq 99m-Tc i.v. ca. 20 Min p.i. angefertigt. Die Daten wurden nach einer Bildvorverarbeitung und -analyse, fusioniert. Insgesamt wurden Bilddaten von 6 Patienten untersucht. Die für die Datenaufbereitung und -fusion erforderlichen Programme wurden in C++ unter Zuhilfenahme des ITK- und VTK-Frameworks für Windows®-Rechner entwickelt.

2.1 Bildvorverarbeitung, Segmentation und 3D-Rekonstruktion der CT-Bilddaten

Im Rahmen einer Bildvorverarbeitung wurden die auf die Schilddrüsenregion beschränkten CT-Bilddaten einer Datenglättung (Median- bzw. Gaußfilter) unterzogen. Empirisch hat sich durch visuelle Kontrolle gezeigt, dass mit einem Curvature Flow Image Filter die besten Ergebnisse erzielt werden konnten. Mit Hilfe einer globalen Grauwert-Schwellwertbildung wurde das Schilddrüsengewebe-Areal binärisiert und anschließend segmentiert (Methode: Region Growing Verfahren). Daraus wurde mit dem bekannten Marching-Cube-Verfahren das Schilddrüsenareal räumlich rekonstruiert und damit ein 3D-Modell der Schilddrüse generiert. Von diesem 3D-Modell der Schilddrüse wurde anschließend eine ebene Parallelprojektion (Topogramm) in frontaler Körperrichtung (Position des Szintigramms) durchgeführt. Dadurch entstand ein zweidimensionales binäres „Schatten"Bild der Schilddrüse (Binärwerte b_T(x,y)), deren Konturen ebenfalls gewonnen wurden (Methode: BinaryContourImageFilter mit Foreground- und Backgroundvalue sowie 8er-Freeman Chain Code). Für die Formcharakterisierung wurde zunächst die Rundheit ($Umfang^2/Fläche$) des SD-Topogramms ermittelt. Anschließend wurden aus den Konturdaten die zugehörigen Fourierdeskriptoren zur Formcharakterisierung der projizierten SD bestimmt [5]. Da die Bildvorverarbeitung und die Segmentation zu atypischen Konturveränderungen bei der Schilddrüse (Zunahme der Kontur-Rauheit) führten, wurden die Konturen durch eine Reduktion höherfrequenter Fourierdeskriptoren geglättet.

2.2 Bildvorverarbeitung und Segmentation der Szintigramme

Die ebenen Szintigramme wurden zunächst von einer unspezifischen Grundaktivität der Nuklidstrahlung befreit. Dazu wurden in Form einer Stichprobe (Anzahl

N_H ca. 20) typische Grauwerte g_H(x,y) aus diesem Bereich interaktiv ausgewählt und daraus ein mittlerer Hintergrundwert g_m bestimmt. Dieser wurde anschließend von den Grauwerten g_S(x,y) des Original-Szintigramms subtrahiert, wobei negative Differenzwerte gleich null gesetzt wurden. Damit konnte die bereinigte Radionuklid-SD-Aktivität als Grauwert g_R(x,y) bestimmt werden. Nachfolgend wurde zur Kontrastverbesserung eine Grauwertspreizung durchgeführt. Schließlich erfolgte eine Binärisierung der Grauwerte g_R mit Hilfe eines konventionellen Schwellwertfilters. Die Konturen dieses binären Szintigramms wurden mit Hilfe eines Kantendetektors ermittelt und daraus schließlich Form bestimmende Parameter (Rundheit, Fourierdeskriptoren) analog zum CT-Topogramm der Schilddrüse bestimmt.

2.3 Datenfusion

Die Datenfusion von CT-Topogramm und Szintigramm wurde auf der Basis der Flächendaten vom binären Topogramm b_T(x,y)) und modifiziertem Szintigramm (g_R(x,y)) und auch auf deren Konturdaten angewendet. Dazu wurde zuerst eine 2D-Kreuzkorrelation (KK) auf die Flächendaten angewendet und die resultierende KK-Funktion $\kappa_\mu(k, l)$ für die Projektion μ ermittelt

$$\kappa_\mu(k,l) = \sum_x \sum_y b_T(x,y) \cdot g_S(x+k, y+l) \tag{1}$$

Diese lieferte für jede vorgegebene Projektion μ jeweils k × l Korrelationswerte, deren Maximum bei bestmöglicher (Flächen-)Übereinstimmung von CT-Topogramm und Szintigramm im Ortsbereich auftritt. Als weitere Prüfgröße einer bestmöglichen Übereinstimmung zwischen CT-Topogramm und Szintigramm für eine Projektion μ diente eine Minimal-Abstandsquadratsummenbildung der Fourierdeskriptoren der Konturen von CT-Topogramm κ_T(r) und binärem Szintigramm κ_S(r)

$$\delta_\mu = \min \sum_{r=0}^{N-1} \left| \kappa_T(r) - \beta \cdot \kappa_S(r+\lambda)e^{j \cdot \Theta} \right|^2 \tag{2}$$

Hier wurden die FD der Schilddrüsenkontur mit der Szintigrammkontur so verglichen, dass unterschiedliche Skalierungen (β), Anfangspositionen (λ) und Rotationen ($e^{j \cdot \Theta}$, $j = \sqrt{-1}$) bei der Minimierung der Abstandsquadratsumme berücksichtigt werden konnten. Mit Hilfe der Größen κ_μ und δ_μ wurde diejenige Projektion μ_0 gefunden, bei der die Größe κ_μ maximal und die Größe δ_μ minimal waren. Diese Projektion wurde verwendet, um die CT-basierten Schilddrüsenkonturen schließlich mit dem Szintigramm zu verknüpfen.

3 Ergebnisse

In einem ersten Schritt gelang die räumliche Rekonstruktion der Schilddrüse aus den CT-Bildsequenzen (Methode: vtkMarchingCube). Die Abb. 1A zeigt exemplarisch die Rohform der 3D-Rekonstruktion, die Abb. 1B die gleiche Rekonstruktion nach erfolgter Oberflächenglättung (Methode: vtkSmoothPolyData). Mit einer vorgegebenen frontaler Projektionsrichtung wurde ein binäres 2D-Topogramm der Schilddrüse erzeugt, welches einen Schattenumriss der Schilddrüse darstellt (Abb. 1C). Aus diesem Topogramm ließ sich die Kontur mit Hilfe eines Kantendetektors (Methode: BinaryContourImageFilter mit Foreground- und Backgroundvalue) bestimmen. Die daraus ermittelten Konturkoordinaten ermöglichen die Bestimmung der zugehörigen Fourierdeskriptoren (FD). Im ausgewählten Beispiel wurden zur vollständigen Beschreibung der Kontur zunächst 128 FD-Paare verwendet (Abb. 1D). Zur Konturglättung erfolgte eine Reduktion auf 10 FD-Paare (Abb. 1E). Abschließend wurde auf der Basis dieser geglätteten Schilddrüsenkontur die projizierte Schilddrüsenfläche als Binärbild mit Hilfe eines Konturfüllungsoperators erzeugt (Abb. 1F). In einem zweiten Schritt wurde das Szintigramm aufbereitet. Dabei wurde das um die Hintergrundstrahlung bereinigte Szintigramm binärisiert (Abb. 1G) und daraus die Kontur bestimmt (Abb. 1H) (verwendete Bildverarbeitungsmethoden analog zum Topogramm). Die Rundheit der Schilddrüsenkontur wurde mit 25, die der geglätteten Kontur mit 20 und die des Binärszintigramms mit 12 ermittelt. In einem dritten Schritt wurde dann die Fusion von SD-Topogramm und Szintigramm durchgeführt, wobei das Szintigramm auf die CT-Größe skaliert wurde.

Danach wurde eine grob frontal vorgegebene Projektionsrichtung für das Topogramm der Schilddrüse zu den Hauptrichtungen der Projektionsebene (links-rechts-oben-unten) hin variiert und die zugehörigen Parameter κ_μ und δ_μ (in

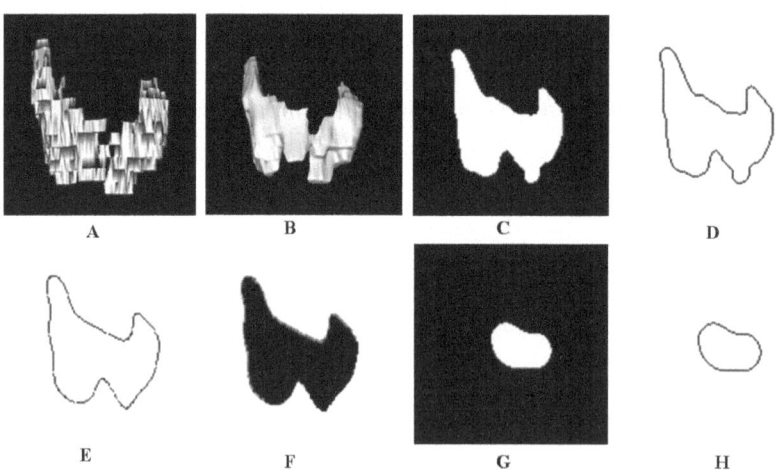

Abb. 1. Datenaufbereitung. 3D-Rekonstruktion der Schilddrüse als Rohversion (A) und nach Konturglättung (B), Projektion der Schilddrüsenumrisse in eine frontoplanare Ebene und Erzeugung sowohl eines zugehörigen SD-Topogramms (C) als auch deren Kontur vor (D) und nach Oberflächenglättung (E) sowie Füllen der geglätteten Kontur (F). Binärisiertes gefiltertes Szintigramm (G) und seine Kontur (H).

relativen Einheiten) ermittelt. Die Abb. 2A und 2 B zeigen zwei typische Beispiele für die Ergebnisse unterschiedlicher Projektionen, wobei gleichzeitig die Lage der Schilddrüsenkontur aus der 3D-Rekonstruktion und die Lage des binären Szintigramms eingeblendet wurden. Mit Hilfe der Parameter κ_μ und δ_μ wurde nun die bestmögliche Projektionsrichtung μ_0 ausgewählt. Die Abb. 2C zeigt die bildliche Überlagerung der Schilddrüsenkontur aus der CT-basierten Projektion und dem binärem Szintigramm, die Abb. 2D die finale Übertragung des Original-Szintigramms auf die Schilddrüsenkontur. Die relativen Werte der Parameter κ_μ und δ_μ in Abhängigkeit von der Projektion μ demonstriert die Abb. 2E. Sie zeigt die systematische Variation der Projektionsrichtung und den jeweiligen Korrelationswert, während der Scatterplot (Abb. 2F) die Zusammenhänge zwischen den Parametern $\max(\kappa_{\mu 0})$ und $\min(\delta_{\mu 0})$ für die insgesamt sechs untersuchten Patienten aufzeigt. Zwischen beiden Größen besteht hier offenbar eine ausgeprägte lineare Korrelation (Korrelationskoeffizient = - 0.914).

4 Diskussion

Nach wie vor spielt gerade in der Routinediagnostik von Schilddrüsenerkrankungen die klassische Szintigrafie eine wichtige Rolle. Die Schilddrüsenszintigrafie ist eine funktionelle Diagnostik und daher nicht immer mit der Anatomie der Drüse deckungsgleich. Klinisch relevant wird diese Problematik bei Patienten, die mehrere Knoten aufweisen und einer dieser Knoten in der Szintigrafie als „kalt"

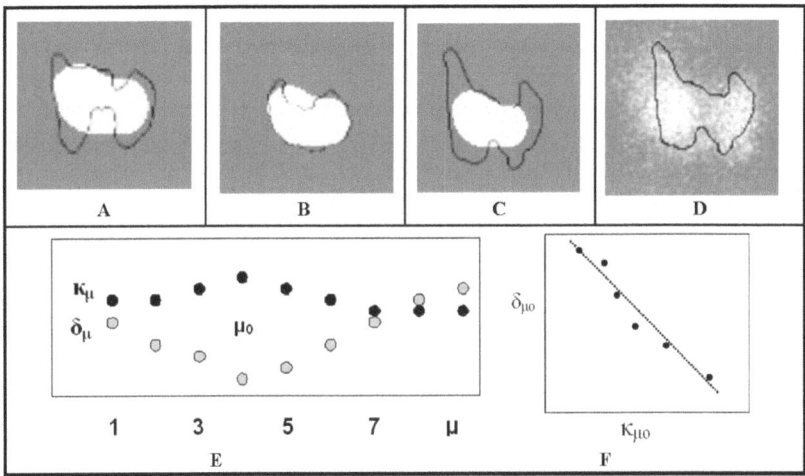

Abb. 2. Datenfusion. Überlagerung von binärem Szintigramm und Kontur des SD-Topogramms bei verschiedenen Projektionsrichtungen (A, B, C). Bestmögliche Projektion (C) und Überlagerung von SD-Kontur und Original-Szintigramm (D). Festlegung der bestmöglichen Projektion μ_0 bei $\mu = 4$ (Maximum von κ_μ und gleichzeitig Minimum von δ_μ) (E). Verteilung (Scatterplot) der Parameter $\kappa_{\mu 0}$ und $\delta_{\mu 0}$ für 6 analysierte Bilddatensätze (F).

und damit suspekt eingestuft wird. Ein solcher Knoten sollte weiter z.B. durch eine Feinnadelpunktion abgeklärt werden. Bei multinodösen Strumen ist jedoch die Identifikation des suspekten Knotens in einer Szintigrafie nicht trivial, da das Bild lediglich die Projektion der Schilddrüse darstellt. Daher ist ein Verfahren erforderlich, das eine Fusion von der Verteilung des radiaktiven Tracers und anatomischer Struktur ermöglicht. Die Computertomografie liefert die anatomische Bildinformation, so dass eine Datenfusion von (projiziertem) 2D-Topogramm der Schilddrüse (SD) und dem planaren Szintigramm möglich ist. Die CT-Bilddaten sind axial zwar mit einer Auflösung von 512x512 Pixel recht groß, die Schichtabstände jedoch relativ weit, so dass die 3D-Rekonstruktion zumindest in der z-Ebene eher ungenau ist. Da aber lediglich die Konturen der SD für die Projektion entscheidend sind und auch die räumliche Auflösung des konventionellen Szintigramms mit 128x128 Bildpunkten ebenfalls eher gering ist, erscheint die gewählte SD-Projektionsmethode ausreichend. Für die Fusion steht eine Reihe von klassischen Methoden zur Verfügung. Ausgewählt wurden die Kreuzkorrelation (KK) von binärem SD-Topogramm und dem Szintigramm und ein Abstandsmaß auf der Basis einer klassischen Gaußschen Abstandsquadratsummen-Minimierung. Mehrdimensionale KK sind häufig sehr rechenintensiv und damit auch zeitaufwändig. Da hier das 2D-Topogramm der Schilddrüse in binärer Form vorliegt, ist die Berechnung der Kreuzkorrelationsfunktion jedoch einfach durchzuführen und benötigt kaum Rechenzeit. Die erzielten Maxima der KK-Funktion sind hingegen nur schwach ausgeprägt. Daher erlaubt diese Methode allein keine sichere Datenfusion. Ergänzend zur KK wurde daher ein Form-basiertes Verfahren verwendet. Da klassische Formparameter, wie die Rundheit der Konturen von projizierter SD und Szintigramm, sich als zu unspezifisch erwiesen, wurde eine Formanalyse mit Hilfe von Fourierdeskriptoren durchgeführt. Dabei zeigte sich empirisch, dass sowohl eine elegante Kantenglättung der SD-Topografie möglich war als auch eine Abstandsquadrat-Minimierung der FD von SD-Topogramm- und Szintigrafie-Kontur durchaus deutliche Minima hinsichtlich einer variierten Projektionsrichtung des SD-Topogramms aufwies. In Kombination mit einer KK lieferte diese Methode brauchbare Ergebnisse für die Datenfusion, so dass eine Routineanwendung im Klinikbetrieb möglich erscheint.

Literaturverzeichnis

1. Völzke H, Lüdemann J, Robinson D, et al. The prevalence of undiagnosed thyroid disorders in a previously iodine-deficient area. Thyroid. 2003;13:803–10.
2. Görges R. The changing epidemiology of thyroid cancer. In: Biersack HJ, Grünwald F (eds). Springer. 2005;13:3–27.
3. Rosa GL, Belfiore A, et al . Evaluation of the fine needle aspiration biopsy in the preoperative selection of cold thyroid nodules. Cancer. 1991;67:2137–41.
4. Dickinson R, Erwin W, Stevens D, et al. Hybrid modality fusion of planar scintigraphy and CT topograms to localize sentinal lymph nodes in breast lymphoscintigraphy. Int J Mol Imaging. 2011.
5. Zahn C, Roskies R. Fourier descriptors for plane closed curves. IEEE Trans Comput. 1972;21(3).

Iterative CT Reconstruction Using Curvelet-Based Regularization

Haibo Wu[1,2], Andreas Maier[1], Joachim Hornegger[1,2]

[1]Pattern Recognition Lab (LME), Department of Computer Science,
[2]Graduate School in Advanced Optical Technologies (SAOT),
Friedrich-Alexander-University Erlangen-Nuremberg
haibo.wu@informatik.uni-erlangen.de

Abstract. There is a critical need to reconstruct clinically usable images at a low dose. One way of achieving this is to reconstruct with as few projections as possible. Due to the undersampling, streak artifacts degrade image quality for traditional CT reconstruction. Compressed sensing (CS) [1] theory uses sparsity as a prior and improves the reconstruction quality considerably using only few projections. CS formulates the reconstruction problem to an optimization problem. The objective function consists of one data fidelity term and one regularization term which enforce the sparsity under a certain sparsifying transform. Curvelet is an effective sparse representation for objects [2]. In this work, we introduce to use curvelet as the sparsifying transform in the CS based reconstruction framework. The algorithm was evaluated with one physical phantom dataset and one in vitro dataset and was compared against and two state-of-art approach, namely, wavelet-based regularization (WR) [3] and total variation based regularization methods (TVR) [4]. The results show that the reconstruction quality of our approach is superior to the reconstruction quality of WR and TVR.

1 Introduction

Computed tomography is used as a common examination tool in diagnosis and interventional procedures. However, increasing concerns about radiation exposure have been raised in recent years [5]. Recently, compressed sensing (CS) theory has been introduced [1]. CS asserts that the signal sampling rate which guarantees accurate reconstruction is proportional to the complexity of signal rather than its dimensionality. Most natural signals are well described by only a few significant coefficients in some domain, where the number of significant coefficients is much smaller than the signal size on an equally spaced grid. As such, the signals that are sparse or compressible can be recovered from very few measurements. Several CS based CT reconstruction algorithms have been proposed [3, 4, 6]. It has been found in these papers that the number of x-ray projections can be significantly reduced with little sacrifice in CT image quality. Thus, CS based reconstruction algorithm can reduce the radiation dose under the assumption that the dose is proportional to the number of x-ray projections.

H.-P. Meinzer et al. (Hrsg.), *Bildverarbeitung für die Medizin 2013*, Informatik aktuell,
DOI: 10.1007/978-3-642-36480-8_41, © Springer-Verlag Berlin Heidelberg 2013

A proper sparsifying transform is critical for CS based reconstruction methods. Recently, Candes, who proposed the CS theory, designed a efficient sparsifying transform which is called curvelet [2, 7]. The curvelet transform is a multi scale pyramid with many directions and positions at each length scale, and needle-shaped elements at fine scales. One feature of curvelet makes it very suitable for CS based reconstruction method. Let f_m be the m-term curvelet approximation to the object f, in other words, to represent object f using m largest curvelet coefficients. Then the approximation error is optimal for curvelet and no other sparsifying transform can yield a smaller error with the same number of terms. Therefore, curvelet transform is optimally sparse representation of objects with edges.

In this paper, we take curvelet transform as the sparsifying transform and compare it against two state-of-art sparsifying transforms, namely wavelet transform and total variation. One physical phantom and one in vitro dataset were used for evaluation.

2   Materials and methods

A discrete version of the CT scanning process can be described as

$$\boldsymbol{Ax} = \boldsymbol{b} \tag{1}$$

Here $A = (a_{ij})$ is the system matrix representing the projection operator, $\boldsymbol{x} = (x_1,..., x_n)$ represents the object and $\boldsymbol{b} = (b_1, ..., b_m)$ is the corresponding projection data. So to reconstruct the object $\boldsymbol{x}$ is to solve the linear system. In our case, the linear system is underdetermined due to the undersampling. There exist infinite solutions. As mentioned above, CS takes sparsity as prior knowledge, which formulates the reconstruction problem as

$$\min_{\boldsymbol{x}} ||\varPhi\boldsymbol{x}||_{\mathrm{L1}} \ s.t. \ ||\boldsymbol{Ax} - \boldsymbol{b}||_2^2 < \alpha \tag{2}$$

Here, α stands for the variance of the noise. $\varPhi$ is the sparsifying transform. In our work, $\varPhi$ is curvelet transform. WR and TVR use wavelet and total variation as the sparsifying transforms. The inequality constraint enforces the data fidelity and the L1 norm term promotes the sparsity. It is well known that the constrained optimization problem (2) can be transformed to an easier unconstrained optimization problem [3]

$$\min_{\boldsymbol{x}} ||\varPhi\boldsymbol{x}||_{\mathrm{L1}} + \beta||\boldsymbol{Ax} - \boldsymbol{b}||_2^2 \tag{3}$$

The dimension of (3) is very high. Therefore, we employed the forward-backward splitting method [3] to split (3)) to two sub-optimization problems which are easy to solve.

- *Step 1:* One step of gradient descent method to minimize $||\boldsymbol{Ax} - \boldsymbol{b}||_2^2$
- *Step 2:* Solve the optimization problem $\boldsymbol{x}' = \min ||\boldsymbol{x} - \boldsymbol{v}||_2^2 + \beta||\varPhi\boldsymbol{x}||_{\mathrm{L1}}$ ($\boldsymbol{v}$ is calculated from step 1 which is the volume estimation from step 1).

- *Step 3:* Repeat step 1 to step 2 until until L2 norm of the difference of the two neighboring estimate is less than a certain value or the maximum iteration number is reached.

To further speed up the optimization process, the SART reconstruction can be applied at Step 1. When the sparsifying transform Φ is invertible, a simple soft thresholding operator can be used to solve the objective function in step 2 [8]. The optimal solution of the objective function in Step 2 is:

a) Apply the sparsifying transform Φ on v, $x^a = \Phi v$.
b) Apply the soft thresholding operator

$$x_i^b = S(x_i^a, \beta) = \begin{cases} x_i^a - \beta & x_i^a > \beta \\ 0 & |x_i^a| < \beta \\ x_i^a + \beta & x_i^a < \beta \end{cases} \tag{4}$$

where $S(x_i^a, \beta)$ is the soft thresholding operator. x_i^b is the i-th element of x^b and x_i^a is the i-th element of x^a. The soft thresholding operator is applied element wisely on x^a to achieve the optimal solution of the objective function in step 2 [3].
c) Apply the inverse sparsifying transform on the results of step b.

When the sparsifying transform Φ is not invertible (e.g. total variation), simply soft thresholding operator could not solve the optimization problem in step 2. Several gradient descent steps are applied to solve the optimization problem in step 2. To sum up, the optimization algorithm for the method using invertible sparsifying transforms as the regularizer is:

- *Step 1:* One step of SART to minimize $||Ax - b||_2^2$
- *Step 2:* Apply the soft thresholding operator:
  - *Step 2.1:* Apply the sparsifying transform on the result of step 1.
  - *Step 2.2:* Apply the soft thresholding operator using (4).
  - *Step 2.3:* Apply the inverse sparsifying transform on the result of Step 2.2.
- *Step 3:* Repeat step 1 to step 2 until L2 norm of the difference of the two neighboring estimate is less than a certain value or the maximum iteration number is reached.

The optimization algorithm for the method using non-invertible sparsifying transforms as the regularizer is:

- *Step 1:* One step of SART to minimize $||Ax - b||_2^2$.
- *Step 2:* Apply k steps of sub-gradient descent method to solve $\min ||x - v||_2^2 + \beta ||\Phi_1 x||_1$ (v is calculated from step 1 which is the volume estimation from step 1).
- *Step 3:* Repeat step 1 to step 2 until L2 norm of the difference of the two neighboring estimate is less than a certain value or the maximum iteration number is reached.

k in Step 2 is usually a fixed number which can guarantee that the solution of Step 2 is accurately enough. We set $k = 3$ as in [4].

3   Results

We evaluate our algorithm on one physical phantom dataset (Siemens Cone-beam Phantom, QRM, Möhrendorf, Germany) and one in vitro dataset. Totally 496 projections within 200 degrees were acquired using a C-arm system (Artis Zeego C-arm systems, Siemens, Forchheim, Germany) for both physical phantom and in vitro dataset. Only 50 and 100 equally spaced projections were used to perform the reconstruction for the physical phantom and for in vitro dataset respectively. The resolution of the projection image is 1248 × 960 pixels with a pixel size of 0.31 × 0.31 mm^2. In the experiment, we reconstructed the center slice with the size of 512 × 512 pixels. The pixel size is 0.49 × 0.49 mm^2. For further evaluation, we also reconstructed the image using WR and TVR. The parameter setting of all methods were chosen according to that the final reconstructions contain the same level of noise. The noise level was denoted by the

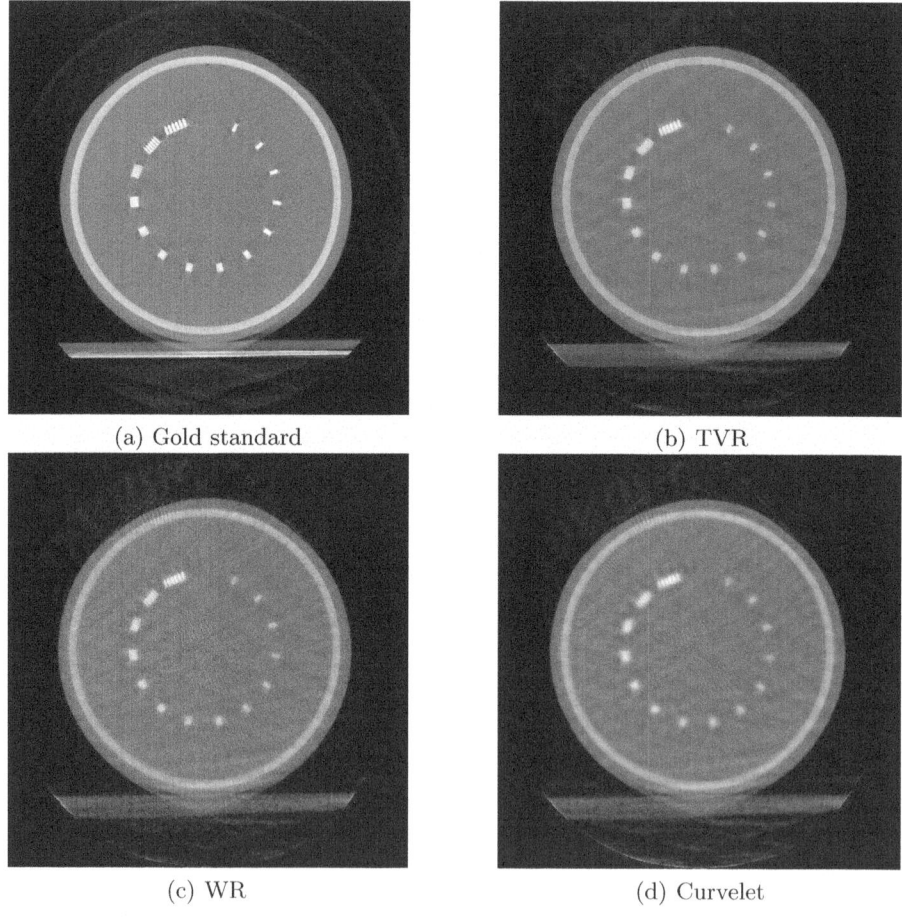

(a) Gold standard   (b) TVR

(c) WR   (d) Curvelet

Fig. 1. Reconstruction results of the physical phantom.

standard derivation of a homogeneous area which is marked with black rectangle in Fig. 1 and Fig. 2. We set parameters in this way because that the datasets used for all methods are the same. Therefore the noise level of the reconstructions should be same. The reconstruction results of the physical phantom are in Fig. 1 and the reconstruction results of in vitro dataset are in Fig. 2. However, TVR introduce the carton-like artifacts. The reconstruction results of WR contains the blocky artifacts (red rectangle in Fig. 2) The reconstruction results of our method do not contain carton-like artifacts.

For qualitative evaluation, we calculated the correlation coefficients of the reconstructions for each method

$$r = \frac{\sum_{n}(x_i - \bar{x})(x_i^{\text{true}} - \bar{x}^{\text{true}})}{\sqrt{\sum_{n}(x_i - \bar{x})^2(x_i^{true} - \bar{x}^{\text{true}})^2}} \tag{5}$$

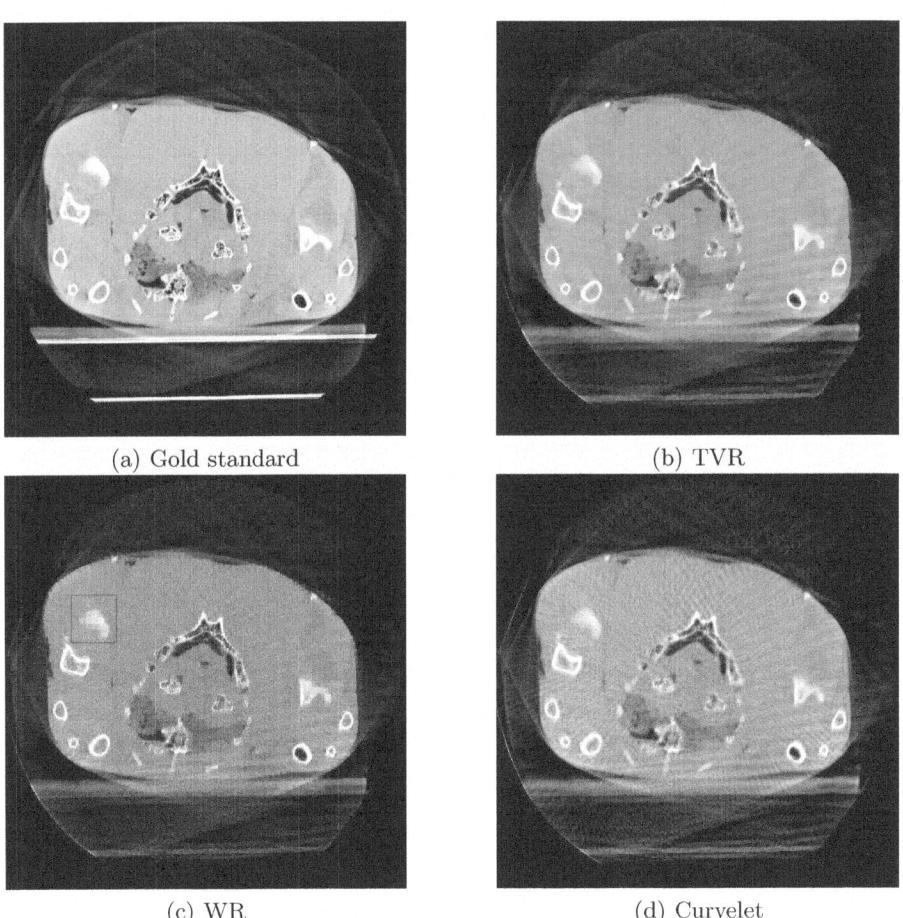

(a) Gold standard   (b) TVR

(c) WR   (d) Curvelet

Fig. 2. Reconstruction results of in vitro dataset.

Table 1. Reconstruction error.

	TVR	WR	Curvelet
Correlation coefficient of physical phantom reconstruction	96.68%	96.59%	96.78%
Correlation coefficient of in vitro dataset reconstruction	94.21%	93.99%	94.34%

x^{true} is the gold standard which is the image reconstructed by FDK using all projections in our experiments. The results can be found in Tab. 1. The similar conclusion can be drawn. The reconstruction results of our approach is superior to the other methods.

4 Discussion

CS uses sparsity as a prior. Therefore, a proper sparse transform is crucial in CS based reconstruction algorithms. Curvelet transform employing directional filter bank is very efficient in encoding images with edges. Often, medical images contain many edges. Therefore, it is quite suitable for CS based reconstruction algorithms. In this work, we introduced the curvelet transform to the CS based reconstruction framework. The experiments show that our approach shows superior image quality compared to the other methods. In addition, since curvelet transform is invertible, the optimization algorithm for our method is simpler than TVR which is the state-of-art CS based reconstruction method.

References

1. Donoho DL. Compressed sensing. IEEE Trans Inf Theory. 2006;52(4):1289–306.
2. Starck JL, Candès EJ, Donoho DL. The curvelet transform for image denoising. IEEE Trans Image Process. 2002;11(6):670–84.
3. Yu H, Wang G. SART-type image reconstruction from a limia fast and accurate method to solveted number of projections with the sparsity constraint. Int J Biomed Imaging. 2010;2010:3.
4. Sidky EY, Pan X, Reiser IS, et al. Enhanced imaging of microcalcifications in digital breast tomosynthesis through improved image-reconstruction algorithms. Med Phys. 2009;36:4920.
5. Brenner DJ, Hall EJ. Computed tomography: an increasing source of radiation exposure. N Engl J Med. 2007;357(22):2277–84.
6. Wu H, Maier A, Fahrig R, et al. Spatial-temporal total variation regularization (STTVR) for 4D-CT reconstruction. SPIE. 2012;8313:83133J.
7. Starck JL, Candès EJ, Donoho DL. The curvelet transform for image denoising. IEEE Trans Image Process. 2002;11(6):670–84.
8. Donoho DL. De-noising by soft-thresholding. IEEE Trans Inf Theory. 1995;41(3):613–27.

Simulationsgestützte Operationsplanung bei angeborenen Herzfehlern

Separation virtueller chirurgischer Eingriffe vom Simulationsmodell

Stefan Kislinskiy[1], Tomás Golembiovský[2,3], Christian Duriez[3],
Eugénie Riesenkampff[4], Titus Kuehne[4], Hans-Peter Meinzer[1], Diana Wald[1]

[1]Deutsches Krebsforschungszentrum Heidelberg, Deutschland
[2]Fakultät für Informatik der Universität Masaryk, Brno, Tschechische Republik)
[3]Inria Lille – Nord Europe, Lille, Frankreich
[4]Deutsches Herzzentrum Berlin, Deutschland
s.kislinskiy@dkfz.de

Kurzfassung. Operationen an angeborenen Herzfehlern bei Kleinkindern sind oft aufgrund komplexer und heterogener Krankheitsbilder sehr herausfordernd. Gegenwärtig können Herzchirurgen lediglich nichtinvasive Bildgebung zur Operationsplanung heranziehen. Wir möchten die Operationsplanung durch ein Simulationssystem verbessern, mit dessen Hilfe Eingriffe simuliert und deren Resultate in ausreichender Genauigkeit schon vor der eigentlichen Operation vorhergesagt werden können. Wir nutzen hierfür eine Simulationsmethode basierend auf finiten Schalenelementen. Um die gesamte Methode unabhängig vom konkreten Simulationsmodell entwickeln zu können, muss diese unabhängig von Eingriffen wie dem Schneiden und Nähen sein. Wir zeigen einen neuen Ansatz zur Trennung dieser bisher voneinander abhängigen Komponenten. Das Simulationssystem kann somit unverzüglich von verbesserten Simulationsmodellen profitieren. Dieser Ansatz führt jedoch zusätzliche Anforderungen beim Neuvernetzen der simulierten Objekte ein.

1 Einleitung

Chirurgische Interventionen bei Kleinkindern mit von Geburt an missgestalteten großen Blutgefäßen und Herzen sind in der Regel sehr anspruchsvoll aufgrund komplexer und heterogener Krankheitsbilder. Herzchirurgen nutzen nichtinvasive Bildgebung zur patientenspezifischen Begutachtung und skizzieren präoperativ verschiedene Ansätze für mögliche Eingriffe. Dennoch wird der erfolgversprechendste Ansatz und dessen Details oft erst während der eigentlichen Operation am offenen Herzen ermittelt, da der Chirurg nun konkretere Vorstellungen der möglichen Resultate hat. Die endgültige Entscheidung bei Verwendung einer Herz-Lungen-Maschine wird dadurch erschwert, dass sich die genaue Formänderung durch den Eingriff nur schwer bildlich vorstellen lässt. Wichtige Entscheidungen müssen in kurzer Zeit getroffen werden und sind von der Erfahrung des Chirurgen abhängig.

H.-P. Meinzer et al. (Hrsg.), *Bildverarbeitung für die Medizin 2013*, Informatik aktuell,   235
DOI: 10.1007/978-3-642-36480-8_42, © Springer-Verlag Berlin Heidelberg 2013

Die Planung für pädiatrische Herzchirurgie kann durch die Verwendung von Herzmodellen verbessert werden, die auf patientenspezifischen Bilddaten basieren. Diese können aufbereitet als Input für entsprechende Simulationssysteme verwendet werden. Der Fokus bisheriger Simulationssysteme im Kontext liegt auf der Ausführung einzelner Schritte wie dem Schneiden und Nähen von Gewebe [1, 2]. Hierbei sind Echtzeitsimulationen höher priorisiert als akkurate Verformung von Gewebe und Blutgefäßen, um die Interaktion mit haptischen Eingabegeräten zu ermöglichen.

Um Resultate komplexer chirurgischer Eingriffe durch Simulationen vorhersagbar zu machen, sind geeignetere Simulationsmethoden wie z.b. die Methode der finiten Elemente (FEM) vonnöten. [3] stellt solch ein Simulationssystem für bidirektionale Glenn-Shunts vor. Die Autoren nutzen ein Hybridmodell zur Simulation von Deformationen der großen Blutgefäße. Dabei wird ein Oberflächen-modell elastisch mit Cosserat-Stäben verbunden, die globale Verformungen der Blutgefäße simulieren. Die Resultate sind vielversprechend, jedoch ist die Methode auf Operationen an relativ gleichförmigen tubulären Strukturen beschränkt und ermöglicht nicht die beliebige Manipulation von deren Oberflächen. Das Nähen von Blutgefäßen und Patchmaterial wird durch das anbringen virtueller, sich zusammenziehender Federn gelöst. Die zugrundeliegende Simulationsmethode muss in ihren Gleichungen angepasst werden, da diese Feder-Hilfskonstrukte u.a. überschüssige Energie erzeugen.

Wir stellen eine neue Methode für die vorhersagende Simulation von Operationen an angeborenen Herzfehlern vor, die ohne Erweiterungen der Gleichungen des zugrundeliegenden Simulationsmodells auskommt und somit komplett unabhängig von dieser ist. Das gesamte Simulationssystem kann somit schnell von neuen und verbesserten Simulationsmodellen profitieren, die nicht erst angepasst oder erweitert werden müssen. Durch die Nutzung von SOFA [4], einem modularen Framework für biomechanische Simulationen, können wir auch praktisch einen Nutzen aus dieser Unabhängigkeit ziehen.

2 Material und Methoden

FEM sind Verfahren, um Verformungen elastischer Körper physikalisch akkurat zu berechnen. Schalenelemente sind zweidimensionale finite Elemente mit festgelegter Dicke, die als Parameter in die Berechnungen einfließt. Aufgrund ihrer Eigenschaften sind sie gut für dünnwandige Strukturen wie Blutgefäße in Kleinkindern geeignet. Detaillierte Beschreibungen können in der Referenzliteratur nachgeschlagen werden [5, 6]. Um einen flüssigen Arbeitsablauf bei einer virtuellen Operation zu erreichen, reduzieren wir die Simulationen auf ein Minimum. Anstatt das Schneiden und Nähen während der Simulation durchzuführen, legen Chirurgen essentielle Eigenschaften der nächsten Manipulation (z.B. Lage und Länge von Schnitten) zwischen den Simulationen fest. An die Simulationen werden nur topologische Veränderungen übergeben und basierend darauf die Verformungen der Blutgefäße berechnet. Der gesamte Prozess ist in Abb. 1 dargestellt.

Die neuartige Methode zum Verbinden der Simulationselemente lässt sich konzeptionell in die Zuordnung der Ausgangsformen des simulierten Objekts vor der Simulation und die Relaxation während der Simulation aufteilen und wird im Folgenden beschrieben.

2.1 Zuordnung von Ausgangsformen vor der Simulation

Wir verbinden die ursprüngliche Ausgangsform x_0 eines Objekts topologisch vor der Simulation durch die Vereinigung der Vertices entlang der zu verbindenden Kanten. Dieses Netz definiert eine künstliche Ausgangsform x und hat durch die Vereinigung zwar weniger Vertices als x_0, jedoch die selbe Anzahl an Elementen. Die 1:n-Zuordnung der Vertices zwischen x und x_0 muss gespeichert werden, so dass adjazente Elemente all ihre Vertices in beiden Netzen x und x_0 referenzieren können.

Die Erstellung einer künstlichen Ausgangsform x und die Zuordnung zu ihrer Ausgangsform x_0 ist in Abb. 2 dargestellt. Aus Gründen der Übersichtlichkeit wurde ein minimales Szenario zur Veranschaulichung gewählt (das Konzept lässt sich auf beliebig komplexe Simulationsszenarien übertragen). Zwei zweidimensionale elastische Bänder, die auf ihren gegenüberliegenden Seiten fixiert sind, sollen miteinander verbunden werden. Die Vertices entlang der zu verbindenden Kante haben 1:2-Zuordnungen, die durch die Pfeile in Abb. 2 angedeutet werden. Durch die Zuordnung kann jedes Element von x auch seine zugehörigen Vertices in x_0 referenzieren.

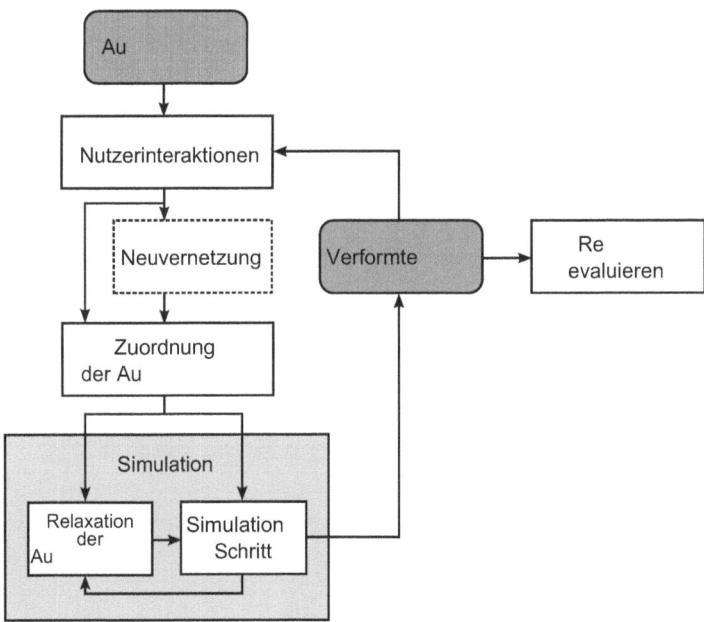

Abb. 1. Übersicht über den kompletten Simulationsprozess.

2.2   Relaxation der künstlichen Ausgangsform während der Simulation

Im Allgemeinen beginnt eine Simulation, in der die Form von x gegen die ursprüngliche Form x_0 strebt, mit einem relativ großen räumlichen Unterschied zwischen x_0 und x. Daraus resultieren unverzüglich sehr hohe interne Kräfte in den Elementen der Umgebung. Um eine exzessive Deformation und numerische Instabilitäten zu vermeiden, generieren wir daher eine zweite künstliche Ausgangsform y_0. Diese ist räumlich deckungsgleich zu x, jedoch topologisch identisch zu x_0, da die Vertices entlang der zu verbindenden Kante nicht miteinander verbunden sind. Die künstliche Ausgangsform y_0 wird der Simulation anstelle der ursprünglichen Ausgangsform x_0 übergeben. Durch die initiale Kongruenz zur ebenfalls künstlichen momentanen Form x befindet sich das Objekt im energetischen Beharrungszustand. Während der Simulation relaxieren wir die Ausgangsform y_0 zurück zu x_0 und die momentane Form x strebt kontrolliert gegen die interpolierte Ausgangsform. Dies geschieht mit linearer Interpolation der Vertexpositionen und linearer sphärischer Interpolation (Slerp) der Vertexorientierungen. Sobald die Relaxation abgeschlossen ist, befindet sich die Simulation in einem Zustand, im dem die Verbindung der Objekte vollends abgeschlossen ist und fährt noch so lange fort, bis nachschwingende Deformationen zur Ruhe kommen und sich das Objekt somit im energetischen Beharrungszustand befindet. Im Unterschied zu einer klassischen Simulation verändern wir also die Ausgangsform jeden Simulationsschritt, anstatt nur zu Beginn eine statische Ausgangsform zu übergeben, gegen die die momentane Form konvergiert.

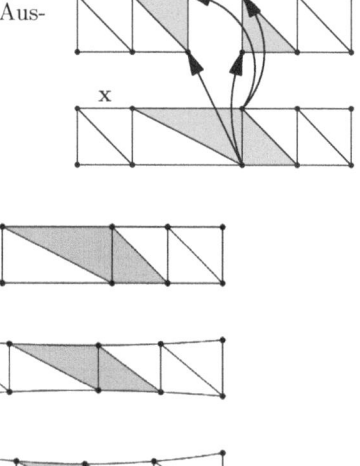

Abb. 2. Erstellung der topologisch verbundenen Ausgangsform x und ihre Zuordnung zur ursprünglichen Ausgangsform x_0.

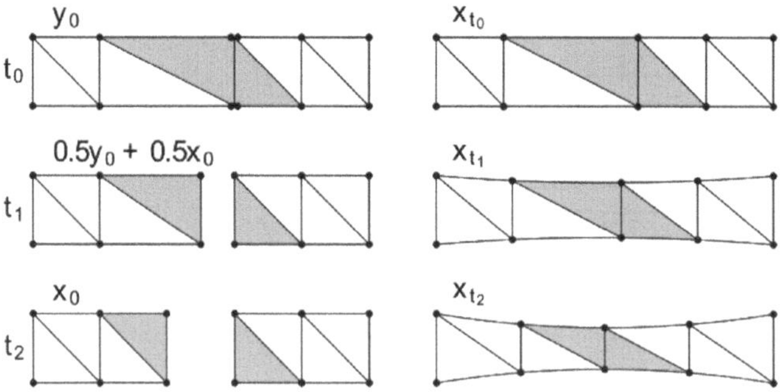

Abb. 3. Ausgangsform (links) und momentane Form (rechts) für drei Zeitschritte t_0 bis t_2 aus der Simulation.

Das Beispiel aus Abb. 2 wird in Abb. 3 fortgesetzt um den Relaxations-
prozess zu veranschaulichen. Die Ausgangsform y_0 und momentane Form x des
Objekts werden jeweils nebeneinander für drei Zeitschritte t_0 bis t_2 gezeigt, die
den Anfang, die Mitte und das Ende des Simulationsdurchlaufs zeigen. Während
y_0 extern manipuliert und für jeden Zeitschritt der Simulation angepasst wird,
strebt die Simulation entsprechend ihres normalen Funktionsprinzips nach einem
energetischen Minimum der Form x bezogen zur Ausgangsform des Objekts (zu
Beginn y_0, am Ende x_0).

3 Ergebnisse

Basierend auf realen Bilddaten einer Koarktation der Aorta eines Kleinkindes haben wir manuell ein sehr regelmäßiges Simulationsobjekt modelliert, mit dessen
Hilfe wir einen praktischen Machbarkeitsnachweis unserer Methode mit einem
ersten Software-Prototypen durchführen können. Eine Neuvernetzung des Objekts zwischen Simulationsdurchläufen kann so vorübergehend vermieden werden. Schnitte können entsprechend nur entlang bereits vorhandener Kanten erfolgen und es können nur Ränder miteinander verbunden werden, die die gleiche
Anzahl an Vertices aufweisen (Abb. 4).

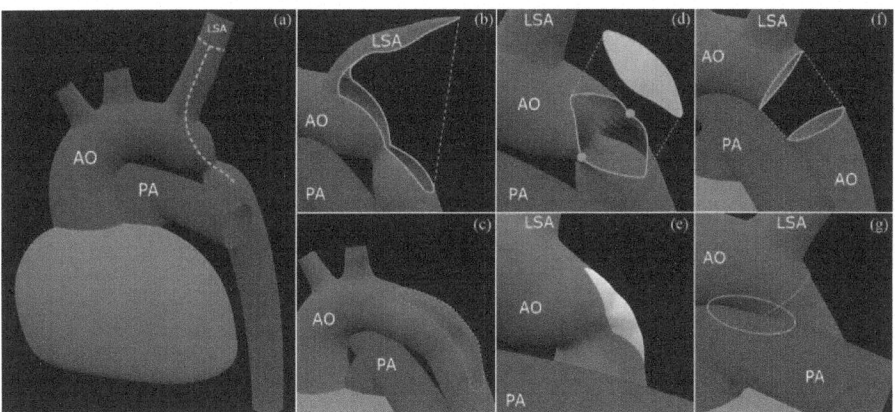

Abb. 4. Mit Skizzen überlagerte Bildschirmaufnahmen unseres Simulationsprototy-
pen für verschiedene Operationen einer Aortenkoarktation. (a) Übersicht der Szene,
bestehend aus Aortenbogen (AO), der linken Ateria subclavia (LSA) und der Pulmo-
nalarterie (PA). (b, c) Waldhausen-Prozedur – Die LSA wird als organischer Patch
verwendet um die Koarktation zu erweitern. (d, e) Patch-Aortoplastie – Ein Patch
wird in die Koarktation eingenäht. (f, g) Ende-zu-Ende-Anastomose – Die Koraktation
wird reseziert und die losen Enden der Aorta zusammengenäht.

4 Diskussion

Wir konnten zeigen, dass unsere neue Methode zum Verbinden von Simulations-objekten praktisch anwendbar und unabhängig vom verwendeten Simulations-modell ist. Nach unserer Kenntnis ist dies das erste Mal, dass das zugrundeliegen-de Simulationsmodell austauschbar ist und unabhängig entwickelt werden kann, was einen immensen Wert für die praktische Entwicklung eines Simulationssy-stems für den klinischen Einsatz darstellt. Auf zurzeit noch fehlende geeignete prä- und postoperative Bilddaten bei Säuglingen und Kleinkindern zu Evalua-tionszwecken kann besser reagiert werden. Auch rheologische Eigenschaften von deren Blutgefäßen müssen erst noch ermittelt werden. Beides hat starken Ein-fluss auf das Simulationsmodell selbst, während alle anderen Komponenten des Simulationssystems bereits parallel entwickelt werden können. Ein für FEM ge-eignetes Verfahren zur Neuvernetzung für die simulierten Objekte muss noch ausgewählt und um die Anforderungen erweitert werden, die unsere vertexba-sierte Methode impliziert – zu verbindende Ränder müssen die gleiche Anzahl an Vertices aufweisen sowie jeweils den gleichen Abstand zwischen den Kanten ent-lang dieser Ränder haben. Würden sich unterschiedliche Kantenlängen während der Relaxation annähern, würde dies zu unerwünschten Verformungen innerhalb der Elemente kommen, da deren innere Kräfte durch die Unabhängigkeit unserer Methode nicht direkt manipuliert werden dürfen.

Literaturverzeichnis

1. Sørensen TS, Greil GF, Hansen OK, et al. Surgical simulation: a new tool to evaluate surgical incisions in congenital heart disease? Interact Cardiovasc Thorac Surg. 2006;5(5):536–9.
2. Mosegaard J. LR–Spring Mass model for cardiac surgical simulation. Proc MMVR. 2004; p. 256–8.
3. Li H, Leow WK, Chiu IS. Predictive Simulation of Bidirectional Glenn Shunt Using a Hybrid Blood Vessel Model. Proc MICCAI. 2009;5762:266–74.
4. Allard J, Cotin S, Faure F, et al. SOFA: an open source framework for medical simulation. Proc MMVR. 2007;15.
5. Comas O, Cotin S, Duriez C. A Shell Model for Real–Time Simulation of Intra–ocular Implant Deployment. Biomed Sim. 2010;5958:160–70.
6. Comas O, Duriez C, Cotin S. Shell model for reconstruction and real-time simulation of thin anatomical structures. Proc MICCAI. 2010;6362:371–9.

Structure-Enhanced Visualization for Manual Registration in Fluoroscopy

Matthias Hoffmann[1], Felix Bourier[2], Norbert Strobel[3], Joachim Hornegger[1,4]

[1]Pattern Recognition Lab, Friedrich-Alexander-Universität Erlangen-Nürnberg, Erlangen, Germany
[2]Krankenhaus Barmherzige Brüder, Regensburg, Germany
[3]Siemens AG, Healthcare Sector, Forchheim, Germany
[4]Erlangen Graduate School in Advanced Optical Technologies (SAOT), Erlangen, Germany
matthias.hoffmann@cs.fau.de

Abstract. Electrophysiology procedures are in many cases performed under fluoroscopic guidance. As the heart is not visible under fluoroscopy, a preoperatively acquired heart model of the patient may be fused with the live X-ray images to provide the physician with a better orientation. This heart model needs to be registered to the fluoroscopic images. Currently, registration is performed manually, e.g., after contrast injection into the left atrium during atrial fibrillation procedures. We propose a novel visualization of the heart model that shows the same structures as the contrast agent and allows an easy identification of corresponding landmarks and features in both the model and the angiography images.

1 Introduction

Pulmonary vein isolation is the standard treatment of paroxysmal atrial fibrillation (Afib) [1]. Afib is the most common heart arrhythmia affecting more than 2.2 million people in the US alone [2]. Ablation is usually performed under fluoroscopic guidance using a C-arm system. Unfortunately, fluoroscopy shows only the catheters, while the left atrium remains invisible without the injection of contrast agent. A mapping system [3] can be used to generate a model of the left atrium and to show the position of the catheters with respect to this model. Their use, however, increases the cost of the intervention. Besides or in addition to using a mapping system, the orientation of the physician can also be improved by fusing the live X-ray images with a 3-D heart model of the patient. A 2D image of this model can be rendered using the same camera perspective as the fluoroscopic system. This image is used as overlay for the fluoroscopic images and provides an outline of the patients heart [4, 5]. The 3-D heart model is in many cases acquired preoperatively using CT or MRI. Since the patient is not positioned exactly the same way during acquisition of the model and intervention, the 3-D heart model has to be registered to the coordinate system

H.-P. Meinzer et al. (Hrsg.), *Bildverarbeitung für die Medizin 2013*, Informatik aktuell,
DOI: 10.1007/978-3-642-36480-8_43, © Springer-Verlag Berlin Heidelberg 2013

of the fluoroscopic system. This applies also if the patient moves during the intervention.

Currently, registration is performed by capturing a biplane fluoroscopic sequence while contrast agent is injected into the left atrium. The contrast agent flows through the heart and outlines the structure of the left atrium. Then, the overlay's position is adjusted until it fits to the structure shown by the contrast agent.

Unfortunately, there may be cases, where the whole shape of the left atrium is not well outlined by the contrast agent. This is because the contrast is used sparingly since contrast puts a burden on the kidneys. So, it may not reach all areas of the left atrium. It also mixes rapidly with the blood inside the left atrium often leaving only a diffuse shadow of its anatomy. The most dominant structures highlighted by the contrast agent are edges in the left atrium.

Current fluoroscopy overlays depict a rendering of the heart model. To reveal internal structures, techniques such as adaptive clipping techniques [6] can be used. The overlay may occlude the view to the fluoroscopic image. Increasing the transparency of the overlay usually improves the visibility of the fluoroscopic image. However, the edges of the pulmonary veins and other important features are more difficult to see such that it predominantly shows the outline of the heart. Also the identification of corresponding parts of the heart model in the two views requires an experienced user.

We present a novel overlay that helps also unexperienced users to achieve reliable alignment of the heart model to the structures highlighted by the contrast agent. The overlay highlights edges that potentially could be outlined by contrast agent. The edges are colored according to their position in 3-D space such that an easy identification of corresponding parts in both views is possible. This overlay method is described for models of the left atrium but can also be applied to other organs. The contribution is structured as follows. In the second section, details on the overlay generation as well as the method for evaluation are provided. The results are presented in section three. In the final section, we discuss our results and draw some conclusions.

2   Materials and methods

The left atrium model is represented as a triangle mesh, information about the camera geometry is provided by a 3×4 projection matrix for both views A and B. In section 2.1 we present which structures are selected for display, in section 2.2 the color scheme is explained.

2.1   Structure selection

The edges that may become visible by a contrast agent injection depend on the viewing direction of the C-arm. The direction is defined by the projection matrix $P \in \mathbb{R}^{3 \times 4}$. The optical center $o \in \mathbb{R}^3$ is given as the null space of the projection matrix

$$o = \mathrm{Null}(P) \tag{1}$$

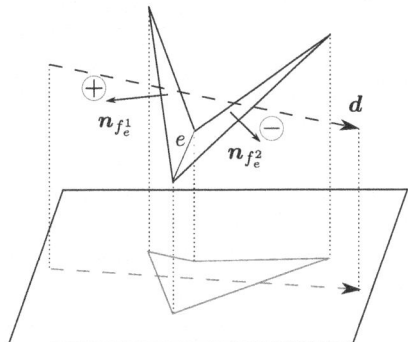

Fig. 1. Depending on the viewing direction d and the normals $n_{f_e^1}$, $n_{f_e^2}$ of the adjacent faces, an edge of the mesh is visible in the 2D. If the results of the scalar products of d with each normal vector have different signs, the edge is visible in 2D.

The viewing direction d_x to a point $x \in \mathbb{R}^3$ can be easily computed by the difference vector (Fig. 1)

$$d_x = x - o \tag{2}$$

To determine, if an edge $e = (e_1, e_2)$ of the mesh, defined by two points $e_1, e_{,2} \in \mathbb{R}^3$ is visible as edge from the perspective of the camera center, the normals $n_{f_e^1}$ and $n_{f_e^2}$ of the two faces f_e^1 and f_e^2 which are adjacent to e are considered. If the results of the scalar products of d with $n_{f_e^1}$ and $n_{f_e^2}$, respectively, have different signs, the edge is visible in the 2D projection [7]. Therefore the set E of visible edges is given by

$$E = \left\{ e \mid \mathrm{sgn}(d_{e_1}^T n_{f_e^1}) \neq \mathrm{sgn}(d_{e_1}^T n_{f_e^2}) \right\} \tag{3}$$

2.2 Color scheme

When the edges are displayed as parts of a fluoroscopy overlay image, they might cross if there are overlapping structures in the heart. This could happen when a pulmonary vein lies before the heart wall. To differentiate between overlapping details, it helps to color edges belonging to the same structures similarly. On possible solution may be coloring depending on the perspective depth of the edge. This would present additional depth information to the physician which is difficult to derive from 2D projections only. However, due to the different orientations of the biplane views, the same structures would be colored differently in both images, since they have different distances to each camera center.

To avoid this kind of confusion, we color edges according to their position in 3-D space. When choosing the color scheme, it is important that an edge does not assume a color with a low saturation, because it would be hard to see it in the grayscale fluoroscopic image. Especially white and black colors should be avoided. We chose a color encoding in which the coordinate of a point along the patients left-right axis corresponds to the green intensity, the coordinate along the front-back-axis corresponds to the blue intensity and the red intensity is fixed. The relationship of 3-D points along the head-feet axis is preserved in the projection. I.e. a 3-D point a that is nearer to the head than a point b will also be located nearer to the top border of the projection images. Therefore, it does not need to be encoded in color. Using this color scheme, colors with a high saturation occur at salient features like pulmonary veins.

2.3 Evaluation method

The goal of the evaluation was to test if people that are familiar with images from EP procedures can do a registration more accurately using the novel overlay compared to an overlay just showing the outline of the heart model. To evaluate this, five people working with these images on a regular basis were asked to do a manual registration on six images acquired during atrial fibrillation procedures using the overlay showing just the overall outline followed by a manual registration of the six images using the edge-enhancing approach. To make the registration easier, also a subtraction image showing only the contrast agent could be displayed. For each biplane image pair, a registration performed by a specialized physician was available as gold standard. The registration is restricted to 3-D translation as it is typically done in clinical practice [8].

3 Results

The results of the evaluation are presented in Fig. 2. The error is given as difference between the registration done by the user and the reference registration. The mean error and the standard deviation for each sequence is given for both overlay types.

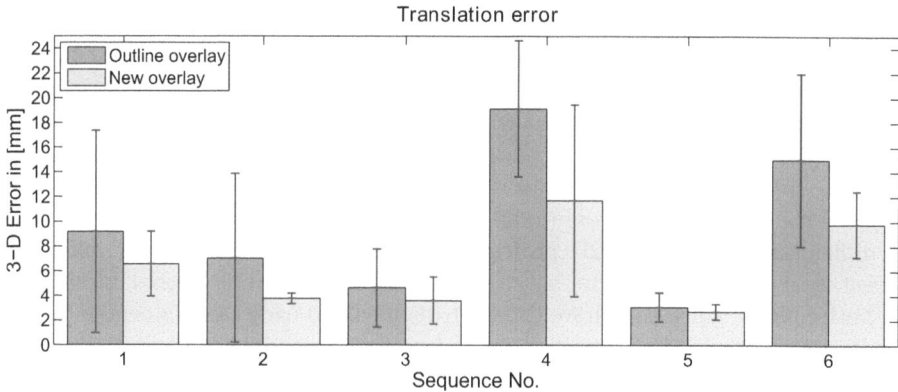

Fig. 2. Mean translational error in mm and standard deviation of the mesh registration using the outline overlay and the structure enhancing mesh overlay.

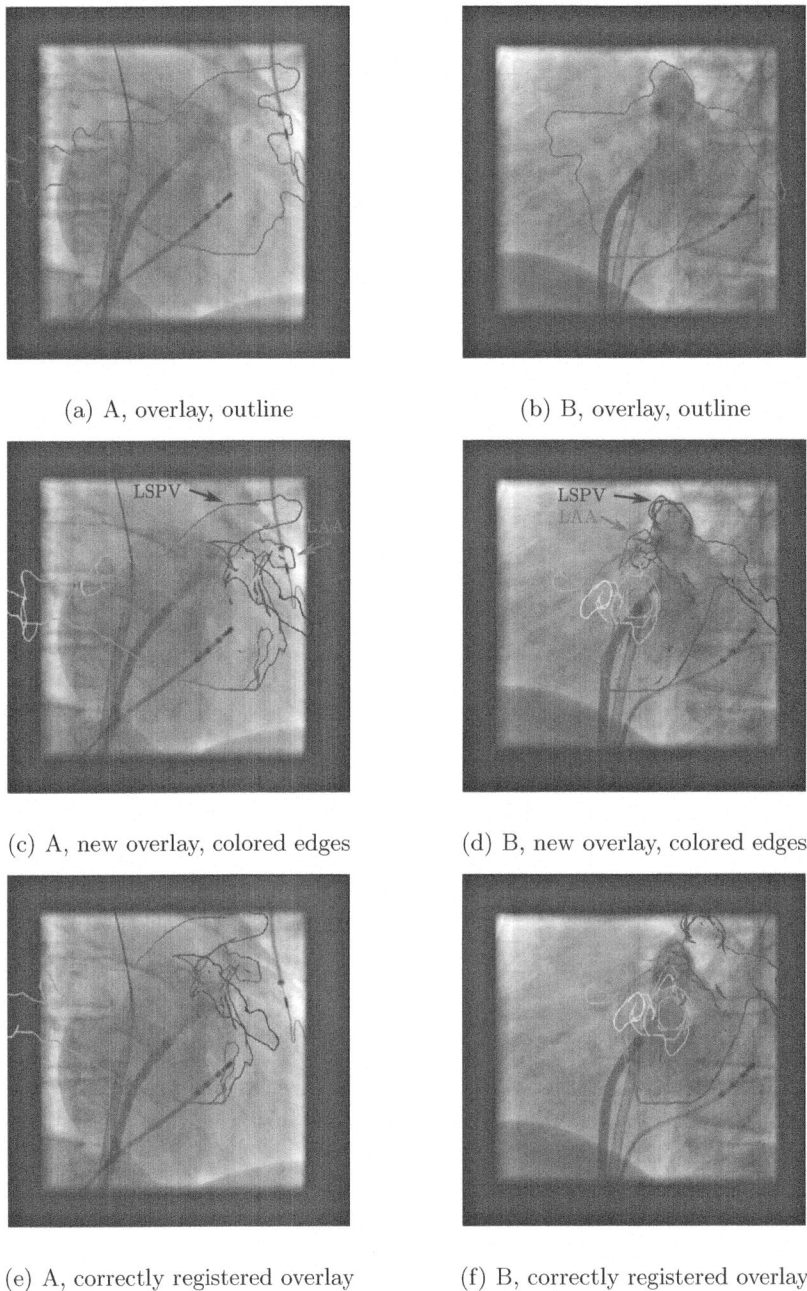

(a) A, overlay, outline

(b) B, overlay, outline

(c) A, new overlay, colored edges

(d) B, new overlay, colored edges

(e) A, correctly registered overlay

(f) B, correctly registered overlay

Fig. 3. Views A and B. Using the overlay showing only the outline, the registration results given in (a) and (b) seem to be correct. When using the structure enhancing overlay, one can see that the left superior pulmonary vein (LSPV) in (c) is uncontrasted while is filled with contrast agent in (d). Instead, the left atrial appendage (LAA) is the contrasted structure. By aligning the overlays such that the LAA is filled with contrast agent in both images, a correct registration is achieved, (e) and (f).

4   Discussion

The results show that the use of the new overlay allows a more precise manual registration. For every sequence the mean error decreased, even if in some cases the error increased for a single user. The least decrease is found at sequence 5. Here, the structure shown by the contrast agent contained a greater part of the overall outline such that it was possible to do a good registration based on the outline overlay. The most decrease can be found for sequence 4. All users made a registration where the contrast agent is registered in one view to the left atrial appendage and in the other view to the left superior pulmonary vein (Fig. 3). The new overlay revealed the shape of the left atrial appendage and by searching for correspondences, two users were able to notice this mistake and correct it.

To conclude, the main contribution of the new overlay are following two features: 1.) The edges shown by the overlay provides the user additional structures he can register to and 2.) the coloring scheme allows the user to check if in both images the same heart region is highlighted by the contrast agent.

Acknowledgement. This work was supported by the German Federal Ministry of Education and Research (BMBF) in the context of the initiative Spitzencluster Medical Valley – Europäische Metropolregion Nürnberg, project grant Nos. 01EX1012A and 01EX1012E, respectively. Additional funding was provided by Siemens AG, Healthcare Sector. Disclaimer: The concepts and information presented in this paper are based on research and are not commercially available.

References

1. Calkins H, Brugada J, Packer DL, et al. HRS/EHRA/ECAS expert consensus statement on catheter and surgical ablation of atrial fibrillation: recommendations for personnel, policy, procedures and follow-up. Europace. 2007;9(6):335.
2. Fuster V, Rydén LE, Cannom DS, et al. ACC/AHA/ESC 2006 guidelines for the management of patients with atrial fibrillation. J Am Coll Cardiol. 2006;48(4):854.
3. Wittkampf FHM, Wever EFD, Derksen R, et al. LocaLisa: new technique for real-time 3-dimensional localization of regular intracardiac electrodes. Circulation. 1999;99(10):1312–7.
4. Dilling-Boer D, van der Merwe N, Adams J, et al. Ablation of focally induced atrial fibrillation:. J Cardiovasc Electrophysiol. 2004;15(2):200–5.
5. De Buck S, Maes F, Ector J, et al. An augmented reality system for patient-specific guidance of cardiac catheter ablation procedures. IEEE Trans Med Imaging. 2005;24(11):1512 –24.
6. Brost A, Bourier F, Kleinoeder A, et al. AFiT: atrial fibrillation ablation planning tool. Proc VMV. 2011; p. 223–30.
7. Möller T, Haines E, Hoffman N. Real-time rendering. AK Peters Limited; 2008.
8. Bourier F, Vukajlovic D, Brost A, et al. Pulmonary vein isolation supported by MRI-derived 3D-augmented biplane fluoroscopy: a feasibility study and a quantitative analysis of the accuracy of the technique. J Cardiovasc Electrophysiol. 2007;115:3057–63.

Dynamic Heart Valve Cusp Bending Deformation Analysis

Sven Friedl[1], Stefan König[1], Michael Weyand[2], Thomas Wittenberg[1], Markus Kondruweit[2]

[1]Fraunhofer-Institut für Integrierte Schaltungen IIS, Erlangen
[2]Herzchirurgische Klinik des Universitätsklinikums Erlangen
sven.friedl@iis.fraunhofer.de

Abstract. Proper hemodynamics is a major issue in research of heart valve bio-prostheses. In the examination of these, the bending deformation and fluttering of heart valve cusps is an interesting and influential aspect. An analysis of the deformation can support the understanding of correlations between hemodynamics and occurring mechanical stress. This contribution describes an approach to determine the dynamic bending deformation of aortic heart valve bio-prostheses in high speed video recordings and to compare different fluttering characteristics. The bio-prostheses are recorded in an artificial circulation setup and observed during the opening and closure of a systolic phase. Based on a segmentation of the orifice area, a distance signal is derived for each cusp relative to a base line given by the commissure points. This distance signal describes the static bending deformation of the cusps in one image frame. By observing the deformation during the phase of maximal flow, the dynamics of the cusps can be determined over time. The resulting fluttering is quantified by a frequency analysis of the time dependent distance signal. Thus, significant fluttering characteristics can be modeled and compared.

1 Introduction

For heart valve transplantations, bio-prostheses are of increasing significance due to the more physiological-like hemodynamics compared to mechanical grafts and the absence of compulsory long term anticoagulation. However, common degeneration of those bio-prostheses during life-time is still an issue in the patient related choice of heart valve prostheses [1]. To avoid re-operations, bio-prostheses are chosen for older patients, whereas for younger patients with higher life expectancy mechanical grafts with longer durability are implanted. The degeneration of bio-prostheses is mainly caused by bio-chemical related processes which is in research in the field of tissue engineering and related domains. However, another significant cause is mechanical stress by non-physiological movements and hemodynamics. One aspect of the movement and correlation with hemodynamics is the bending deformation of heart valve cusps. The fluttering during the phase of maximal flow is an indicator for hemodynamic issues and influences it vice versa. An analysis of these aspects can support the understanding of correlations between hemodynamics and occurring mechanical stress.

Different efforts have been made, examining deformation and fluttering of heart valves. Rishni et al. [2] analyzed echocardiography sequences to determine fluttering of heart valves of dogs as analogy to the situation in humans. Erasmi at al. [3] extracted a static bending deformation index at the state of maximum opening of the heart valves. Hahn et al. [4] presented a segmentation based approach to analyze the fluttering of the heart valve orifice boundaries. This approach is developed further by Condurache et al. [5], where the segmentation is the basis for different aspects of flutter determination. Another method has been introduced by Friedl et al. [6] who analyzed the movements by determining the illumination depending pixel frequency.

This contribution aims to proceed with the approach of Condurache et al. [5] to determine the bending deformation dynamically and to analyze the related fluttering. By quantifying the fluttering characteristics, a model of different grades shall be derived to which hemodynamic aspects can be compared.

2 Materials and methods

2.1 High speed video recordings of heart valves

To observe the movements of heart valve bio-prostheses, an artificial circulation setup has been built in a laboratory environment. The prostheses are streamed by a replacement liquid, precisely water, to obtain systolic cycles. In a replaceable container, the valve is fixated to be streamed in flow direction. The container is connected by a tube to an artificial heart ventricle which invokes the flow. Vertically on top of the container is a reservoir connected by another straight tube, where the liquid is collected before returned to the ventricle. The reservoir represents the atrium in the heart circulation. An artificial heart pump, connected to the ventricle, regulates the systolic and diastolic parameters and an invasive pressure sensor controls the pressure during the circulation.

Through an opening in the reservoir, an endoscope can be introduced and guided close to the prosthesis. Attached to the endoscope is a digital high speed video camera, which observes the valve movements and records them with 2000 frames per second. This recording rate allows to observe also high frequency movements. The spatial resolution of the camera is 256×256 pixel. Using this setup, currently 17 recordings of four different aortic heart valve bio-prostheses are obtained. Each recording consist of two to four complete systolic cycles. The movement characteristics are influenced by the type of the prosthesis and the hemodynamic parameters of the systole. Thus, the recordings contain different grades of cusp bending deformation and fluttering. An example image of one of those recordings is shown in Fig. 1(a).

2.2 Extraction of the bending deformation

The core aspect of the determination of the bending deformation is the extraction of a signal which describes the deformation along the cusp boundary. Basic prerequisites for this signal are two anatomical landmarks. The first one is the annulus which encloses the heart valve. This defines the general location of the valve and can serve as a reference structure for further calculations. Due to the ring structure of the annulus, a circular Hough transform is applied to detect and track the annulus as an anatomical landmark as described by König et al. [7]. The second landmarks used as reference are the commissure points, where the cusps join together. As per Condurache et al. [5], those can be determined utilizing a linear Hough tranform on a skeletonized segmentation of the orifice. However, this works only for some of the available recordings. Since, with the detection of the annulus, a fixed reference is given and thus relative motion can be disregarded, a one-time manual selection of the commissure points will be sufficient accurate.

The detected landmarks can construct a region of interest (ROI) to detect and to describe the cusp boundaries by a segmentation of the orifice. For each cusp, a straight line is defined between the both relevant commissure points. Centric to this line, the normal is determined and extracted to the border of the annulus. With the commissure points and the intersection of the normal with the annulus, a triangle is constructed as can be seen in Fig. 1(b). The areas of the given triangles can now serve as a ROI to limit the segmentation. For the given recordings, a threshold based region growing is the fastest and most stable approach. Starting with a seed point along the normal line, the orifice is extracted for each cusp resulting in a segmentation of the interesting movement phase. The complete processing chain is shown in Fig. 1 including the regional segmentation in Fig. 1(c).

The segmentation of the cusp related orifices is now used to extract a distance signal which describes the bending deformation of the cusp boundaries. The line between the commissure points is defined as a base line. For each point of this base line, the perpendicular euclidean distance to the segmented cusp border is determined as shown in Fig. 2. By mapping these distance vectors, a signal is derived representing the deformation of the boundaries.

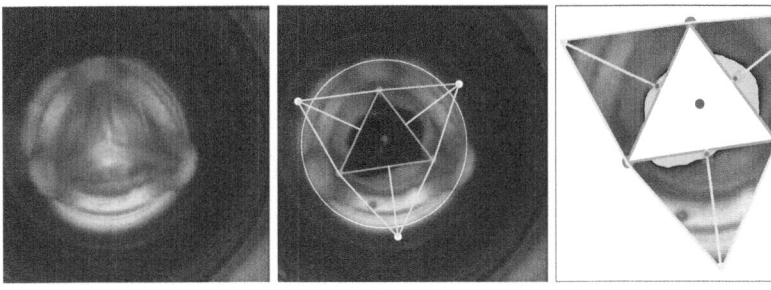

(a) Sample image of an aortic heart valve bio-prosthesis

(b) Geometric construc-tion of the cusp related ROI

(c) Segmentation of cusp related orifices

Fig. 1. Processing chain to extract cusp boundary deformation.

Fig. 2.   Generation
of the distance sig-
nal from the cusp re-
lated orifice segmenta-
tion with the base line
onto the x-axis and the
distance onto the y-
axis.

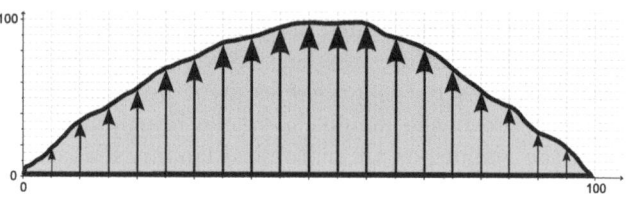

2.3   Determination of fluttering characteristics

The interesting phase during a systolic cycle, regarding the fluttering characteristics, is the phase of maximal flow. During this phase of a recording, the cusp
related distance signal is determined for each relevant frame. Thus, the time
dependent bending deformation can be examined. As shown in Fig. 3(a), the
fluttering can be visualized by plotting the distance along the base line onto a
time axis. To quantify the fluttering, the frequency spectrum of the deformation
variance along the time can be determined. Therefor, the distance is considered
along the time axis for each single base line point. A Fourier transform is applied
to this signals to determine occurring frequencies. By realigning the spectra according the base line, the distribution of frequencies can be visualized as shown
in Fig. 3(b). Here, the occurring frequencies can be examined along the base
line.

3   Results

The methods described above determine the dynamic cusp bending deformation
during the phase of maximal flow. The visualization of the plotted distance signal

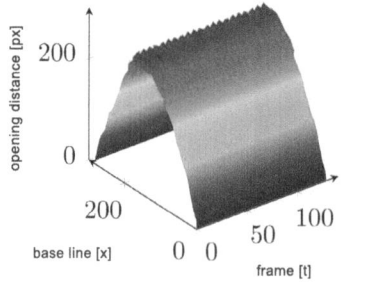

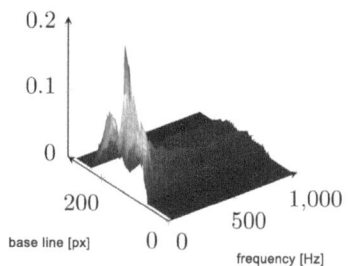

(a) Distance signals of the base line (b) Fourier spectrum of the distance
along the time axis   variance for each base line point

Fig. 3. Visualization of fluttering characteristics.

along the time allows a comparison of the deformation variances for different fluttering grades. Those differences can be examined and interpreted regarding types and architectures of heart valve bio-prostheses. The determination of the Fourier spectrum of distance variances for each point of the base line, leads to a quantification of the fluttering and its distribution. The available recordings used in this contribution are classified in three different grades of fluttering by a visual inspection of the video sequences. The grades are distinguished as no, little and strong fluttering. For all sequences of one grade classification, the average of the Fourier spectra over all base line points is calculated. The result is one mean frequency spectrum considering the distribution along the base line which models a specific grade of fluttering. Those three models of mean spectra are shown in Fig. 4. The blue line describes the spectrum of non fluttering sequences, while the red line describes light, and the green line strong fluttering. It can be seen, that the slope differs significantly for the different grades. For non fluttering sequences, the frequency amplitude declines fast after a first peak. For light and strong fluttering grades, the slope declines with higher frequencies. A significance level at the amplitude of 0.1 can be determined to distinguish between fluttering and non fluttering grades.

4 Discussion

The bending deformation and fluttering characteristics of heart valve cusps is an interesting aspect in research regarding heart valve bio-prostheses. By proceeding with the approach firstly presented by Condurache et al. [5], the adopted

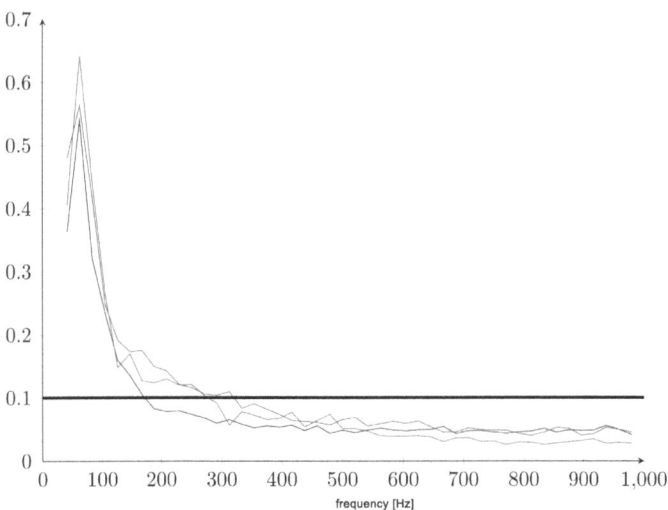

Fig. 4. Fourier model of different fluttering characteristics. Non fluttering (blue); light fluttering (red); strong fluttering (green).

methods stated in this contribution have shown that a dynamic analysis of the bending deformation is possible and lead to the identification of fluttering characteristics. By visualizing the time dependent deformation, different appearances can be illustrated. With a determination of the frequency spectra, specific grades of fluttering can be modeled. These methods and models shall be fundamental for experiments, analyzing different types and architectures of aortic heart valve bio-prostheses. Those results shall then be compared to long term studies observing degeneration processes to determine correlations between fluttering, hemodynamics and corresponding mechanical stress.

References

1. Bloomfield P. Choice of heart valve prosthesis. Heart. 2002;87(6):583–9.
2. Rishniw M. Systolic aortic valve flutter in 6 dogs. Vet Radiol Ultrasound. 2001;42(5):446–7.
3. Erasmi A, Sievers HH, Scharfschwerdt M, et al. In vitro hydrodynamics, cusp-bending deformation, and root distensibility for different types of aortic valve-sparing operations: Remodeling, sinus prosthesis, and reimplantation. J Thorac Cardiovasc Surg. 2005;130(4):1044–9.
4. Hahn T, Condurache AP, Aach T, et al. Automatic in-vitro orifice area determination and fluttering analysis for tricuspid heart valves. Procs BVM. 2006; p. 21–5.
5. Condurache AP, Hahn T, Scharfschwerdt M, et al. Video-based measuring of quality parameters for tricuspid xenograft heart valve implants. IEEE Trans Biomed Eng. 2009;56(12):2868–78.
6. Friedl S, Herdt E, König S, et al. Determination of heart valve fluttering by analyzing pixel frequency. Procs BVM. 2012; p. 87–91.
7. König S, Kondruweit M, Weyand M, et al. Detection and compensation of relative motion in endoscopic heart valve recordings by circular hough transform. Procs GMDS. 2012; p. 242–3.

3D Lung Surface Analysis Towards Segmentation of Pleural Thickenings

P. M. Kengne Nzegne[1], P. Faltin[1], T. Kraus[2], K. Chaisaowong[1,3]

[1]Institute of Imaging and Computer Vision, RWTH Aachen University, Germany
[2]Institute and Out-patient Clinic of Occupational Medicine, University Hospital Aachen, Germany
[3]King Mongkut's University of Technology North Bangkok, Thailand
Pierre.Kengne@rwth-aachen.de

Abstract. Pleural thickenings are connective tissue propagations caused also by a long time exposure to asbestos. They can be an early stage indicator of the malignant pleural mesothelioma. Its diagnosis is time-consuming and underlies the physician's subjective judgment. In order to speed-up the diagnosis and to increase the objectivity of the analysis, three fully automatic methods to detect pleural thickenings from CT data are described and compare in this paper. We apply normal vector analysis, second derivate analysis or curvature scale space computation to analyze the lung surface. In the second step we combine a hysteresis-thresholding with the principle of the convex hull to segment localized thickenings precisely. These new approaches are presented in order to allow precise and robust detection of pleural mesothelioma in early stage.

1 Introduction

Pleural mesothelioma is a malignant tumor of the pleura that can be caused by long time exposure to asbestos. Due to the long latency time of 35 years a peak of pleural mesothelioma morbidity and mortality is expected during 2018 [1]. High risk patients undergo a regular check-up including CT imaging. A diagnosis is time consuming and subject to strong inter- and intra-reader variability.

An older approach [2] detects thickenings by generating the healthy lung model using 2D convex hull. Pleural thickenings are founded by calculating the difference between the convex hull and the existing contour. Drawbacks of this method are the high number of false detections and unsteady fusion of thickenings in different slices. A semi-automatic method for pleural mesothelioma assessment during therapy is presented in [3]. The method requires manual adjustment and is time consuming. In order to increase the objectivity and to speed-up the diagnosis we developed three 3D methods to detect and segment pleural thickenings automatically.

The first step consists of extracting the lungs contours by using a two-step supervised range-constrained Otsu thresholding [2]. The second step is the thickening localization using surface analysis methods. In the last step a hysteresis-thresholding is combined with the convex hull to segment the detected thickenings. A consensus classification made by medical expert is used to evaluate the

H.-P. Meinzer et al. (Hrsg.), *Bildverarbeitung für die Medizin 2013*, Informatik aktuell,
DOI: 10.1007/978-3-642-36480-8_45, © Springer-Verlag Berlin Heidelberg 2013

implemented algorithms and to compare our results with the method in [2]. This
paper provides detailed description of the two last steps of thickening detection.

2   Materials and methods

Pleural thickenings cause strong indention and bumpy structures in the detected
lung surface. Fig. 1 shows examples of pleural plaques in the lung. Normal vector, second derivate analysis and curvature scale space computation are applied
and compared to identify strong variations of the lung surface. Input for the
surface analysis is a binary volume of the lung surface generated by the lung
contour extraction [2].

2.1   Normal vector analysis of lung surface

For a binary segmentation normal vector can be computed at a point $p = (x, y, z)$
of a discrete surface S in any adjacent neighborhood N [4]. By considering all
points of the neighborhood N_n of size $2n_n + 1$, the three components $n_x(p), n_y(p)$
and $n_z(p)$ of the normal vector $n(p)$ are computed

$$n_q(p) = \sum_{i=-n_n}^{n_n} \sum_{j=-n_n}^{n_n} \sum_{k=-n_n}^{n_n} \frac{w \cdot i_q \cdot \alpha(x+i, y+j, z+k)}{\sqrt{i^2 + j^2 + k^2}} \qquad (1)$$

where $q = \{x, y, z\}$, $\alpha(x+i, y+j, z+k)$ is the value of the binary mask and w is a
weighting factor defined as the inverse of the Euclidean distance [4]. Thereafter,
the deviation d_q of each component n_q of the normal vectors is computed in a
defined region of interest N_d of size $2n_d + 1$, in order to localize strong variations

$$d_q(p) = |\max(n_q(\tilde{p})) - \min(n_q(\tilde{p}))| \ \forall \ \tilde{p} \in N_d \qquad (2)$$

The variation of the lung surface is finally defined by the product of the deviation
components $d_q(p)$

$$v(p) = d_x(p) \cdot d_y(p) \cdot d_z(p) \qquad (3)$$

Fig. 3(a) shows an example of the localization of strong variations using normal
vector computation.

Fig. 1. Pleuraplaque as strong indention (left) and as strong variation of the lung surface (right).

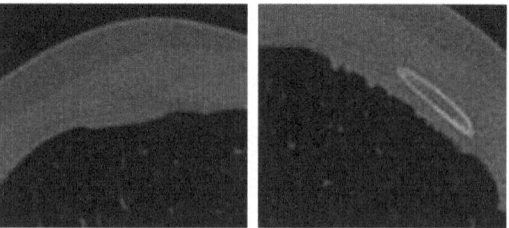

2.2 Second derivate analysis with parameterization of surface

An alternative approach to detect high variation is a second derivate analysis. Due to the small range of binary values $\{0, 1\}$, the second derivate analysis on binary masks is subject to strong noise. Therefore we developed a new parameterization of the lung surface. For the parameterization we computed the Euclidean distance $d(\boldsymbol{p})$ of each lung point $\boldsymbol{p} = (x, y, z)$ to the lung center $\boldsymbol{c} = (x_c, y_c, z_c)$

$$d(\boldsymbol{p}) = \sqrt{(x - x_c)^2 + (y - y_c)^2 + (z - z_c)^2} \qquad (4)$$

The computed distances $d(x, y, z)$ are mapped to $d(i, z)$ in a 2D surface S'. The surface S' can be seen as a 2D matrix with $n \times m$ points, where m represents the number of slices in the given 3D mask and n represents the maximum number of contour points in one slice. The distances $d(i, z)$ of all contour points of slice z are sorted in the corresponding column of S' with respect to their connection. The columns of S' are aligned considering the relationship between contour points from different slices. As shown in Fig. 2, the parameterization represents an opening and unfolding of the lung surface.

After parameterization, the surface S' is smoothed with a 2D Gaussian function $g(i, z, \sigma)$ in order to remove noises

$$d_\sigma(i, z) = d(i, z) * g(i, z, \sigma) \qquad (5)$$

where σ is the standard deviation of the Gaussian function. We then computed the second derivative of the smoothed surface for each parameter i and z

$$\ddot{d}_l(i, z) = \frac{\partial^2 d_\sigma(i, z)}{\partial l^2} \qquad (6)$$

where $l = \{i, z\}$. The localization is then performed by applying Eq. (2) and Eq. (3). Fig. 3(b) shows an example of the localization of strong variations using second derivate analysis.

2.3 Curvature scale space

The curvature scale space is a gradient based method that analyses the curvature of surfaces at different scales. The lung surface is parameterized similarly to the

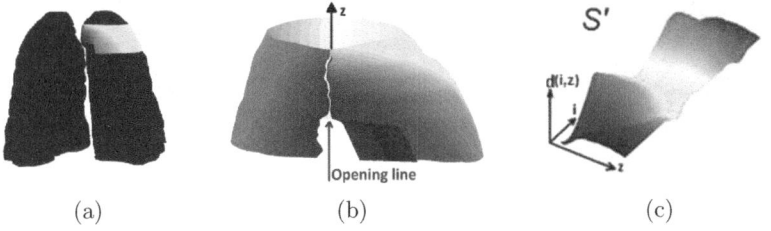

(a)   (b)   (c)

Fig. 2. 3D surface of the left and right lung (a); Cutout of the left lung (b); Parameterization of a cutout of the left lung (c). The color represents the position of the surface points from the start- to the endpoint after opening.

second derivate analysis with the difference, that the x and y coordinates instead of the Euclidean distances are mapped in two 2D surfaces $\Gamma(x(i, z), y(i, z))$. The parameterized surfaces are then smoothed with a 2D Gaussian function in order to remove noises $\Gamma_\sigma(X_\sigma(i, z), Y_\sigma(i, z))$.

The curvature of the parameterized surface is computed [5]

$$k_l(i, z, \sigma) = \frac{\dot{X}_l(i, z)\ddot{Y}_l(i, z) - \ddot{X}_l(i, z)\dot{Y}_l(i, z)}{\dot{X}_l(i, z)^2 + \dot{Y}_l(i, z)^2} \tag{7}$$

where $l = \{i, z\}$. The localization is finally determined with Eq. (2) and Eq. (3). Fig. 3(c) shows an example of the localization of strong variations using the curvature scale space.

2.4   Segmentation of thickenings

The segmentation of thickenings is carried out through hysteresis-thresholding. Two thresholds t_{High} and t_{Low} are used to extract lung regions of high variation. All surface points $\boldsymbol{p} = (x, y, z)$ with variation $v(\boldsymbol{p}) \geq t_{\text{High}}$ (strong points) as well as all points with variation $t_{\text{High}} \geq v(\boldsymbol{p}) \geq t_{\text{Low}}$ (weak points), that are connected to a strong point are extracted. The surface analysis does not differ between convex and concave structures. In addition, the hysteresis-thresholding does not always manage to segment thickenings completely. To refine the thickenings border and remove the convex structures, we combine the hysteresis-thresholding with the convex hull computed separately for the left and right lung in transversal plane. The similarity of the final segmentation of the three methods in Fig. 4 is a consequence of the refinement function that uses the convex hull of the lung to correct the thickening border.

3   Results

No gold standard regarding the volume of thickenings was available. Therefore the experiments are carried out using CT data from eight lungs from different

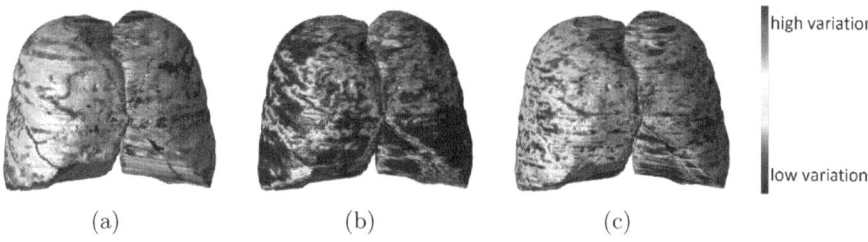

(a)   (b)   (c)

Fig. 3. Variation of the lung surface computed with (a) normal computation in a cubic neighborhood N_n with $n_\text{n} = 3$, (b) second derivate analysis on parameterized surface by scale parameter $\sigma = 2$, (c) curvature scale space by scale parameters $\sigma = 2, 6$ and deviation for all three methods by a cubic neighborhood N_d with $n_\text{d} = 1$. High variations are represented in red and low variations in blue.

patients with focus on maximum detection. These scans of the lung typically contain 80 to 700 images-slices. In order to determine the optimal parameters, we varied the parameter n_n of the cubic neighborhood N_n for normal vector, the scale parameter σ for second derivate and curvature scale space, and the parameter n_d of the cubic region of interest N_d for deviation computation from 1 to 10. Fig. 5 shows the variability of the detection in function of the parameters.

In a second experiment we use a consensus classification of thickenings made by two medical experts and compared the results of the implemented tools with the results of another fully automatic detection system [2] based on the principle of the convex hull. The classification of the detected thickenings, the sensitivity and the precision of all algorithms are given in Tab. 1. The true negative (TN) part of the lung is difficult to quantify without errors, therefore further quality criteria like specificity and efficiency were not determined.

4   Discussion

We have presented three approaches for thickenings detection. The normal vector achieves the highest sensitivity of 74, 49% but the lowest precision of 24, 47%. Contrariwise the gradient achieved the highest precision of 30% and only 2% more sensitivity than the principle of the convex hull. The curvature scale space offers the best compromise between more detections for less errors by achieving

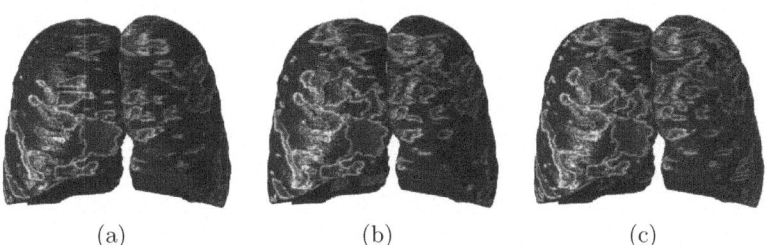

Fig. 4. Segmentation and refinement of detected thickenings using (a) normal vector, (b) second derivate analysis and (c) curvature scale space. Lung surface is represented in blue and segmented thickenings are represented in red.

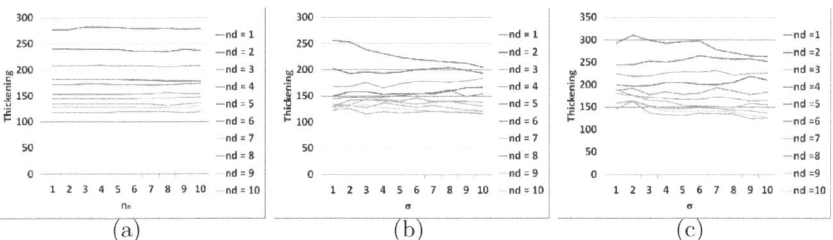

Fig. 5. Number of detected thickening using (a) normal vector, (b) second derivate analysis and (c) curvature scale space.

Table 1. Classification of detected thickenings. TP = true positive, FN = false negative, FP = false positive and NE = new detected thickenings that does not match the consensus classification. Used parameters n_i, n_r and σ are the same as in Fig. 4.

Algorithm	TP	FN	FP	NE	NE+FP	Sensitivity	Precision
Convex hull [2]	741	388	2108	-	2108	66%	26%
Normal vector	841	288	1498	1097	2595	74,49%	24,47%
Second derivate	767	362	1286	527	1813	68%	30%
Curvature scale space	825	304	1516	293	2099	73,07%	28,21%

a sensitivity of $73,07\%$ and a precision of $28,21\%$. Furthermore, several new detected thickenings, that did not match the consensus classification, have been classified as false positive. New investigation of the results by medical experts will probably improve the results of the three implemented algorithms.

All three algorithms improve the thickening detection. However the segmentation of the rear of the thickenings is approximated by the convex hull. Approaches like [6] offer a tissue-oriented segmentation method in order to separate detected thickenings from surrounding tissues. Furthermore the localization can be improved by adaptive methods or wavelet-analysis instead of the maximum deviation.

References

1. Pistolesi M, Rhusthoven J. Malignant pleural mesothelioma: update, current management, and newer therapeutics strategies. Chest. 2004;126(4):1318–29.
2. Chaisaowong K, Knepper A, Kraus T, et al. Application of supervised range-constrained thresholding to extract lung pleura for automated detection of pleural thickenings from thoracic CT images. Proc SPIE. 2007;6514:65143M.
3. Frauenfelder T, Tutic M, Weder W, et al. Volumetriy: an alternative to asses therapy response for malignant pleural mesothelioma. ERJ. 2011;38:162–8.
4. Thürmer G, Würthrich CA. Normal computation for discrete surface in 3D space. Proc EuroGraphics. 1997;16(3).
5. Abbasi S, Mokhtrian F, Kittler J. Curvature scale space image in shape similarity retrieval. CVSSP. 1999;7:467–76.
6. Buerger C, Chaisaowong K, Knepper A, et al. A topology-oriented and tissue-specific approach to detect pleural thickenings from CT data. Proc SPIE. 2009;7258:72593D–11.

Verfahren zur Referenzmodellerstellung für die Evaluierung CT-basierter Segmentierung des Kortikalis-Spongiosa-Überganges im Femur

Timm Surup[1], Anna Hänler[1], Annika Homeier[1], Andreas Petersik[1], Geert von Oldenburg[1], Rainer Burgkart[2]

[1]Stryker Trauma GmbH, Schönkirchen
[2]Klinikum rechts der Isar Technische Universität München, München
timm.surup@stryker.com

Kurzfassung. In der Implantatentwicklung werden zunehmend 3D-Modelle von Knochen eingesetzt, um anatomische Charakteristika umfassender untersuchen zu können. Eine detaillierte Kenntnis der Knochensubstanzen ist die Grundlage für die heutige Entwicklung von Marknägeln und Gelenkendoprothesen. Um Implantaten eine anatomisch optimale Passform verleihen und somit das klinische Ergebnis langfristig verbessern zu können, sollte zukünftig auch 3D-Wissen zum inneren Kortikalis-Spongiosa-Übergang in den Entwicklungsprozess einfließen. Für die Segmentierung dieses Grenzbereichs werden bereits unterschiedliche Methoden angewendet. Oft wird bei der Evaluierung dieser Segmentierungsverfahren auf sogenannte Expertensegmentierungen zurückgegriffen. In der vorliegenden Arbeit wird ein Prozess vorgestellt, eine Referenz für Segmentierungsverfahren mittels industrieller Computertomographie zu identifizieren ohne die Präparate zu zerstören. Es wird gezeigt, dass die entwickelte Methode valide Referenzmodelle erzeugt.

1 Einleitung

Der Entwicklungsprozess von Implantaten zur Frakturversorgung von Knochen greift zunehmend auf Daten von 3D-Knochenmodellen zurück. Im patientenorientierten Implantatdesign finden zum Teil bereits große anatomische Datenmengen Anwendung [1]. Die 3D-Knochenmodelle werden dabei aus CT-Scans der klinischen Routine generiert.

Für die Knochensegmentierung aus CT-Scans gibt es diverse Automatisierungsansätze, welche eine effiziente Erstellung von 3D-Knochenmodellen ermöglichen [2, 3]. So werden aktive Konturmodelle, wie zB. Snake-Algorithmen, eingesetzt [4, 5]. Bei nahezu allen automatisierten Verfahren wird auf eine manuelle Segmentierung des Knochens durch einen Experten referenziert. Dabei wird die Genauigkeit der Segmentierung häufig nicht beschrieben oder bewertet. Darüber hinaus bleibt das Vorgehen bei einer Expertensegmentierung zumeist ungenannt [6, 7, 8]. Hinzu kommt, dass die Referenzmodelle häufig aus den CT-Scans generiert werden, die auch für die Testsegmentierungen verwendet werden [3, 6, 7, 8]. Oft sind aber gerade diese Testfälle in ihrer Qualität schlecht oder haben kein realitätsgetreues Setup [3]. Sie sind daher nicht optimal, um die wahren Verhältnisse zu beschreiben. Die Genauigkeit der Referenz muss nachvollziehbar evaluiert sein, um die Korrektheit der automatisch generierten 3D-Modelle zu gewährleisten und die Vergleichbarkeit mit anderen Segmentierungsverfahren zu sichern.

Aamodt et al. [9] greift nicht auf manuelle Expertensegmentierungen aus CT-Scans, sondern auf fotografierte anatomische Schnittbilder von Knochen zurück, um die Kontur des Kortikalis-Spongiosa-Überganges abzuleiten. Dies ermöglicht die Herstellung einer Referenz, die unabhängig von Artefakten und Auflösungsdefekten eines klinischen CT ist. Abb. 1 gibt einen Überblick über die unterschiedlichen Knochenmaterialübergänge im proximalen Femur.

Zu erkennen sind auch die klare Abgrenzung der äußeren Kortikalisoberfläche sowie der graduelle Übergang der Kortikalis zur Spongiosa (siehe auch Abb. 4). Die vorliegende Studie stellt einen nicht-destruierenden Referenzgenerationsprozess vor und vergleicht die Ergebnisse mit [9].

2 Material und Methoden

Um die Referenz zu erstellen, wurden zwölf humane Femurpräparate (frisch, tiefgefroren, ohne Weichteilmantel) mit einem Alter von 75 Jahren im Median (Bereich: 20 − 85 Jahre) in einem Industrie-Computertomographen eingescannt (Metrotom 1500, CarlZeiss Industrielle Messtechnik GmbH, Aalen, Deutschland). Mit dem Industrie-CT ist es möglich, Voxelgrößen von unter 0,2 mm zu erreichen. In einem klinischen CT sind Auflösungen für den Femurbereich von lediglich 1 mm üblich. Die hohe Auflösung eines Industrie-CTs ermöglicht die Detektierbarkeit von feinsten Strukturen und Unterschieden zwischen dichtem kortikalem und spongiösem Gewebe (Abb. 2).

Durch die räumliche Begrenzung im Industrie-CT wurden die Präparate in drei Abschnitten gescannt: Proximaler, distaler Bereich und Schaftbereich (Dia-

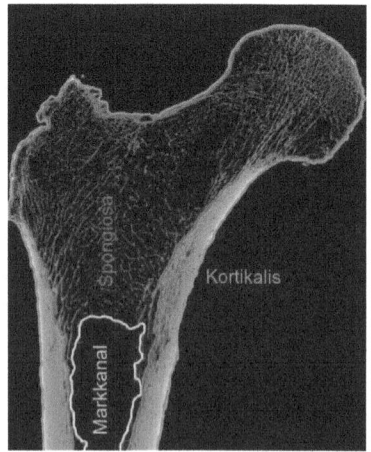

Abb. 1. Übersicht der unterschiedlichen Knochenmaterialien, Koronarschnitt des proximalen Femurs im Industrie-CT. Der Kortikalis-Spongiosa-Übergang ist rot markiert.

physe). Dadurch konnten durchschnittliche Voxelkantenlängen von 0,16 mm proximal und distal sowie 0,23 mm im Schaftbereich erreicht werden (isotrope Voxel).

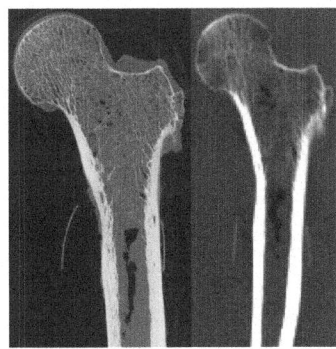

Abb. 2. Koronarschnitt des proximalen Femurs im Industrie-CT (links, 0,2 mm Voxelgröße) und klinischen CT (rechts, 1 mm Voxelgröße).

Anschließend wurden aus den Industrie-CT-Scans mittels manueller Expertensegmentierung Referenzmodelle generiert. Dafür wurde zunächst die äußere Kortikalisoberfläche markiert. Daraufhin wurde dieses Volumen um ein Voxel in 26er-Nachbarschaft geschrumpft (3D-Volumenschrumpfen). Das so erhaltene Volumen stellt die äußere Begrenzung für das eigentliche Spongiosamodell dar. Dieser Schritt ist notwendig, um sicherzustellen, dass die Kortikalis in jedem Fall eine Dicke von über 0 mm aufweist. Dann wurden die Spongiosamodelle von einem medizinischen Experten generiert. Sämtliche Segmentierungsschritte wurden mit der Software Amira (Version 5.4.0, Visage Imaging, Inc. und Konrad-Zuse-Zentrum Berlin) durchgeführt. Das nachträgliche Zusammenfügen der Einzelteile (proximaler und distaler Bereich, Diaphyse) geschah mit Hilfe der Standardsoftware Geomagic Studio 2012 (Geomagic, Inc., Morrisville, USA). Um die Testmodelle zu erzeugen, wurden die Femurpräparate in einem Weichteilphantom (bestehend aus Gelatine und Wasser) in einem klinischen CT-Scanner erfasst (Philips Brilliance 16-slice, Philips Healthcare, DA Best, Niederlande). Dabei wurde eine in der Klinik übliche Auflösung von 1 mm Voxelkantenlänge (isotrop) gewählt.

Der Kortikalis-Spongiosa-Übergang wurde dann grauwertbasiert segmentiert und mit den erstellten Referenzmodellen verglichen. Die gewählten Grenzwerte betrugen 300 − 1.100 HU in 100 HU Inkrementen. Anstelle von 600 HU wurden 580 HU verwendet, da dieser Wert von Aamodt et al. [9] als optimal für die Segmentierung des Übergangs identifiziert wurde. Die Modellerzeugung erfolgte auch hier mittels Amira.

Daraufhin wurden die generierten Oberflächen der jeweiligen Modelle mit der Standardsoftware Geomagic Qualify 2012 dreidimensional miteinander verglichen. Dafür wurde das jeweilige Testmodell mittels Iterative Closest Point Algorithmus auf das entsprechende Referenzmodell registriert. Die Punktewolken zur Registrierung waren pro Modell auf 100.000 gleichmäßig verteilte Punkte be-

Tabelle 1. Übersicht der Volu-	Grenzwert (HU)	VF (%)	OA (mm)
menfehler und des Oberflächen- abstandes der Test- gegenüber	300	− 17,5	− 1,7 ± 1,2
den Referenzmodellen der zwölf	400	− 9,5	− 0,7 ± 0,6
verwendeten humanen Femora;	500	− 5,1	− 0,3 ± 0,3
negative Werte bedeuten ein klei- neres Testmodell als das Refe-	580	− 3,1	− 0,2 ± 0,2
renzmodell (HU = Hounsfield-	700	− 1,4	− 0,1 ± 0,2
Einheit; VF = Volumenfehler;	800	0,3	0,0 ± 0,2
OA = mittlerer Oberflächenab- stand ± Standardabweichung).	900	2,2	0,2 ± 0,1
	1.000	4,2	0,3 ± 0,1
	1.100	6,4	0,5 ± 0,1

grenzt, bei denen iterativ der minimalste mittlere Abstand zwischen den beiden Punktwolken gesucht wird. Nach der Registrierung wurde der kürzeste Abstand eines Testpunktes (auf der Oberfläche des Testobjektes) zur Referenzoberfläche bestimmt. Pro Testmodell wurden ebenfalls 100.000 gleichmäßig verteilte Testpunkte generiert. Aus dem 3D-Oberflächenabstand eines jeden Testmodells wurde dann jeweils der mittlere Oberflächenabstand (OA) für jeden verwendeten Grenzwert ermittelt. Zusätzlich wurde der durchschnittliche Volumenfehler (VF) berechnet.

3 Ergebnisse

Tabelle 1 zeigt die Abweichungen aus den vorliegenden Testsegmentierungen in Bezug auf die generierten Referenzmodelle.

Es ergeben sich Werte von − 1,7 mm bis + 0,5 mm in der Oberflächenabweichung. Im Volumen sind die Testmodelle zwischen 17,5 % kleiner und 6,4 % größer als die Referenzmodelle. Dabei werden die Werte mit ansteigendem Grenzwert höher.

Abb. 3 zeigt den Abweichungsverlauf über die verwendeten Grenzwerte für die Segmentierung mit dazugehörigen 95 %-Konfidenzintervallen sowie die durchschnittlichen Volumenfehler.

Es zeigt sich, dass eine minimale mittlere Abweichung sowie Volumenfehler bei einem Grenzwert von 800 HU erreicht wird. Werte von unter 800 HU haben zu kleine Knochenmodelle zur Folge, wohingegen Werte darüber zu große Knochenmodelle generieren. Insgesamt korrespondieren mittlerer Oberflächenabstand und Volumenfehler.

4 Diskussion

Um Implantate zukünftig noch besser auf die natürliche Anatomie abzustimmen, sind hochgenaue und in der Abweichung wenig streuende Verfahren zur Generierung von 3D-Knochenmodellen notwendig und sinnvoll [1]. Aussagen über die

Abb. 3. Durchschnittlicher Oberflächenabstand der segmentierten Testmodelle für die jeweiligen Grenzwerte. Die Fehlerbalken zeigen jeweils das 95 %-Konfidenzintervall. Negative Werte bedeuten, dass das Testmodell kleiner als das Referenzmodell ist.

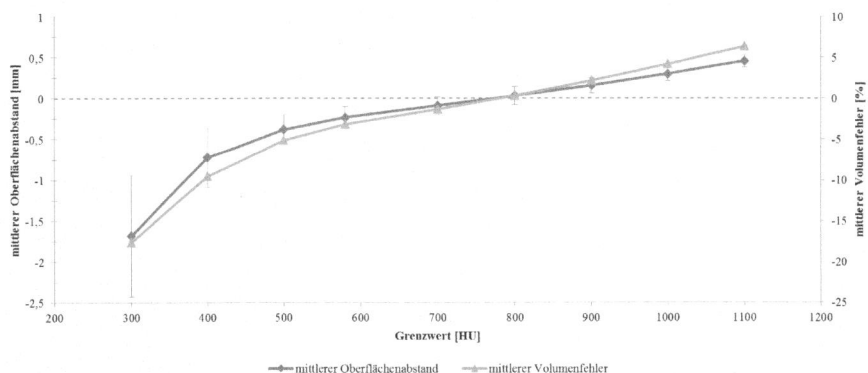

Genauigkeit dieser Modelle hängen entscheidend von den verwendeten Referenzmodellen ab. Daher ist es unerlässlich, Referenzmodelle zu erzeugen, die eine der realen Geometrie nahe liegende Form und Dimension haben. Insbesondere für die Entwicklung intramedullärer Implantate ist es essentiell, die Genauigkeit von Segmentierungen des Kortikalis-Spongiosa-Übergangs exakt zu kennen [9].

Die Ergebnisse aus dieser Studie zeigen einen identischen Verlauf des Oberflächenabstandes wie in [9] beschrieben. Allerdings sind einige Unterschiede sowohl in den Ergebnissen, als auch in der Methodik zu beachten. So wurden die Femurpräparate in dieser Studie in einem Weichteilphantom gescannt, wohingegen in [9] die Präparate in Epoxidharz eingebettet wurden. Zudem wurde hier eine CT-Auflösung von 1 mm Voxelgröße gewählt (hier 0,3 mm). Allein diese Umstände können dazu führen, dass die Ergebnisse aus dieser Studie unterschiedliche Werte von etwa 0,2 mm im Bereich zwischen 500 HU und 1.100 HU aufweisen. 0,2 mm entsprechen dem zu erwartenden Fehler bei einer CT-Voxelauflösung von 1 mm. Die Unterschiede zwischen dieser Studie und der in [9] beschriebenen können also durch die gröbere Auflösung der Test-CT-Scans und Umgebungsmedien der Präparate nachvollzogen werden. Zusätzlich wurde bei dieser Studie der 3D-Abstand der resultierenden 3D-Knochenmodelle betrachtet (lediglich 2D-Abstand in jeder einzelnen Schicht in [9]). Des Weiteren wurde in dieser Studie der gesamte Femur in die Analyse einbezogen. Die Einbeziehung des gesamten distalen Teiles kann zu der erhöhten Streuung geführt haben. Die Verschiebung der in Abb. 3 vorliegenden Kurve hin zu höheren Grenzwerten kann durch die Berücksichtigung des gesamten Schaftbereiches erklärt werden, in denen die Grenzwerte generell im Vergleich zu den Gelenkbereichen erhöht sind.

Dennoch zeigt die hier vorliegende Studie einen deutlich vergleichbaren Trendverlauf der durchschnittlichen Oberflächenabweichung. Es kann also davon ausgegangen werden, dass die vorliegende Methode zur Referenzmodellerstellung dazu geeignet ist, als Grundlage für die Beurteilung der Qualität von segmentierten 3D-Modellen des Kortikalis-Spongiosa-Übergangs verwendet zu werden.

Ein sehr großer Vorteil der vorgestellten Methode liegt darin, dass die Präparate nicht zerstört werden. Abschließend muss erwähnt werden, dass der Kortikalis-Spongiosa-Übergang keine starre Grenze, sondern vielmehr ein gradueller Übergang ist und Schwankungen bei den Referenzmodellen hervorrufen kann (Abb. 4).

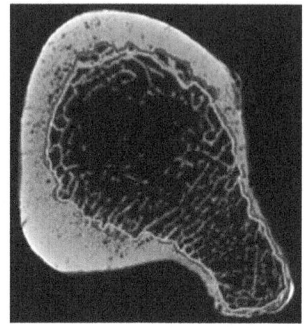

Abb. 4. Darstellung des Kortikalis-Spongiosa-Übergangs auf Höhe des Trochanter Minor in Transversalschnitt im Industrie-CT. Die blaue Linie zeigt einen aggressiven, die grüne Linie einen konservativeren Ansatz zur Beschreibung des Kortikalis-Spongiosa-Übergangs. Die Referenzen dieser Studie wurden mit einem aggressiveren Ansatz erstellt.

Zukünftig sollen die für den Femur gewonnenen Erkenntnisse auch für die Tibia und den Humerus verifiziert werden.

Literaturverzeichnis

1. Kozic N, Weber S, Büchler P, et al. Optimization of orthopaedic implant design using statistical shape space analysis based on level sets. Med Image Anal. 2010;14(3):265–75.
2. Westin CF, Bhalerao A, Knutsson H, et al. Using local 3D structure for segmentatino of bone from computer tomography images. Proc CVPR. 1997; p. 794–800.
3. Kang Y, Engelke K, Kalender WA. A new accurate and precise 3-D segmentation method for skeletal structures in volumetric CT data. IEEE Trans Med Imaging. 2003;22(5):586–98.
4. Pardo JM, Cabello D, Heras J. A snake for model-based segmentation of biomedical images. Pattern Recognit Lett. 1997;18:1529–38.
5. van Ginneken B, Frangi AF, Steel JJ, et al. Active shape model segmentation with optimal features. IEEE Trans Med Imaging. 2002;21(8):924–33.
6. Wang LI, Greenspan M, Ellis R. Validation of bone segmentation and improved 3-D registration using contour coherency in CT data. IEEE Trans Med Imag. 2006;25(3):324–34.
7. Calder J, Tahmasebi AM, Masouri AR. A variational approach to bone segmentation in CT images. Proc SPIE. 2011;7962.
8. Krčah M, Székely G, Blanc R. Fully automatic and fast segmentation of the femur bone from 3D-CT images with no shape prior. Proc ISBI. 2011; p. 2087–90.
9. Aamodt A, Kvistad K, Andersen E, et al. Determination of the hounsfield value for CT-based design of custom femoral stems. J Bone Joint Surg Br. 1999;81(1):143–7.

Untersuchung der Normalverteilungsannahme bei der statistischen Formmodellierung

Florian S Burmester, Sebastian T. Gollmer, Thorsten M. Buzug

Institut für Medizintechnik, Universität zu Lübeck
burmester@imt.uni-luebeck.de

Kurzfassung. In der medizinischen Bildanalyse werden häufig statistische Formmodelle zur Segmentierung von Organen verwendet. Dabei wird im Standardansatz der Formmodellierung davon ausgegangen, dass eine Normalverteilung der Trainingsdaten vorliegt. In dieser Arbeit werden „klassische" medizinische Segmentierungsobjekte auf diese Normalverteilungsannahme hin untersucht. Dazu werden zwei statistische Tests auf Leber- und Milzdaten angewendet. Die Ergebnisse der beiden Tests belegen erstmals, dass die Variabilität dieser Organe nicht normalverteilt ist. Die Untersuchung von Trainingsdaten mit dem hier vorgestellten Ansatz stellt somit eine Möglichkeit dar, bereits im Vorfeld zu entscheiden, ob die Verwendung von z.b. nichtlinearen Verfahren die tatsächliche Formvariabilität eines bestimmten Organs potenziell besser beschreibt.

1 Einleitung

In den letzten beiden Jahrzehnten wurden Segmentierungsansätze auf der Basis von dreidimensionalen statistischen Formmodellen (SFM) (z.B. Heimann [1]) entwickelt, welche zu einem wichtigen Bestandteil der medizinischen Bildverarbeitung geworden sind. SFM basieren auf einer punktbasierten Repräsentation einer gewissen Anzahl von Trainingsformen mit dem Ziel, die zu erwartende Formvariabilität einer bestimmten Objektklasse zu modellieren. Beim linearen statistischen Formmodell wird davon ausgegangen, dass die zu betrachtenden Formen normalverteilt sind. Deshalb verwendet man in diesem Fall die Hauptkomponentenanalyse (engl.: Principle Component Analysis, PCA) um die mögliche Formvariation zu beschreiben. Es finden sich allerdings in der Praxis mehrere medizinische Beispiele, Kirschner et al. [2] führen als Illustration Wirbelknochen an, die keiner Linearkombination der Trainingsdaten folgen. Diese Wirbelknochen stammen allerdings aus verschiedenen Objektklassen (z.B. Lenden- und Brustwirbel) und sind somit offensichtlich nicht normalverteilt. Dementsprechend wird in [2] die Verwendung der nichtlinearen Kernel-PCA vorgeschlagen. Letztere wurde bereits in [1] als mögliche Erweiterung des SFM diskutiert. Für die Modellierung einer bestimmten Objektklasse, wie z.B der Leber, greifen punktbasierte SFM jedoch insbesondere auf die PCA zurück, während im Level-Set-Ansatz auch zunehmend nichtlineare Formmodelle eingesetzt werden [3]. Eine quantitative Analyse im Bezug auf die Normalverteilung der Trainingsdaten

H.-P. Meinzer et al. (Hrsg.), *Bildverarbeitung für die Medizin 2013*, Informatik aktuell,
DOI: 10.1007/978-3-642-36480-8_47, © Springer-Verlag Berlin Heidelberg 2013

wurde im Zusammenhang mit statistischen Formmodellen von Organen unseres Wissens nach bislang nicht durchgeführt. Ziel dieser Arbeit ist es, zu untersuchen, ob die Normalverteilungsannahme der PCA bei „klassischen" Segmentierungsobjekten wie Milz und Leber sinnvoll ist. Dieses wird mittels zweier statistischer Tests realisiert. Dieser Ansatz bietet den Vorteil, dass anhand der Verteilung der Trainingsdaten eine begründete Entscheidung für oder gegen den linearen Modellierungsansatz getroffen werden kann.

2   Material und Methoden

2.1   Statistische Formmodelle (SFM)

Im punktbasierten SFM werden $n_s \in \mathbb{N}^+$ Trainingsformen durch n_p korrespondierende Landmarken repräsentiert. Diese werden für jedes Objekt zu einem Formvektor $\mathbf{x}_i \in \mathbb{R}^{3n_p}$ verknüpft. Es ergibt sich eine mittlere Objektform $\overline{\mathbf{x}} = \frac{1}{n_s} \sum_{i=1}^{n_s} \mathbf{x}_i$.

Im linearen Fall benutzt das SFM die PCA zur Darstellung der verschiedenen Formen. Man berechnet die Eigenvektoren $\mathbf{p}_1, \ldots, \mathbf{p}_{3n_p}$ und die dazugehörigen Eigenwerte $\lambda_1 \geq \ldots \geq \lambda_{3n_p}$ der Kovarianzmatrix der Trainingsformen. Verworfen werden nun die Eigenvektoren mit Index $i > t$, wobei $t = \min \{t' | \sum_{i=1}^{t'} \lambda_i / \sum_{i=1}^{3n_p} \lambda_i > 0.98\}$. Die $3n_p \times t$-Matrix der verbliebenen Eigenvektoren wird als $\mathbf{P} = (\mathbf{p}_1, \ldots, \mathbf{p}_t)$ bezeichnet. Das lineare SFM repräsentiert die Formen $\{\mathbf{x} = \overline{\mathbf{x}} + \mathbf{P}\mathbf{b} \mid \mathbf{b} \in \mathbb{R}^t, \mathbf{b}_i \in [-3\sqrt{\lambda_i}, 3\sqrt{\lambda_i}]\}$ mit $\mathbf{b}$ als Formparameter.

2.2   Multivariate Normalverteilung

Mardia [4] definiert die multivariate Normalverteilung folgendermaßen:

Definition 1. *Ein Zufallsvektor* $\mathbf{y}$ *ist p-variat normalverteilt ($p \in \mathbb{N}^+$), wenn* $\mathbf{a}^T\mathbf{y}$ *univariat normalverteilt ist für jeden beliebigen aber festen p-wertigen Vektor* $\mathbf{a}$.

Das bedeutet, man müsste dies für jede beliebige Linearkombination überprüfen, um einen formalen Beweis zu führen. Eine Einschränkung bei statistischen Tests ist, dass bei einer Stichprobe lediglich geprüft wird, ob die Stichprobe aus einer Normalverteilung mit einer Fehlerwahrscheinlichkeit α entstammen kann. Deswegen wurden im folgenden zwei Tests auf multivariate Normalverteilung verwendet. Zum einen Mardias Test [5] und zum anderen ein BHEP-Test [6]. Aufgrund des Zentralen Grenzwertsatzes kann man nicht die Summation verschiedener Dimensionen untersuchen. Dimensionsweise Tests liefern andererseits keine verlässlichen Ergebnisse, da ein solcher Schätzer nicht suffizient wäre (vgl. Rencher [7]):

1. Die Verwendung von p univariaten Tests, erhöht den Fehler erster Art.
2. Die univariaten Test ignorieren die Korrelation zwischen den Variablen.
3. Multivariate Tests haben in vielen Fällen eine höhere Teststärke (Power).

2.3 Testmethoden

Es seien $\mathbf{y}_1, ..., \mathbf{y}_n$ n unabhängig identisch verteilte Beobachtungen mit einer unbekannten Verteilungsfunktion $F(\mathbf{y})$ ($\mathbf{y} \in \mathbb{R}^p, p \geq 2$). Es wird die Nullhypothese

$$H_{0p} : F(\mathbf{y}) \in \mathcal{N}_p \tag{1}$$

getestet, wobei $\mathcal{N}_p$ die Klasse aller nicht degenerierten p-dimensionalen Normalverteilungen $N_p(\overline{\mathbf{y}}, \mathbf{C})$, $\mathbf{C} > \mathbf{0}$ die Kovarianzmatrix und $\overline{\mathbf{y}}$ der Mittelwert ist.

Mardias Test. Es wird betrachtet, inwiefern die Schiefe und Wölbung (Kurtosis) der Testdaten, unabhängig voneinander berechnet, denen einer Normalverteilung entsprechen. Man berechnet zunächst die invarianten Kenngrößen g_{rs}

$$g_{rs} = (\mathbf{y}_r - \overline{\mathbf{y}})^T \mathbf{C}^{-1}(\mathbf{y}_s - \overline{\mathbf{y}}); r, s = 1, 2, ..., n \tag{2}$$

und damit die Schiefe $b_{1,p} = n^{-2} \sum_{r,s}^n g_{rs}^3$ und die Kurtosis $b_{2,p} = n^{-1} \sum_r^n g_{rr}^2$.

Zur Überprüfung der Hypothese verwendet man jeweils eine Teststatistik für die Schiefe und die Kurtosis. Die Teststatistik

$$A = \frac{1}{6} n b_{1,p} \tag{3}$$

für die Schiefe ist χ^2-verteilt mit $p(p+1)(p+2)/6$ Freiheitsgraden. Für die Kurtosis wird die der Standardnormalverteilung folgenden Teststatistik B berechnet,

$$B = \frac{b_{2,p} - p(p+2)}{\sqrt{\frac{8p(p+2)}{n}}} \sim N(0,1) \tag{4}$$

BHEP Tests. Diese Tests sind eine Klasse von praktisch affin invarianten und universell konsistenten Tests, die auf gewichteten Integralen der quadrierten Differenz zwischen empirischer charakteristischer Funktion der skalierten Residuen und der charakteristischen Funktion der Standardnormalverteilung beruhen [6]. Diese Klasse von Tests kann folgende Teststatistik verwenden

$$T_{n,\gamma} := \begin{cases} 4n, & \text{falls } \mathbf{C} \text{ singulär} \\ nW_{n,\gamma}, & \text{falls } \mathbf{C} \text{ nicht singulär} \end{cases} \tag{5}$$

Der Glättungsparameter γ wurde nach Henze und Zirkler [6] gewählt als

$$\gamma := \frac{1}{\sqrt{2}} \left(\frac{2p+1}{4} \right)^{\frac{1}{p+4}} n^{\left(\frac{1}{p+4} \right)} \tag{6}$$

Mit der Dichte einer bestimmten Normalverteilung als Gewichtungsfunktion [6] ergibt sich

$$W_{n,\gamma} = \frac{1}{n^2} \sum_{j,k=1}^n \exp\left(-\frac{\gamma^2}{2} \|Y_j - Y_k\|^2 \right) - 2(1 + \gamma^2)^{-p/2} \cdot$$
$$\frac{1}{n} \sum_{j=1}^n \exp\left(-\frac{\gamma^2 \|Y_j\|^2}{2(1 + \gamma^2)} \right) + (1 + 2\gamma^2)^{-p/2} \tag{7}$$

mit den skalierten Residuen $Y_k := \mathbf{C}^{-1/2}(\mathbf{y}_k - \bar{\mathbf{y}}), (k = 1, 2, ..., n)$. Man geht bei dieser Form des BHEP-Tests nun davon aus, dass die Teststatistik $T_{n,\gamma}$ der Log-Normalverteilung folgt.

2.4 Experimente

Es wurden zwei Organe (Leber und Milz) von jeweils 82 Probanden (Stichprobengröße) auf Normalverteilung getestet. Die Leberdaten verwenden 2562 Landmarken. Die Milzdaten bestehen jeweils aus 1002 Punkten. Die Korrespondenzfindung wurde sowohl nach dem Distmin-Ansatz [8] als auch nach dem MDL-Ansatz [9] durchgeführt. Letzterem liegt die Annahme eines Gaußmodells zugrunde, wobei versucht wird, die Landmarken bezüglich dieser Annahme möglichst optimal auf den Trainingsformen zu verteilen.

Das Signifikanzniveau wurde für beide Tests auf 1 % festgelegt, um das Verwerfen einer tatsächlichen Normalverteilung möglichst unwahrscheinlich zu machen. Aufgrund der Hochdimensionalität der Daten und weil relativ dazu wenige Stichproben vorliegen, wurde eine Dimensionsreduktion mittels PCA durchgeführt. Liang et al. [10] haben gezeigt, dass dies ein valider Ansatz ist, und verwenden z.b. 95 % der Varianz der Eigenwerte zur Bestimmung einer sinnvollen Zieldimension. Während die PCA eine potenziell vorhandene Normalverteilung der Daten erhält, ist der Umkehrschluss nicht zulässig: Aus einer Normalverteilung nach PCA-Transformation kann nicht auf die Normalverteilung der Originaldaten geschlossen werden [10]. Ferner wurde sogar gezeigt, dass die Teststärke des Tests durch die Dimensionsreduktion mittels PCA eher höher als geringer wird. Wir folgen diesem Ansatz und testen die PCA-transformierten Stichproben auf Normalverteilung, sodass die zu testenden Beobachtungen (Gl. (1)) den Formparametern $\mathbf{b}$ (Abs. 2.1) entsprechen. In [1] wurde festgestellt, dass Werte von mindestens 90 % für die kumulierte Varianz der Eigenwerte im Zusammenhang mit SFM sinnvoll sind. Wir haben unabhängig vom Organ und der Korrespondenzfindung 20 Eigenwerte benutzt, wodurch für alle vier SFM mindestens 90 % der kumulierten Varianz abdeckt wird.

Bei Mardias Test wird sowohl auf die Schiefe als auch auf die Kurtosis getestet. Wird bei einem der beiden Teiltests zum Signifikanzniveau 1 % die Nullhypothese verworfen, so wird die Nullhypothese für Mardias Test insgesamt verworfen und es wird davon ausgegangen, dass die Daten nicht normalverteilt sind. Schiefe und Kurtosis sind allerdings nicht unabhängig voneinander, da beide die Kenngrößen aus Gl. (2) verwenden. Deshalb erhöht sich der Fehler erster Art, also die Wahrscheinlichkeit, eine tatsächliche Normalverteilung fälschlicherweise abzulehnen. Um eine Abschätzung für diesen Fehler zu erhalten wurde mit jeweils 10.000 Testläufen von randomisierten normalverteilten Daten der Dimension 20 getestet, wie sich der α-Fehler von Mardias und vom BHEP-Test für unterschiedliche Stichprobengrößen verhält. Der α-Fehler für beide Teststatistiken wurde als 1 % vorgegeben.

Tabelle 1. P-Werte der statistischen Tests.

	Leber$_{\text{MDL}}$	Leber$_{\text{Distmin}}$	Milz$_{\text{MDL}}$	Milz$_{\text{Distmin}}$
Mardia Schiefe	$6,0 \cdot 10^{-14}$	$< 10^{-16}$	$< 10^{-16}$	$< 10^{-16}$
Mardia Kurtosis	$1,0 \cdot 10^{-4}$	$6,7 \cdot 10^{-16}$	$< 10^{-16}$	$< 10^{-16}$
BHEP	$8,6 \cdot 10^{-3}$	$< 10^{-16}$	$6,3 \cdot 10^{-6}$	$2,8 \cdot 10^{-9}$

3 Ergebnisse

In Tab. 1 werden die p-Werte der beiden Tests für die Leber und die Milz angegeben. Alle Test lehnen eine Normalverteilung der beiden Organe zum Signifikanzniveau α ab, wobei dies für die Distmin-Modelle noch deutlicher ist.

Aufgrund der Tatsache, dass bei Mardia zwei Tests durchgeführt werden, erhöht sich der gesamte α-Fehler des Tests für den Stichprobenumfang $n = 82$ empirisch für die gemäß Abs. 2.4 durchgeführten Testläufen auf ca. 7,9 % (Abb. 1 links). Um den β-Fehler des Tests zu schätzen, wurde auf 10.000 gleichverteilten Daten getestet. Von diesen wurden nur ca. 1,3 % der Testdaten fälschlicherweise positiv auf Normalverteilung getestet. Beim BHEP-Test beträgt der α-Fehler empirisch ca. 1,5 % (Abb. 1 rechts). Dies zeigt, dass der α-Fehler bei $p = 20$ für die gegebene Stichprobengröße $n = 82$ im Vergleich zu einer deutlich größeren Stichprobengröße (z.B. $n = 1000$) akzeptabel ist.

4 Diskussion

Die Auswertung der Daten mit zwei verschiedenen Tests auf multivariate Normalverteilung verwirft die Nullhypothese aus Gl. (1). Es ist zu vermuten, dass sich diese Erkenntnisse auch auf andere Organe übertragen lassen, was durch weitere Experimente untersucht werden muss. Die Ergebnisse für die verschiedenen Korrespondenzfindungsverfahren sind nachvollziehbar: Die MDL-Optimierung

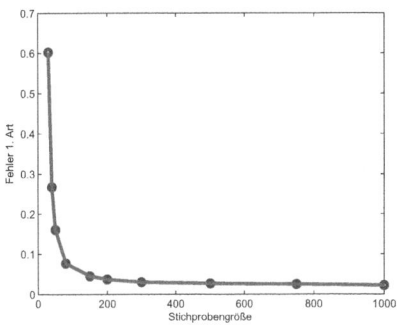 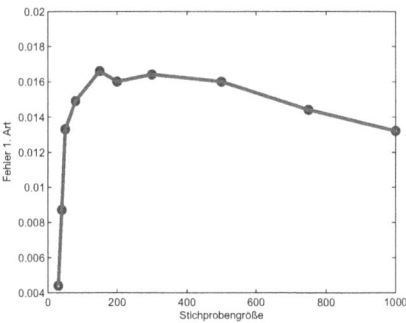

Abb. 1. α-Fehler von Mardias Test (links) und dem BHEP-Test (rechts).

verschiebt die Landmarken zu einer Normalverteilung, was sich in kleineren p-Werten widerspiegelt (Tab. 1). Im Hinblick auf die Anwendung statistischer Formmodelle motivieren unsere Ergebnisse die Verwendung von nichtlinearen Ansätzen wie z.B. der Kernel-PCA. In diesem Zusammenhang könnte der vorgestellte Ansatz bereits bei der Erstellung eines statistischen Formmodells zur Beurteilung der multivariaten Normalverteilung eingesetzt werden, um dann, in Abhängigkeit vom Testergebnis, ein lineares oder nichtlineares Formmodell für die jeweilige Objektklasse zu verwenden. Im Fall von nicht normalverteilten Daten könnte ein nichtlineares Modell die Formvariabilität besser beschreiben als ein auf der linearen PCA basierendes SFM, und damit auch potenziell bessere Segmentierungsergebnisse erzielen. Dies im Rahmen einer tatsächlichen Segmentierung zu untersuchen ist Gegenstand aktueller und zukünftiger Arbeiten.

Danksagung. Wir danken M. Simon, UKSH, Institut für Neuroradiologie, A. Bischof, IMAGE Information Systems Ltd. und Prof. J. Barkhausen, UKSH, Klinik für Radiologie und Neuroradiologie für die Bereitstellung der Daten.

Literaturverzeichnis

1. Heimann T, Meinzer HP. Statistical shape models for 3D medical image segmentation: a review. Med Image Anal. 2009;13:543–63.
2. Kirschner M, Becker M, Wesarg S. 3D active shape model segmentation with nonlinear shape priors. Lect Notes Computer Sci. 2011;6892:492–9.
3. Wimmer A, Soza G, Hornegger J. A generic probabilistic active shape model for organ segmentation. Lect Notes Computer Sci. 2009;5762:26–33.
4. Mardia KV, Kent JT, Bibby JM. Multivariate Analysis. New York: Academic Press; 1979.
5. Mardia KV. Measures of multivariate skewness and kurtosis with applications. Biometrika. 1970;57:519–30.
6. Henze N, Zirkler B. A class of invariant consistent tests for multivariate normality. Commun Statist Theory Meth. 1990;19:3595–617.
7. Rencher AC, Christensen WF. Methods of Multivariate Analysis. Wiley Series in Probability and Statistics; 1995.
8. Kirschner M, Gollmer ST, Wesarg S, et al. Optimal initialization for 3D correspondence optimization: an evaluation study. Lect Notes Computer Sci. 2011;6801:308–19.
9. Davies RH, Twining CJ, Cootes TF, et al. Building 3-D statistical shape models by direct optimization. IEEE Trans Med Imaging. 2010;29(4):961–81.
10. Liang J, Lic R, Fanga H, et al. Testing multinormality based on low-dimensional projection. J Stat Plan Inference. 2000;86:129–41.

Robust Feature for Transcranial Sonography Image Classification Using Rotation-Invariant Gabor Filter

Arkan Al-Zubaidi[1], Lei Chen[1,3], Johann Hagenah[2], Alfred Mertins[1]

[1]Institute for Signal Processing, University of Luebeck,Germany
[2]Department of Neurology, University Hospital Schleswig-Holstein, Germany
[3]Graduate School, University of Luebeck, Germany
chen@isip.uni-luebeck.de

Abstract. Transcranial sonography is a new tool for the diagnosis of Parkinson's disease according to a distinct hyperechogenic pattern in the substantia nigra region. In order to reduce the influence of the image properties from different settings of ultrasound machine, we propose a robust feature extraction method using rotation-invariant Gabor filter bank. Except the general Gabor features, such as mean and standard deviation, we suggest to use the entropy of the filtered images for the TCS images classification. The performance of the Gabor features is evaluated by a feature selection method with the objective function of support vector machine classifier. The results show that the rotation-invariant Gabor filter is better than the conventional one, and the entropy is invariant to the intensity and the contrast changes.

1 Introduction

Transcranial sonography (TCS) was first used in 1995 to distinguish between a group of Parkinson's disease (PD) patients and healthy controls by Becker et al. [1]. For the healthy controls, the hyperechogenicity of the substantia nigra (SN) was significantly decreased compared to PD patients. It is possible to determine the structure of the idiopathic from of Parkinsonism at an early state by means of TCS technique [2]. However, the structural abnormalities were not detected on CT and MRI scans [3]. Three feature analysis algorithms were implemented based on the ipsilateral mesencephalon wing, which is close to the ultrasound probe as shown in Fig. 1. First, the moment of inertia and Hul-moment were calculated based on manually segmented half of mesencephalon (HoM) for separating control subjects from Parkin mutation carriers [4]. Then, a hybrid feature extraction method, which includes statistical, geometrical and texture features for the early PD risk assessment, was proposed [5], It showed a good performance of texture features, especially Gabor features. Third, a texture analysis method that applied a bank of Gabor filters and gray-level co-occurrence matrices (GLCM) was used on TCS images [6]. In this paper, we used three datasets that were acquired by different examiners with in different

H.-P. Meinzer et al. (Hrsg.), *Bildverarbeitung für die Medizin 2013*, Informatik aktuell,
DOI: 10.1007/978-3-642-36480-8_48, © Springer-Verlag Berlin Heidelberg 2013

periods. These datasets include the TCS images from the healthy controls (HC) and PD patients. The properties of the TCS images, such as the contrast and brightness, are effected by different setting of the US machine used by different examiners. Furthermore, the challenge of the classification of the TCS images using Gabor filters is that orientations and shapes of the HoM are different from one PD patient to another.

2 Methods

Our goal is to develop Gabor features that are invariant to the direction of HoM, the brightness and the contrast changes from the different settings. Therefore, we propose a texture analysis method that applies a rotation-invariant Gabor filter bank on the HoM area and computes the histogram feature from the filtered images for the TCS image classification.

2.1 Conventional gabor filter bank

The performance of conventional Gabor filters becomes poor if texture can occur with arbitrary orientations [7, 8]. Let $I(x, y)$ be an image, its discrete Gabor wavelet transform is defined by a convolution

$$G_{mn}(x, y) = \sum_{\xi} \sum_{\eta} I(x - \xi, y - \eta) g_{mn}^*(\xi, \eta) \tag{1}$$

where parameters m and n specify the scales and orientations, respectively, and $*$ indicates the complex conjugate of g_{mn} [9]. The 2D Gabor function $g(\xi, \eta)$ is

$$g(\xi, \eta) = \frac{1}{2\pi\sigma_\xi\sigma_\eta} \exp[-\frac{1}{2}(\frac{\xi^2}{\sigma_\xi^2} + \frac{\eta^2}{\sigma_\eta^2})] \cdot \exp[2\pi jW\xi] \tag{2}$$

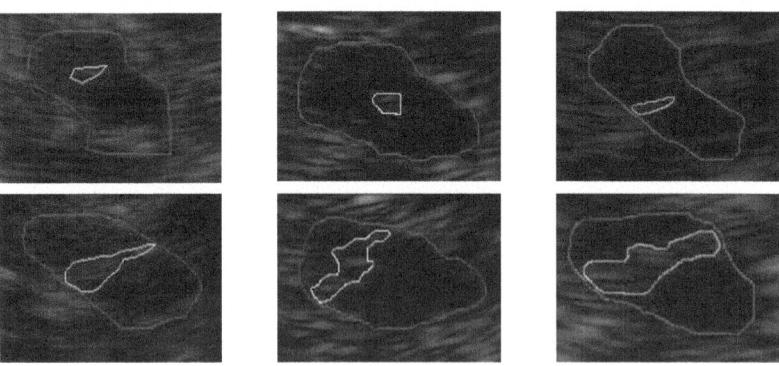

Fig. 1. Manually segmented TCS images with Philips SONOS 5500. The first and second row are from healthy control subjects and PD patients, respectively. The red marker indicates the upper HoM. Yellow/green markers show the SN area.

where W is called the modulation frequency, the other parameters are chosen as in [6]. It is assumed that the SN region in the ROI (HoM) has homogeneous texture, therefore the mean μ_{mn} and the standard deviation σ_{mn} of the coefficients' magnitudes are used to represent the texture features in the conventional Gabor feature vector f_c as in [6]. The filter mask size is 61×61, five scales and six orientations have been used in the experiments.

2.2 Rotation-invariant gabor filter design

Han et al. [7] proposed the summation of all the Gabor filter responses under different orientations, but along the same scale, could yield a rotation-invariant Gabor filter

$$g_m^{(R)}(\xi, \eta) = \sum_{n=0}^{K-1} g_{m,n}(\xi, \eta), m = 0, 1, ..., S - 1 \qquad (3)$$

Zhang et al. [8] suggested to sort the Gabor features by the total energy of the filtered images over the orientation with the same scale. The orientation of filtered image with the highest total energy is defined as the dominant direction. An example texture image and the energy map are shown in Fig. 2 (a) and (b), respectively. The rotated image (90° of the first image) and the corresponding energy map are shown in Fig. 2 (c) and (d), respectively. Fig. 2 (b) shows that image (a) has a dominant direction at orientation 5 (150°), while for image (c), the dominant direction has moved to orientation 2 (30°). Using the same concept, the filtered image G_{ij} with the dominant direction j is moved to be at the first position at scale i, and the other filtered images are circularly shifted accordingly. As a result, the feature elements μ_{ij}, σ_{ij} in conventional Gabor feature vector f_c are shifted as in the rotation-invariant Gabor feature vector f_r. For example, if f_c is (A,B,C,D,E,F) and (C) is at the dominant direction, then f_r is (C,D,E,F,A,B).

2.3 Robust feature extraction

In gerenal, the conventional Gabor features, the mean and the standard deviation are calculated from the intensity values of the filtered image directly. In this section, we compute the entropy from the histogram of the filtered image. Shannon entropy can be used to measure the randomness of the image histogram.

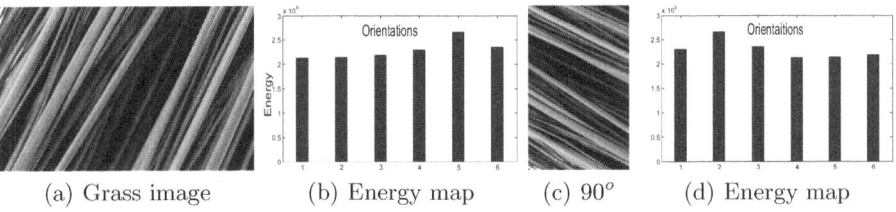

(a) Grass image   (b) Energy map   (c) 90° (d) Energy map

Fig. 2. Texture image and the energy map of the filtered images at each orientation.

In other words, the entropy measures the uniformity of the filtered image. In Fig. 3, the TCS images were normalized to the range [0,255], then the method of Zhang et al. was used to extract the features from HoM region. The result shows that the mean and standard deviation features from ROI are changed but the entropy feature of the histogram is more stable. Actually, the symbol alphabet of filtered image is in general not finite. Therefore, a proper measurement of entropy is differential entropy [10]. The entropy of the histogram image is given

$$H(X) = -\sum_{x \in S} \text{hist}_{\text{norm}}(x) \log_2(\text{hist}_{\text{norm}}(x)) \tag{4}$$

where S is the support set of the random variable x and $\text{hist}_{\text{norm}}(x)$ is the histogram properly normalized to fit a probability density function. The summation of the probability density function $\text{hist}_{\text{norm}}(x)$ is one. In our case, the complete feature vector F of the rotation-invariant Gabor filter has 90 dimensions: $F(1,...,60)$ are 60 Gabor features μ_{ij}, σ_{ij} in feature vector $f_r(1, 2, ..., 60)$; $F(61, ..., 90)$ are 30 features of entropy $f_{re}(1, 2, ..., 30)$.

3   Method of evaluation

The normalization process is used to simulate different user settings. Brightness and contrast changes were applied to the TCS images. In this paper, three normalization methods are tested on the TCS images. The first normalization is zero mean and unit variance ($\frac{X-\mu}{\sigma}$). Second, all TCS images are rescaled to full gray level range [0,255]. Third, we applied the contrast-limited adaptive histogram equalization (CLAHE) [11] to match the histogram of ROI with a desired shape. The exponential and Rayleigh distributions were used in this experiment. Furthermore, the Gabor features were evaluated by the sequential forward floating selection (SFFS) method. The accuracy of the SVM classifier was used as a criterion function of SFFS. The sequential minimal optimization (SMO) method

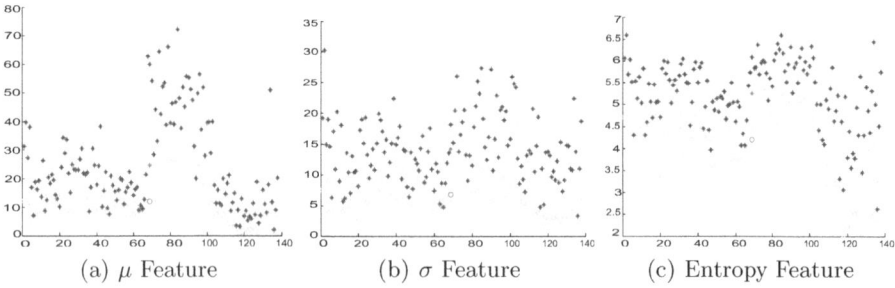

(a) μ Feature   (b) σ Feature   (c) Entropy Feature

Fig. 3. Green circles: Features of the original images. Blue stars: Features of the rescaled images ([0,255]). Red points: Mean value of the features. Under the rescaling the mean value of the μ and the σ features are shifted from 11 to 26, and shifted from 7 to 14, respectively. But the entropy features are more stable than μ, and the σ features, the corresponding mean value only shifted from 4.1 to 5.2.

Table 1. Performance of Gabor filter banks on the public dataset [12].

SVMs cross-validation	Conventional Gabor	Zhang et al. [8]	Han et al. [7]
Accuracy	72%	76%	72%
Confusion matrix	$\left(\begin{smallmatrix}39 & 1\\21 & 19\end{smallmatrix}\right)$	$\left(\begin{smallmatrix}40 & 0\\19 & 21\end{smallmatrix}\right)$	$\left(\begin{smallmatrix}38 & 2\\20 & 20\end{smallmatrix}\right)$

and the linear kernel were specified to find the separating hyperplane. The cross validation was set with the leave-one-out method.

We compared the rotation-invariant Gabor filter algorithms according to the UIUC database [12]. We selected T01(bark1) and T15(brick2) from that database. These are two rotated texture sets, each one containing 40 samples. The results in Tab. 1 show that the method of Zhang et al. [8] works better than the method of Han et al. [7] and the conventional Gabor filter method.

4 Experimental results

The classification results were based on three datasets of TCS images, which were obtained using Philips SONOS 5500 by different examiners. Dataset 1 includes 36 TCS images from 21 healthy subjects and 42 TCS images from 23 PD patients. Dataset 2 includes 8 control TCS images from 4 healthy subjects and 15 PD TCS images from 10 patients. The last dataset consisted of 27 control TCS images from 14 healthy subjects and 10 PD TCS images from 5 patients. Totally, this dataset includes 67 PD images from 38 PD patients and 71 control images from 39 healthy subjects. The Gabor filter bank was applied to the ROI of TCS images. Then, the rotation-invariant Gabor features were extracted and shifted by the dominant direction. The feature extraction from the manual segmentation of HoM, which was marked by the physicians as shown in Fig. 1. The feature analysis results in Tab. 2 show that the entropy features $F(61, 77)$ are more stable than the mean and the standard deviation features $F(1, 5, 7)$. The feature subset $F(66, 3)$ obtained by $SFFS$ gave the highest classification rate of 81.88% ($F(66)$ is the entropy feature $f_{re}(6)$ and $F(3)$ is the mean feature $f_r(3)$). The results in the right two columns of Tab. 2 show the performance of the feature sets with different methods of image normalization, and the confusion matrices for the feature set $F(66, 3)$. At last, based on this dataset, the features of the conventional Gabor filter in [6] achieved 69.56% classification rate. In this paper, the accuracy reached 81.88% which is better than the method of Chen et al. [6], and the histogram feature is more stable.

5 Conclusions

This paper has concentrated on the texture analysis of the HoM and even the SN area by using rotation-invariant Gabor filters and selecting good combinations of features for PD detection. The accuracy of the classification results shows

Table 2. Classification results of rotation-invariant Gabor filter banks (Zhang et al.) based on different normalization methods for TCS images.

Normalized dataset	$F(1,5,7)$	$F(61,77)$	$F(66,3)$	Confusion matrix
$\frac{X-\mu}{\sigma}$	67.39%	60.08%	70.29 %	$\left(\begin{smallmatrix} 66 & 1 \\ 40 & 31 \end{smallmatrix}\right)$
$[0,255]$	65.94%	61.59 %	70.29%	$\left(\begin{smallmatrix} 60 & 7 \\ 34 & 37 \end{smallmatrix}\right)$
Exponential	63.76%	60.14%	78.26%	$\left(\begin{smallmatrix} 61 & 6 \\ 24 & 47 \end{smallmatrix}\right)$
Rayleigh	30.43%	68.84%	77.53%	$\left(\begin{smallmatrix} 60 & 7 \\ 24 & 47 \end{smallmatrix}\right)$

that the rotation-invariant Gabor filter is better than the conventional Gabor filter. In addition, the rotation-invariant Gabor filter helps the SVM to separate between PD patients and healthy controls. In particular, the entropy feature is more stable than the mean and the standard deviation features in the monotonic change of the gray scale. One of the factors that determine the accuracy of the results is the manual segmentation of HoM area by physician. In our future work, we plan to develop an automatic segmentation algorithm for localization of the HoM area.

References

1. Becker G, Seufert J, Bogdahn U, et al. Degeneration of substantia nigra in chronic Parkinson's diseasevisualized by transcranial color-coded real-time sonograph. Neurology. 1995;45:182–4.
2. Behnke S, Berg D, Becker G. Does ultrasound disclose a vulnerability factor for Parkinson's disease? J Neural. 2003;250 Suppl 1:I24–I2.
3. Hagenah JM, Hedrich K, Becker B, et al. Distinguishing early-onset PD from dopa-responsive dystonia with transcranial sonography. Neurology. 2006;66:1951–52.
4. Kier C, Seidel G, Bregemann N, et al. Transcranial sonography as early indicator for genetic Parkinson's disease. Proc IFMBE. 2009; p. 456–9.
5. Chen L, Seidel G, Mertins A. Multiple feature extraction for early Parkinson risk assessment based on transcranial sonography image. Proc Int Conf Image Proc. 2010.
6. Chen L, Hagenah J, Mertins A. Texture analysis using gabor filter based on transcranial sonography image. Proc BVM. 2011; p. 249–53.
7. Han J, Ma KK. Rotation-invariant and scale-invariant gabor features for texture image retrieval. Image Vis Comput. 2007;25:1474–81.
8. D Zhang MI A Wong, Lu G. Content-based image retrival using gabor texture features. IEEE Trans Trans Pattern Anal Mach Intell. 2000; p. 13–5.
9. Manjunath BS, Ma WY. Texture features for browsing and retrieval of image data. IEEE Trans Pattern Anal Mach Intell. 1996;18:837–42.
10. Cover TM, Thomas JA. Elements of information theory. USA: John Wiley; 2006.
11. Zuiderveld K. Contrast limited adaptive histogram equalization. In: Heckbert PS, editor. Graphics gems IV. San Diego, CA, USA: Academic Press Professional, Inc.; 1994. p. 474–85.
12. Lazebnik S, Schmid C, Ponce J. A sparse texture representation using local affine regions. IEEE Trans Pattern Anal Mach Intell. 2005;27:1265–78.

Automatic Histogram-Based Initialization of K-Means Clustering in CT

Mengqiu Tian[1,2], Qiao Yang[1,2], Andreas Maier[2], Ingo Schasiepen[1], Nicole Maass[1], Matthias Elter[1]

[1]Siemens AG, H CP CV ME, Erlangen, Germany
[2]Pattern Recognition Lab, Friedrich-Alexander-University Erlangen-Nuremberg, Erlangen, Germany
tianmengqiu@gmail.com

Abstract. K-means clustering [1] has been widely used in various applications. One intrinsic limitation in K-means clustering is that the choice of initial clustering centroids may highly influence the performance of the algorithm. Some existing K-means initialization algorithms could generally achieve good results. However, in certain cases, such as CT images that contain several materials with similar gray-levels, such existing initialization algorithms will lead to poor performance in distinguishing those materials. We propose an automatic K-means initialization algorithm based on histogram analysis, which manages to overcome the aforementioned deficiency. Results demonstrate that our method achieves high efficiency in terms of finding starting points close to ground truth so that offers reliable segmentation results for CT images in aforementioned situation.

1 Introduction

Segmentation plays a critical role in many medical image processing applications, such as beam hardening correction in CT images. However, in practical cases, accurate object identification and separation are non-trivial tasks due to data acquisition and reconstruction artifacts.

Global thresholding has been widely used for object segmentation. However, most thresholding methods suffer from inaccurate detection of shapes and peaks in histogram due to noise and artifacts, thus leading to the process being difficult to fully automate. On the other hand, K-means clustering, which accepts classes with different shapes, has an intrinsic limitation that the computational efficiency highly depends on cluster initialization. Authors of [2] and [3] respectively compared 14 and 4 approaches for K-means clustering initialization. In [2] the scrambled midpoints and in [3] the Kaufman initialization algorithm have been reported to perform the best. However, in certain cases, the above two initialization methods for K-means clustering have the limitation to accurately distinguish materials with similar gray-levels in CT images. For example, in application such as segmenting hearing aid containing air, plastic and metal components, those methods are not sensitive enough to separate air and plastic

H.-P. Meinzer et al. (Hrsg.), *Bildverarbeitung für die Medizin 2013*, Informatik aktuell,
DOI: 10.1007/978-3-642-36480-8_49, © Springer-Verlag Berlin Heidelberg 2013

which have much closer densities compared to metal. We propose a novel K-means initialization algorithm, which offers better sensitivity in distinguishing similar materials, and meanwhile yields better performance for general datasets . The new algorithm achieves automatic initialization of cluster centroids for K-means with prior-knowledge from histogram. In Section 3, we compare the proposed algorithm with the scrambled midpoints and the Kaufman initialization algorithms with respect to initialization accuracy, and Otsu's method, a classical histogram-based thresholding method, to compare segmentation performance [4, 5].

2   Materials and methods

The algorithm's main idea is to detect the peaks in histogram and to employ the corresponding gray-levels as initial cluster centroids for K-means clustering. For the first centroid, the gray-level of the highest peak in the histogram is selected. Then the local maximum with the largest weighted distance to all other known centroids is chosen as a new centroid.

2.1   Algorithm

For the distance metric, the product of the gray-level difference $d_{n,i}$ between centroid C_n and local maximum i, and the height h_i of the local maximum is used. This process is iteratively repeated until the desired number of centroids is found. We use the product (instead of the sum) of all weighted distances as criterion, since iff. all ($h_i \cdot d_{n,i}$) were large, the product would be maximized. The flowchart of our algorithm is depicted in Fig. 1.

1. Calculate the image histogram.
2. Detect all local maxima in the histogram. We assume a total number of I local maxima are detected.
3. Choose the global maximum of the histogram as the first centroid C_1.
4. Identify the remaining centroids as follows:
   (a) Calculate
   $$P_{N+1}(i) = \prod_{n=1}^{N} (h_i \cdot d_{n,i}) \tag{1}$$

   for each local maximum ($i = 1, 2, ..., I$). N is the number of already found centroids. The computational complexity can be reduced by using a recursive implementation

   $$P_2(i) = h_i \cdot d_{1,i} \tag{2}$$
   $$P_{N+1}(i) = P_N(i) \cdot (h_i \cdot d_{N,i}) \tag{3}$$

   which employs similar idea of Viterbi algorithm [6].
   (b) Then the new centroid $C_{N+1} = \arg\max_i(P_{N+1}(i)), N = N + 1$.
5. Repeat 4 until N equals the user-specified number of classes K.

2.2 Experiments

The proposed method was evaluated with ten datasets containing simulated data and CT scans. Three simulated datasets were obtained using DRASIM (Siemens Healthcare, Forchheim, Germany), and seven real CT datasets were obtained from industrial and medical CT scanners (industrial datasets: Siemens Healthcare, Munich, Germany; medical datasets: Siemens Healthcare, Erlangen, Germany; Dataset I: jaw phantom; II: head phantom; III: aluminum and iron cylinders phantom IV: hearing-aid; V: computer mouse; VI: aluminum component; VII: CD spindle; VIII: elbow; IX: knee; X: head) All datasets were reconstructed using filtered back projection (FBP) on a $512 \times 512 \times 512$ grid, except for dataset IX which uses FBP on a $384 \times 384 \times 384$ grid. We segmented all these ten datasets, and read out the segmentation results.

We use the normalized sum of absolute difference (NSAD) to measure the proximity of initial cluster centroids to ground truth. The smaller the NSAD value is, the closer the initial cluster centroids are to the ground truth. If NSAD is too large, it can happen that K-means clustering algorithm does not converge to ground truth.

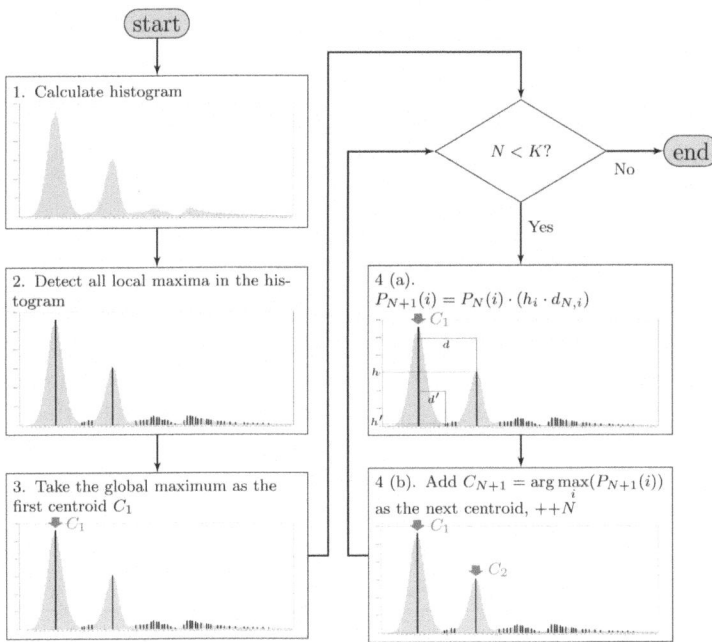

Fig. 1. Flowchart of the proposed algorithm (X-axis of histogram: bin index; Y-axis of histogram: number of pixels).

We first calculated the normalized distance between the initial cluster centroids given by initialization algorithms and ground truth:

$$d[k] = \frac{|\text{Ground truth}[k] - \text{Initial cluster centroid}[k]|}{\Delta t} \qquad (4)$$

Δt is the width of each histogram bin: $\Delta t = (v_{\max} - v_{\min})/L$, where $v_{\min}$ and $v_{\max}$ are the minimal and maximal gray-levels of the image respectively, and L is the number of histogram bins. 512 bins are applied in our experiments for all datasets. Then we have

$$\text{NSAD} = \sum_{k=1}^{K} d[k] \qquad (5)$$

3   Results

In this section, we present the results from a series of experiments, comparing our algorithm with alternative approaches in terms of segmentation accuracy and the proximity of starting points to ground truth.

3.1   Analysis of segmentation result

The percentage of misclassified pixels (pMP) are used to measure the performance of three initialization algorithms and multi-level Otsu's method. Fig. 2 shows that our proposed method results in the best clustering results with minimal pMP in our datasets.

3.2   Analysis of proximity of starting points to ground truth

Tab. 1 shows a summary of NSAD for ten datasets ranging from simulated data to experimental CT data. For experimental datasets, human observers selected a given number of peaks from histograms, and used the average value of corresponding gray values as ground truth. The highlighted terms show the

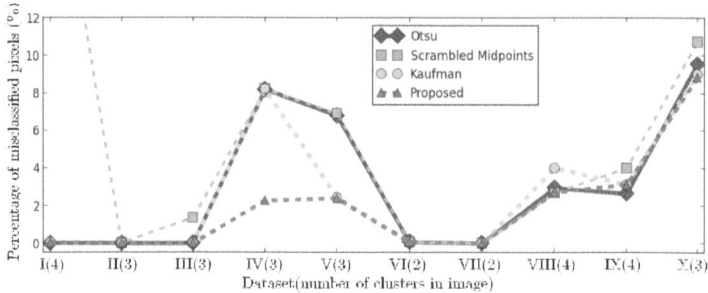

Fig. 2. Number of misclassified pixels in each dataset (%).

Table 1. Normalized Sum of Absolute Difference (NSAD).

Dataset	I	II	III	IV	V	VI	VII	VIII	IX	X
Scrambled midpoints	525	122	331	633	690	90.8	135	514	484	307
Kaufman	30.9	36.3	55.5	331	77.6	**1.67**	30.2	41.5	**50.9**	**46.8**
Proposed	**4.48**	**0.00**	**0.00**	**17.0**	**1.0**	10.0	**2.0**	**1.0**	212	105

smallest NSAD value for each dataset. It can be seen that, for most datasets the proposed algorithm outperforms others.

We depict the segmentation results from initial cluster centroids of three datasets (one simulated dataset I and two real datasets IV and VIII) in Fig. 3, in order to compare the performance of selected initial centroids with ground truth. It can be seen that the segmentation results of proposed algorithm are already very close to the segmentation results based on ground truth, while scrambled midpoints and Kaufman method could not perform as well as expected. The reason is when datasets consisting of similarly dense objects, the latter two methods have lower sensitivity to detect histogram peaks. For example, in hearing-aid dataset, air and plastic have close density values, resulting in the peaks of air and plastic (orange arrows 1 and 2) located very close to each other compared

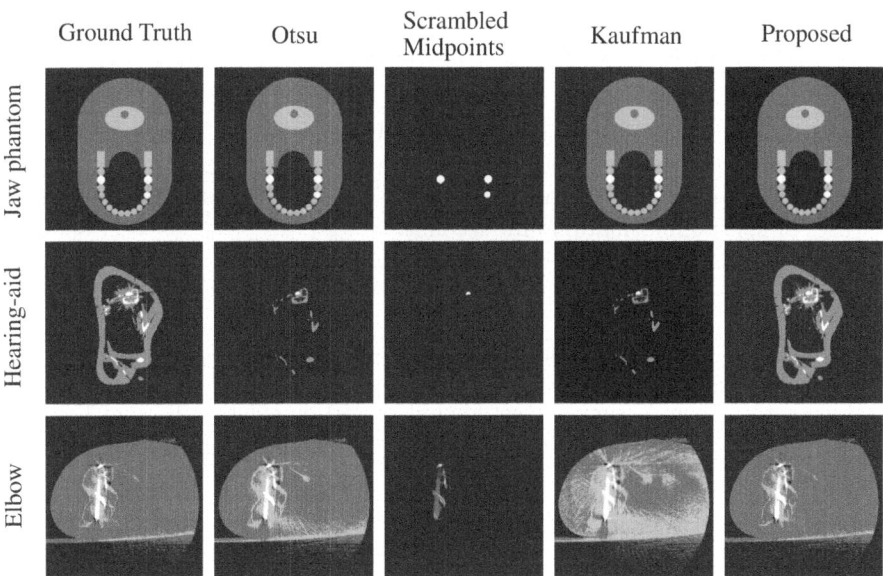

Fig. 3. Segmentation results analysis: Column 1: Segmentation results based on ground truth; Column 2: Segmentation results of multi-level Otsu Method; Column 3-5: Segmentation results of K-means initial clustering centroids for scrambled midpoints, Kaufman and proposed method.

Fig. 4. Logarithm histogram of hearing-aid.

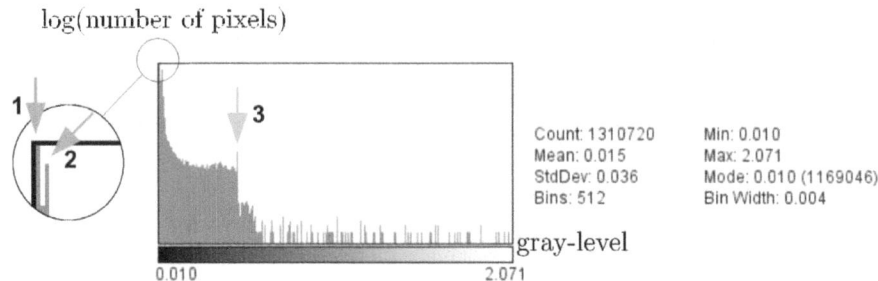

to the peak of metal (green arrow 3) (Fig. 4). Moreover, our algorithm leads to better segmentation results than multi-level Otsu's algorithm, while multi-level Otsu's algorithm is very time consuming. The computational complexity of the proposed algorithm is $\mathcal{O}(KL)$, while it is $\mathcal{O}(L^{K-1})$ for multi-level Otsu's method [5].

4   Discussion

In this paper, we compared the proposed method with several existing initialization methods on a variety of datasets. Experimental results demonstrate that the proposed algorithm achieves better accuracy and closer proximity of initial centroids to ground truth. However, even if K-means algorithm is properly initialized, it might be insufficient for medical purpose since in medical CT images, different organs at different location could yield same gray levels. In such cases, the segmentation could not based only on gray levels, but also should take features or spatial information into account.

References

1. MacQueen J. Some methods for classification and analysis of multivariate observations. Proc BSMSP. 1967;1:281–97.
2. Robinson F, Apon A, Brewer D, et al. Initial starting point analysis for K-means clustering: a case study. Proc ALAR Conference on Applied Research in Information Technology. 2006.
3. Pena JM, Lozano JA, Larranaga P. An empirical comparison of four initialization methods for the K-Means algorithm. Pattern Recognit Lett. 1999;20:1027–40.
4. Otsu N. A threshold Selection method from gray-level histograms. IEEE Trans Syst Man Cybern. 1979;SMC-9:62–6.
5. Liao PS, Chen TS, Chung PC. A fast algorithm for multilevel thresholding. J Inf Sci Eng. 2001;17:713–27.
6. Huang X, Acero A, Hon HW. Spoken language processing: a guide to theory, algorithm, and system development. 1st ed. Upper Saddle River, NJ, USA: Prentice Hall PTR; 2001.

Extraction of Partial Skeletons for Semi-Automatic Segmentation of Cortical Structures

Eduard Fried, Tony Pilz, Stefan van Waasen, Gudrun Wagenknecht

Multimodal Image Processing Group, Electronic Systems, ZEA-2,
Forschungszentrum Jülich GmbH
e.fried@fz-juelich.de

Abstract. Volume-of-interest segmentation is an important part in the functional analysis of multimodal data (MRI, PET). The usual approach of manually segmenting structures in single 2D slices is cumbersome and prone to errors. The authors present an extension of a semiautomatic approach, which allows the user to define a volume of interest on a 3D visualization of the cortical surface. The volume of interest is computed with a volume growing approach, in which a partial sulcal skeleton serves as a boundary. A new 3D algorithm computes a partial skeleton that is more compact and complete compared to 2D algorithms applied in three orthogonal orientations. This method allows us to simplify the subsequent postprocessing steps and thus to compute a more precise segmentation.

1 Introduction

Volume-of-interest (VOI) segmentation of multimodal data (e.g., MRI, PET) is an important part in the functional analysis of cortical structures. The usual approach is to create a segmentation by manually labeling structures in several 2D slices of a 3D data set. Toolkits, such as 3D Slicer [1], speed up this segmentation process, e.g., by defining polygons or labeling single voxels with a brush-like widget. Nevertheless, this procedure is often time-consuming and prone to inter-user variability.

Automatic segmentation of the sulcal structure of the brain was computed by Mangin et al. [2] and Lohmann et al. [3]. Their goal was to compute a parcellation of the whole gray matter area and to identify and describe the sulcus structure. Wagenknecht et al. [4] presented a semiautomatic approach that computes cortical volumes of interest based on classified MR images. The VOI boundaries are computed from the class borders, user-defined 3D live-wire (3DLW) contour paths on the 3D visualization of the cortical surface, and a partial skeleton marked by 2D algorithms applied in three orthogonal orientations on a 3D sulcal skeleton. In this paper, a 3D skeleton marking algorithm is presented.

H.-P. Meinzer et al. (Hrsg.), *Bildverarbeitung für die Medizin 2013*, Informatik aktuell,
DOI: 10.1007/978-3-642-36480-8_50, © Springer-Verlag Berlin Heidelberg 2013

2   Materials and methods

The 3D skeleton marking algorithm is integrated into the semiautomatic segmentation approach [4] summarized in this paragraph. This approach requires a classified image with five classes as input: background (B), extracerebral region (C), cerebrospinal fluid (CSF), gray matter (GM), and white matter (WM). This information is obtained from a T1-weighted MR image. From this image, a skeleton **S** of the sulci (inside the merged area of the classes C, CSF, GM) and a 3D visualization of the cortical surface are computed. The user sets points inside the sulci on the cortical surface, which are then connected by a 3D livewire algorithm (3DLW) generating a closed contour path on the brain surface. This 3DLW contour intersects the skeleton **S** and is used as a feature to extract the desired part **PS** of the skeleton with 2D algorithms applied in orthogonal orientations. The partial skeleton and the class borders serve as a boundary for the following volume growing process, which computes the VOI inside the GM class. Since the skeleton does not connect with the WM class and does not exist where the 3DLW contour crosses gyri, the VOI surface contains gaps, which are closed by postprocessing steps such as interpolation or dilation to prevent leakage during volume growing.

Due to the complex 3D skeleton geometry, 2D algorithms cannot always follow its structure, even if they are applied in each of the three orientations (transaxial, coronal, sagittal). The two 2D algorithms used in [4] have inherent problems, as the clockwise approach (Fig. 1a) can get "stuck" in small side branches. The tracing approach (Fig. 1c) can grow too far away from the desired branches, thus marking a partial skeleton that is too large, which in turn might result in cutting off parts of the VOI in a subsequent closing process (e.g., dilation).

In order to solve these problems, a new 3D skeleton marking algorithm was implemented. The skeleton consists of branches reaching into the sulci and a hull completely covering the brain. Since the VOI is a gray matter region and

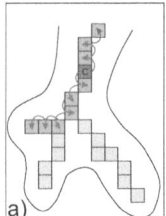 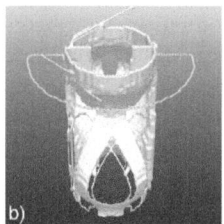 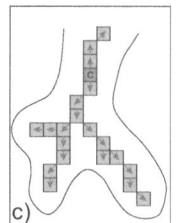 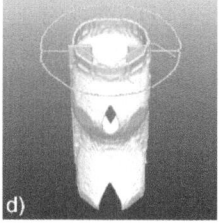

Fig. 1. Principle of the 2D algorithms. a) *Clockwise* algorithm, which marks skeleton voxels starting at the 3DLW contour voxel C and successively choosing the first voxel when iterating the neighborhood in a clockwise or anticlockwise manner. This algorithm can get stuck in small branches. c) *Tracing* algorithm, which marks all neighbors. b,d) 3D visualization of the marked partial skeleton for the *Clockwise* and *Tracing* algorithms shown for the phantom data set of Fig. 4.

is bounded by the classes CSF and WM, only the skeleton branches inside the GM are required for the VOI boundary. Thus, in a preprocessing step, the hull is separated from the full skeleton and is used as a feature in the following steps.

The 3D marking algorithm used to compute the desired **PS**, which is a partial surface containing parts of the 3DLW contour, is executed in six steps:

1. A partial skeleton **PS1** is computed by a distance transform on the skeleton **S** starting from the 3DLW contour voxels that intersect the skeleton. The growing process successively adds neighbor skeleton voxels to the result. Additionally, a pointer is stored for each result voxel pointing to its predecessor voxel. Thus, for each voxel, a "reversed" path of minimal distance can be determined, which points to a start voxel on the 3DLW contour (Fig. 2a). The growing process stops when a user-defined maximum distance is reached. Since the 3D algorithm grows in all directions, the resulting partial skeleton **PS1** also contains undesired skeleton branches that have to be removed in subsequent steps.
2. The **PS1** is a thin curved structure comprising inner and border voxels. The border voxels are computed as topologically simple points, i.e., they can be removed without changing the topology of **PS1** [5]. Border voxels that have a neighbor voxel in the skeleton hull are referred to as *top points*.
3. A second growing process is computed in a similar manner to step 1, but uses the top points from step 2 as starting points and **PS1** as the computation domain. The new partial skeleton **PS2** thus consists of the same voxels as **PS1**, but the distance values and minimal paths are different (Fig. 2b).
4. All paths of **PS1** reach the 3DLW contour voxels. In **PS2**, however, only a fraction of the paths pass through the 3DLW contour voxels. Therefore, paths that directly lead to a top point are discarded (Fig. 2c).
5. The desired partial skeleton **PS** contains voxels on paths that do not pass through a 3DLW contour voxel, due to a closer connection to one of the top points lying outside of **PS**. Such paths are discarded in step 4. However, subpaths can be restored, if they contain a neighbor voxel of the marked skeleton after step 4. In Fig. 3a, for example, subpath $q \rightarrow k$ is restored, because k is a neighbor of voxel j on the marked skeleton.
6. Paths on the partial skeleton **PS2** that lie between the top points and the 3DLW contour are discarded in step 4. To recover these paths, the list of top

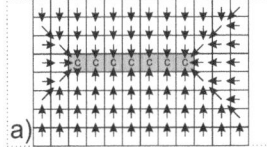 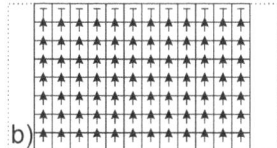 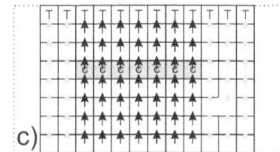

Fig. 2. Idealized view of a skeleton patch as a 2D plane. a) Minimal paths pointing to the 3DLW voxels **C** as computed in step 1. b) Minimal paths pointing to the top points **T** (step 2) as computed in step 3. c) Paths that do not pass through the 3DLW voxels are discarded in step 4 (shown in light gray).

points is separated into valid points (top points in the partial skeleton after step 4) and candidate points (all other top points). The valid points are connected by a searching process that starts with a valid point and successively adds neighbors from the set of candidate points to build candidate paths. When another valid point is reached, then the points on the candidate path are also added to the list of valid points. Thus, a candidate path that does not reach another valid point partially lies on an undesired skeleton branch and can be discarded. This process is repeated for all initial valid points. The updated list of valid points is used to recover paths from **PS2** and thus to build the desired partial skeleton **PS** (Fig. 3d, Fig. 5).

3   Results

Since the skeleton geometry for MR brain data sets is very complex, it is difficult to evaluate the marking algorithms. Therefore, we created a phantom data set to model a small region of the brain (Fig. 4). It consists of two cylindrical structures that are shifted on a sine curve in the z direction and rotated by 45 degrees around the z axis. These objects represent the gray matter part of a curved sulcus. Between the gray matter regions, a white matter region is modeled as a cylinder that is also shifted on a sine curve. Additionally, the phantom contains two cuboids of gray matter connecting the two "simulated sulci". The gray and white matter regions are enclosed by regions of CSF and C to ensure correct computation of the full skeleton. The results of the 2D and 3D algorithms are shown in Fig. 1b, Fig. 1d and in Fig. 3c, Fig. 5d. The problems solved in step 6 of the algorithm are shown on a classified T1-weighted MRI data set in Fig 5. The presented algorithm was successfully applied to 38 clinical MRI

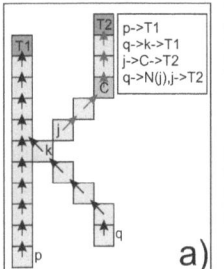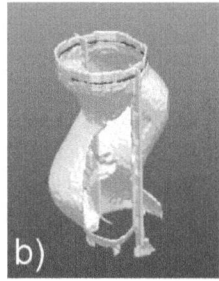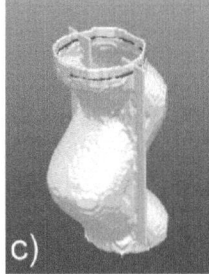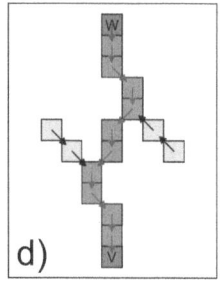

Fig. 3. a) 2D view of a skeleton with computed paths. Only path $j \rightarrow C \rightarrow T2$ is marked in step 4, because the path from q leads to $T1$ and not to the valid top point $T2$. In step 5, path $q \rightarrow k$ is added to the result, because k is a neighbor of the previously marked voxel j ($k \in N(j)$). b) Marked partial skeleton (yellow) after step 4 for a phantom data set. c) Marked skeleton after step 5. The 3DLW contour is shown in red. d) Idealized view of top points in a 2D plane. Path between valid top points **V** and **W** is computed in step 6. Points on other paths (light gray) are discarded.

data sets. With 8 cortical VOIs per data set to segment, a total of 246 from 306 (80.1%) partial skeletons were successfully marked with the new 3D algorithm.

4   Discussion

A 3D marking algorithm to extract a partial sulcal skeleton was implemented. It is based on the fact that the partial VOI Surface can be built using paths on the skeleton starting from a skeleton hull point, passing through a 3DLW contour voxel and reaching the bottom of a sulcus. This idea is implemented in step 2 and step 3 of the algorithm. Step 1 is required to restrict the computation to a smaller volume, as the paths far from the desired partial skeleton will be discarded in step 4. This is achieved using a growing process that stops after a maximum distance value is reached. This value is defined by the user and has to be large enough to completely cover the depth of the skeleton from the hull to the bottom of a sulcus. The value also depends on the intersection position of the 3DLW contour with the skeleton (red line in Fig. 5).

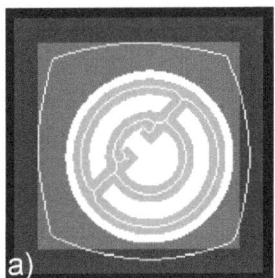 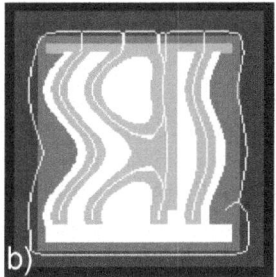 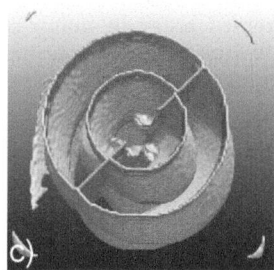

Fig. 4. a,b) Phantom data set (classes: B (black), C (dark gray), CSF (gray), GM (light gray), WM (white)) with skeleton (yellow)) shown in transversal and sagittal orientations. The skeleton is computed in the merged area of the classes C, CSF and GM. c) Skeleton surface without hull. The inner curved cylinder containing the 3DLW contour path (red) serves as ground truth (desired partial skeleton).

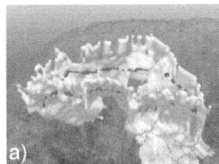 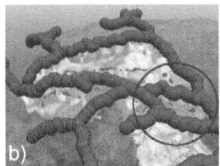 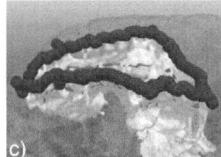 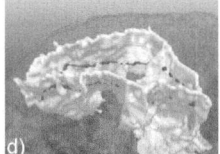

Fig. 5. a) Marked partial skeleton after step 4 in a classified T1-weighted MRI data set (BrainWeb: http://www.bic.mni.mcgill.ca/ServicesAtlases/Colin27). The 3DLW contour is shown as a thin, red line. b) All top points. A potential circle inside the top points is outlined in blue. c) Valid points and their connections. d) Marked skeleton with all recovered paths containing the new valid top points.

As the growing process in step 1 is undirected, i.e., growth occurs in all directions, high maximum distance values result in many undesired skeleton branches being marked. These branches are removed in step 4 by discarding all paths that do not pass through a 3DLW contour voxel. Due to the complex skeleton geometry, the desired partial skeleton **PS** also contains voxels on paths without a 3DLW contour voxel, which are also discarded, thus leaving a hole in the boundary. Two categories of such paths can be identified. The first category contains paths that only lie in part on the desired **PS** and start at a top point that lies outside. This usually occurs in the lower parts of the skeleton close to the bottom of a sulcus. The second category contains paths that do not reach a 3DLW contour voxel during the growing process in step 3. This is the case when the number of top points on the desired **PS** is larger than the number of 3DLW contour voxels. This causes some paths to stop growing, because all possible neighbor voxels can be reached from other top points with smaller path lengths. Such paths lie between the 3DLW contour and the skeleton hull.

These problematic paths are restored in step 5 and step 6. In step 5, all partial paths passing through a neighbor voxel of the previously marked skeleton are recovered. The neighborhood is defined as a sphere with a user-defined radius. A radius of three voxels was heuristically determined to produce a partial surface free of holes in many cases, while adding only a few undesired paths. This approach also partially solves the problem in step 6, as it also recovers the top points and their paths in the neighborhood of the marked skeleton. However, when the distance between the valid top points obtained in step 4 is larger than the selected neighborhood size, some paths cannot be recovered in step 5. This occurs more frequently when the 3DLW contour is located deeper in a sulcus. In step 6, the top points on the desired **PS** are computed by connecting valid top points from step 4 to other top points. This process is independent of the distance between the valid top points, but it is prone to compute "circles" if there are multiple connections within the set of all top points (Fig. 5b).

The 3D marking algorithm together with the recovering steps 5 and 6 is able to mark partial skeletons more completely and more compactly than the 2D algorithms used previously. To obtain a closed VOI boundary, 3D algorithms will be developed in future work to close the gap between the marked **PS** and the WM class and to close gaps where the 3DLW contour crosses gyri. The computation of undesired circles in step 6 will also be addressed in further development.

Acknowledgement. This work was supported by BMBF (grant no. 01EZ0822) and the Helmholtz-Validierungsfond (grant no. HVF-0012).

References

1. Pieper SD, Halle M, Kikinis R. 3D slicer. ISBI'04. 2004 04; p. 632–5.
2. Mangin JF, Rivère D, Cachia A, et al. A framework to study the cortical folding patterns. NeuroImage. 2004;23(Supplement 1):129–38.
3. Lohmann G, von Cramon DY. Automatic labelling of the human cortical surface using sulcal basins. Med Image Anal. 2000;4(3):179–88.

4. Wagenknecht G, Winter S. Volume-of-interest segmentation of cortical regions for multimodal brain analysis. Conf Record IEEE NSS/MIC. 2008 10; p. 4368–72.
5. Bertrand G. Simple points, topological numbers and geodesic neighborhoods in cubic grids. Pattern Recognit Lett. 1994 Oct;15(10):1003–11.

Automatic Conjunctival Provocation Test Using Hough Transform of Extended Canny Edge Maps

Suman Raj Bista[1,3], Serkan Dogan[2], Anatoli Astvatsatourov[2], Ralph Mösges[2], Thomas M. Deserno[1]

[1]Department of Medical Informatics, RWTH Aachen University,Aachen,Germany
[2]Department of Medical Statistics, Informatics and Epidemiology, University of Cologne, Cologne Germany
[3]Centre Universitaire Condorcet, University of Burgundy, Le Creusot, France
sumansrb@gmail.com

Abstract. Computer-aided diagnosis is developed for assessment of allergic rhinitis/rhinoconjunctivitis measuring the relative redness of sclera under application of allergen solution. The patient's eye images are taken from commercial digital camera. The iris is robustly localized using a gradient-based Hough circle transform. From the center of the pupil, the region of interest within the sclera is extracted using geometric anatomy-based a-priori information. The red color pixels are extracted thresholding in the hue, saturation and value color space. Then, redness is measured by taking mean of saturation projected into zero hue. Evaluation is performed with 92 images taken from 13 subjects, 8 responders and 5 non-responders, which were classified according to an experienced otorhinolaryngologist. Provocation is performed with 100, 1,000 and 10,000 AU/ml allergic solution and normalized to control images without provocation. The evaluation yields redness of 1.14, 1.30, 1.60 and 1.04, 1.12, 1.11 for responders and non-responders, respectively. This indicates that our method is suitable as reliable endpoint in controlled clinical trials.

1 Introduction

Atopic diseases such as allergic rhinitis/rhinoconjunctivitis, allergic asthma, and food allergy have increased worldwide [1]. This has been attributed to environmental factors, modulating genetic predisposition, and the natural course of underlying allergic immune responses [2]. Preventive measures and immuno-modulatory treatment play an important role in the management of allergic diseases. Therefore, after establishing a tolerated dose range, a dose-response relationship for clinical efficacy must be established. Provocation tests (e.g. conjunctival, nasal or bronchial provocation or allergen exposure in allergen challenge chambers) and/or clinical endpoints may be used as primary endpoints in controlled clinical trials. The conjunctival provocation test (CPT) has been introduced recently to document the course of allergic diseases and the effects of

H.-P. Meinzer et al. (Hrsg.), *Bildverarbeitung für die Medizin 2013*, Informatik aktuell,
DOI: 10.1007/978-3-642-36480-8_51, © Springer-Verlag Berlin Heidelberg 2013

disease modifying treatments [3]. CPT is performed with grass pollen solutions of three different strengths. However, qualitative inspection of conjunctiva and sclera is highly observer-specific and too subjective as it could be used as a primary endpoint. In this paper, we present a novel method based on automatic processing of color images that is fast, reproducible, accurate, and applicable – at least in principle – to any photographic imaging device.

2   Materials and methods

2.1   CPT protocol

The CPT has been standardized into four consecutive steps.

1. *Preparation*: Firstly, the subject is adapted to the room climate for 10 minutes. Test solutions (expiry date, control temperature, body temperature required) are checked and it is confirmed that the eye is not irritated. Contraindications for CPT (eye diseases except for anomalies of refraction or allergic conjunctivitis, contact lenses, anti-allergic therapy) are excluded. The subject is informed to avoid rubbing his/her eyes during the entire procedure.
2. *Control*: 50 μl of control solution identical to the allergen solution except for allergen content is administered into the lower conjunctival sac of one eye (control eye).
3. *Provocation*: Immediately after application of control solution, administer 50 μl of low-concentrated allergen solution (100 AU/ml) in the lower conjunctival sac of the opposite eye (provocation eye). 10 minutes wait time is taken.
4. *Evaluation*: The response is assessed. If positive, topical antihistamine (e.g. levocabastine, azelastine, emedastine) is administered. If negative, the provocation step is repeated with medium (1,000 AU/ml) and, if again negative, with high concentrated solution (10,000 AU/ml). If it is still negative, CPT is stopped.

2.2   Image acquistion

To derive quantitative measurements, a standard digital SLR (Olympus E3, Japan) with ring light (Hama LED Macro Light, DSLR, Germany) is used to record the eye of the patient. The light is composed of a ring with 12 LEDs for shadow-free illumination of subjects at color temperature of 5500 K. The camera is used with automatic white adjustment disabled. Since the ambient light is dimmed during imaging, the illumination is defined by the LED source. Color calibration patterns are not yet applied, but can be integrated in the process easily. Fig. 1 shows some examples of images. Variations in pupil positioning, focus and blur must be taken into account when designing robust segmentation.

Fig. 1. Images acquired for CPT.

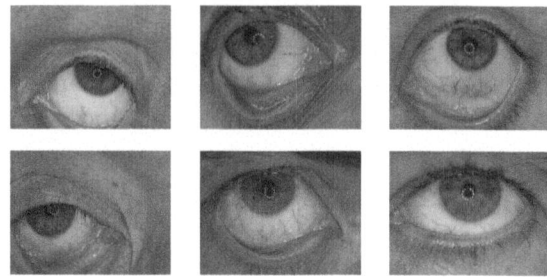

2.3 Image processing

Roughly 20 years ago, the circular Hough transform has been applied robustly by one of the authors for iris localization measuring the angle of squint [4]. Since then, it has been broadly applied in eye pattern analysis and biomedical authentication. Therefore, we rely on a Hough-based strategy for segmentation. The scheme for computer-aided diagnoses (CAD) is illustrated in Fig. 2 and corresponding images are depicted in Fig. 3. At a large scale, we apply pre-processing, segmentation and measurement. All steps have been implemented in Java and plugged into ImageJ.

Fig. 2. Image processing chain.

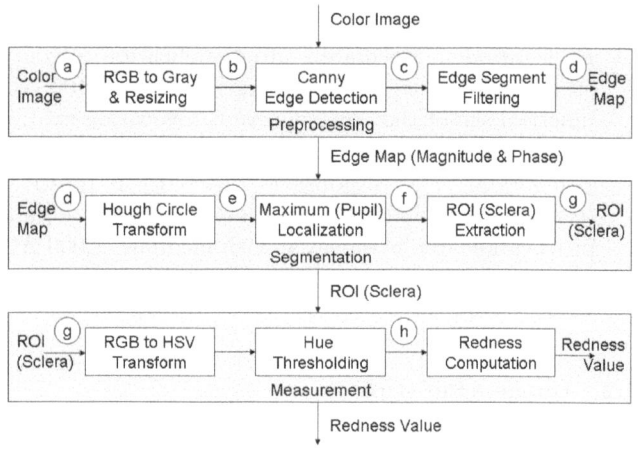

Pre-processing aims at normalization and speeding up the segmentation procedure. After color to 8 bit gray transform, the images are reduced from 3648 x 2736 pixels (Fig. 3a) down to 256 x 192 pixel (Fig. 3b) using linear interpolation [5]. A modified Canny edge detection approach is used to extract prominent edges, where – in addition to the original Canny algorithm – the direction of gradient is captured in a separate phase map [4]. The magnitude is then thresholded according to the hysteresis approach introduced by Canny, and a binary edge image is obtained (Fig. 3c). Applying connected components analysis, short

ments are removed automatically (Fig. 3d). A minimum segment length of
pixels is applied, but this threshold is not critical. Segmentation aims at
:omatic extraction of the sclera ROI. As derived from Fig. 1, the iris forms a
,minent circle that is usable as landmark. The center of the iris corresponds
the center of the pupil and is detected using a directive circular Hough trans-
m [4]. Fig. 3e illustrates the resulting three-dimensional accumulator array,
ich has been sliced at the corresponding radius r. The peak in the Hough
,ce is clearly indicated even if the iris is partly covered by the eyelid. Af-
peak localization, center and radius are projected back to the original scale.
;. 3f illustrates two circles, $(r + \alpha)$ and $(\beta \cdot r)$, where the thresholds α and β
,e been determined heuristically as global constant from known geometry of
ly grown human eyes.

According to the pupil positioning, two angles α_l and α_r for left and right
e, respectively, are used to extract the final ROI, which is completely posi-
ned within the sclera and the parameters α, β, and γ are selected such that
, area of the ROI is maximized (Fig. 3g). Measurement aims at quantitatively

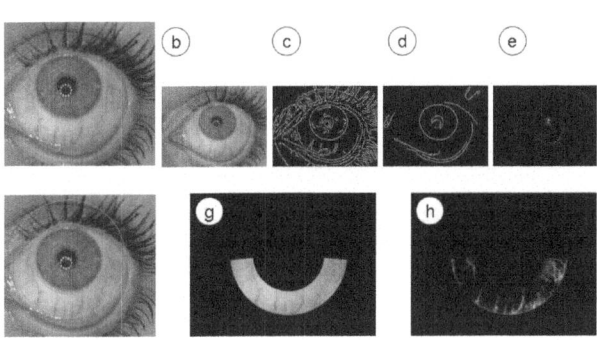

Fig. 3. Results according to image processing chain of Fig. 2.

ermine the redness of the sclera, since the blood vessels expand in response
the provocation. Red, green and blue (RGB) color space is converted into the
,, saturation, value (HSV) space, which better corresponds to semantic color
,cepts. Disregarding the value (indication of brightness), color is represented
a disc of radius S. A symmetric section around H_0 is extracted, where H_0
,resents the color red. In addition, all pixels with low saturation are excluded
m further evaluation (Fig. 4). The resulting amount of red pixels is visualized
Fig. 3h. The redness R is measured by taking mean of saturation projected

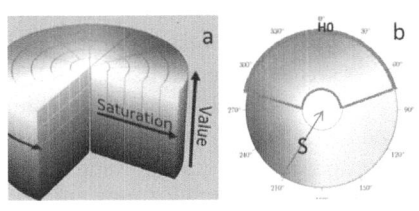

Fig. 4. Thresholding in HSV color space.

into zero hue according to 1, where N denotes the total number of red pixels after thresholding

$$R = \frac{1}{N} \sum_{n=0}^{N-1} (S_n \cdot \cos H_n) \qquad (1)$$

2.4 Evaluation study

In a first evaluation study, 13 patients have been applied to 50 μl of 100, 1000, and 10,000 AU/ml concentrated allergen solution, consecutively. Visual inspection by an otorhinolaryngologist categorizes the subjects into two groups, responder vs. non-responder, and 8 vs. 5 subjects resulted for each of the classes, respectively. N repeated measurements were made at each step (Tab. 1). In total, 92 images have been acquired. Mean and standard deviation of redness for responders and non-responders were computed according to (1) and normalized to the control image (Step 2 of CPT protocol).

3   Results

Fig. 3 illustrates the step-wise processing of images. All photographs were processed successfully. The Hough transform and iris center as well as radius detection performed errorless and accurate for all images disregarding partial occlusion, blur, and noise. This indicates the robustness of image processing. For the group of responders, the relative redness is measured as 1.14, 1.30, and 1.60 for 100, 1000 and 10,000 AU/ml respectively. The group of non-responders yields 1.04, 1.12, and 1.11, respectively (Tab. 1).

4   Discussion

A simple and robust image processing chain has been developed that quantifies CPT making it applicable as primary end point in controlled clinical trials and for quantitative assessment of allergic diseases. Accordingly, a pilot study is planned with 100 subjects using this measure.

So far, we do not apply color pattern and color calibration. This is likely to lower the standard deviation of the redness measure and enable also absolute color assessment. Also, the parameters α, β, and γ will be determined automatically in future. This can be done adding some heuristics into the chain of image processing. Then, the entire process becomes fully automatic.

However, our small evaluation study has already shown that the relative redness is increased significantly for the group of responders, whilst a rather constant redness is obtained for those subjects that have been rated as non-responder. The outlier in Table 1a (subject 2118) is due to incomplete opening of the eye, where the important area is covered by the lower eyelid (Fig. 1, bottom right). In summary, we conclude that the proposed image processing chain is suitable for computer-aided diagnosis in allergic rhinitis/rhinoconjunctivitis.

Table 1. Redness measurement. Dose: a = 0, b = 100, c = 1,000, d = 10,000 AU/ml.

Responders				ID	Dose	N	R	Non-responders			
ID	Dose	N	R					ID	Dose	N	R
A	a	1	1.000	E	a	2	1.000	I	a	1	1.000
	b	2	1.364		b	1	1.242		b	2	1.364
	c	2	1.440		c	1	1.254		c	2	1.440
	d	3	1.494		d	1	1.330		d	3	1.494
B	a	1	1.000	F	a	1	1.000	J	a	1	1.000
	b	1	1.023		b	1	1.065		b	2	1.079
	c	3	1.037		c	2	1.083		c	2	1.199
	d	3	2.018		d	2	1.091		d	2	1.078
C	a	1	1.000	G	a	1	1.000	K	a	1	1.000
	b	4	1.134		b	3	1.243		b	1	1.070
	c	2	1.240		c	2	1.666		c	1	1.001
	d	5	1.423		d	2	1.988		d	2	0.937
D	a	1	1.000	H	a	1	1.000	L	a	1	1.000
	b	2	1.548		b	1	0.525		b	2	1.089
	c	2	1.648		c	2	1.034		c	2	1.140
	d	2	2.139		d	2	1.334		d	2	2.171
								M	a	1	1.000
									b	1	0.940
									c	2	1.023
									d	1	1.056
Total					a	9	1 ± 0		a	5	1 ± 0
					b	15	1.143 ± 0.30		b	8	1.108 ± 0.16
					c	16	1.299 ± 0.26		c	9	1.161 ± 0.18
					d	20	1.602 ± 0.39		d	10	1.147 ± 0.21

References

1. Ait-Khaled N, Pearce N, Anderson H, et al. Global map of the prevalence of symptoms of rhinoconjunctivitis in children-the international study of asthma and allergies in childhood (ISAAC) Phase Three. Allergy. 2009;64(1):122–48.
2. Mösges R, Klimek L. Today's allergic rhinitis patients are different: new factors that may play a role. Allergy. 2007;62(9):969–75.
3. Riechelmann H, Epple B, Gropper G. Comparison of conjunctival and nasal provocation test in allergic rhinitis to house dust mite. Int Arch Allergy Immunol. 2003;130(1):51–9.
4. Kaupp A, Lehmann T, Effert R, et al. Automatic measurement of the angle of squint by Hough-transformation and covariance-filtering. Proc IAPR Int Conf Pattern Recogn. 1994;1:784–6.
5. Lehmann TM, Gönner C, Spitzer K. Addendum: B-spline interpolation in medical image processing. IEEE Trans Med Imaging. 2001;20(7):660–5.

3D-Segmentierungskorrektur unter Berücksichtigung von Bildinformationen für die effiziente und objektive Erfassung pleuraler Verdickungen

Hendrik Hachmann[1], Peter Faltin[1], Thomas Kraus[2], Kraisorn Chaisaowong[1,3]

[1]Lehrstuhl für Bildverarbeitung, RWTH Aachen University
[2]Institut für Arbeitsmedizin und Sozialmedizin, UK Aachen
[3]King Mongkut's University of Technology North Bangkok
tom.hendrik.hachmann@rwth-aachen.de

Kurzfassung. Für die Vermessung asbestbedingter pleuraler Verdickungen in CT-Lungendaten ist eine präzise Segmentierung essentiell. Vollautomatische Verfahren erfordern häufig eine manuelle Nachkorrektur. In dieser Arbeit wird ein speziell hierfür weiterentwickeltes Live-Wire-Werkzeug vorgestellt. Im Vordergrund steht die Effizienzsteigerung des semi-automatischen Werkzeugs, mittels dreidimensionaler Ausweitung der zweidimensionalen Manipulation, geführter Navigation durch die Schichtbilder und der Kombination mit einem Ausbeulwerkzeug. Das durch Benutzerinteraktion eingebrachte a priori Wissen des Anwenders wird im Segmentierungsprozess mit den Bildinformationen verknüpft. Hierdurch erreicht das Live-Wire-Werkzeug hohe Reproduzierbarkeit und geringe Intra- und Inter-Reader-Variabilität.

1 Einleitung

Pleurale Verdickungen der Thorawand und des Zwerchfells können ein Indikator für das aggressive, asbestverursachte Pleuramesotheliom sein (Abb. 1(a)). Das Auftreten hat sowohl diagnostische als auch gutachterliche Relevanz für die Anerkennung als Berufskrankheit. Eine therapeutische Beeinflussung des Pleuramesothelioms ist nur in der Frühphase des Krankheitsverlaufs möglich, wofür eine frühzeitige Diagnose der Verdickungen und deren exakte Beobachtung im zeitlichen Verlauf mit Erfassung einer Wachstumstendenz entscheidend ist [1]. Eine voll-automatisierte Detektion und Segmentierung kann fehlerbehaftet sein und erfordert häufig Korrekturen. Eine schichtbasierte Segmentierung ist zeitintensiv und der Aufwand wird in Zukunft durch höher aufgelöste Bilddaten steigen. Eine Effizienzsteigerung interaktiver Segmentierungswerkzeuge zur Begrenzung des Arbeitsaufwands ist daher essentiell und kann durch die vorgestellten Ansätze erreicht werden.

Die zugrundeliegende Idee ist der Übergang von schichtbasierten Werkzeugen wie das Add/Substract-Tool oder das Paint/Wipe-Tool aus dem MITK-Segmentierungsmodul [2] zu dreidimensional arbeitenden Segmentierungswerkzeugen, die den Arbeitsaufwand reduzieren.

H.-P. Meinzer et al. (Hrsg.), *Bildverarbeitung für die Medizin 2013*, Informatik aktuell,
DOI: 10.1007/978-3-642-36480-8_52, © Springer-Verlag Berlin Heidelberg 2013

2 Material und Methoden

2.1 Live-Wire-Werkzeug

Das Live-Wire-Werkzeug ist ein Zugwerkzeug, dessen Funktionsweise in Abb. 1 aufgezeigt ist. Der Mauscursor führt permanent eine kugelförmige ROI mit, deren Größe über das Mausrad anpassbar ist (Abb. 1(b)). Die Schnittpunkte der Kugel mit der Segmentierungskontur begrenzen den zu verändernden Konturabschnitt, welcher über den Live-Wire- bzw. den Dijkstra-Algorithmus [3] berechnet wird. Der Live-Wire-Algorithmus bestimmt auf einem über den Gradienten detektierten Kantenbild den kürzesten Pfad zwischen den beiden Schnittpunkten. Hierdurch schnappt der Konturabschnitt an der nächstliegenden Kante ein.

2.2 Laplacian Framework

Das Laplacian Framework, vorgestellt von Yaron Lipman und Olga Sorkine [4], berechnet die Position von Knoten in einem Polygonnetz über simulierte Kräfte zu den mit Kanten verbundenen Nachbarknoten. Innerhalb des Frameworks können unveränderbare Ankerknoten bestimmt werden. Durch das Verschieben von Punkten entsteht ein widersprüchliches Gleichungssystem, dass sich über lineare Ausgleichsrechnung mit Euklidischer Norm lösen lässt. Der Fehler im Gleichungssystem wird über das Polygonnetz verteilt und die beteiligten Polygone verformen sich im gleichen Ausmaß.

Die Dijkstra-Kontur gibt Ankerpunkte für das Laplacian Framework vor. Um das Polygonnetz mit der Kontur zu verknüpfen ist eine Knotenzuordnung notwendig. Die Anzahl der Knoten in der Dijkstra-Kontur entspricht in der Regel nicht der Anzahl der betroffenen Knoten im Polygonnetz. Die Anzahl N_K der

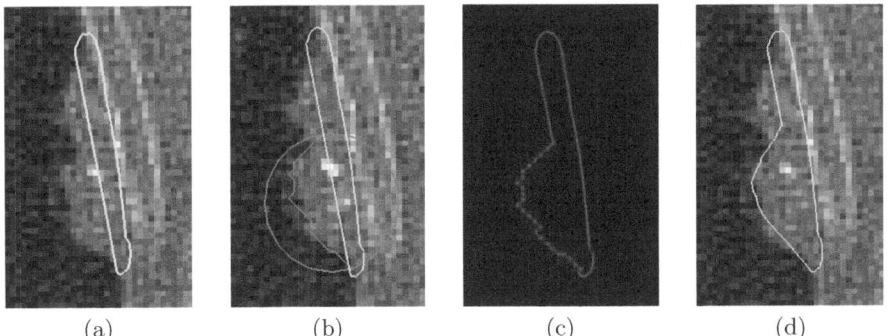

(a)   (b)   (c)   (d)

Abb. 1. Funktionsweise des Live-Wire-Werkzeugs. (a) Pleurale Verdickung und initiale Segmentierung in einem CT-Lungendatensatz. (b) Kugelförmige ROI und herausgezogene Dijkstra-Kontur. (c) Aufgeschnittene initiale Segmentierung und Dijkstra-Kontur. (d) Nachziehen des Polygonnetzes über das Laplacian Framework.

Knoten in den Konturen $K = \{\text{kurz}, \text{lang}\}$ wird eingesetzt um die Lückengröße

$$L = \left\lfloor \frac{N_{\text{lang}} - N_{\text{kurz}}}{N_{\text{kurz}} + 1} \right\rfloor \tag{1}$$

zu berechnen. Diese wird für eine gleichmäßige verteilte Zuordnung, wie exemplarisch in Abb. 2.2 gezeigt, eingesetzt. Im Beispiel wurde von links nach rechts eine durchschnittliche Lückengröße von 1 errechnet, wodurch sich für den restlichen Konturabschnitt ab Knoten G (Abb. 2.2) eine Lückengröße von 2 ergibt.

Das Laplacian Framework verschiebt alle Punkte, die nicht wie die Dijkstra-Konturpunkte und die Randpunkte der ROI als Ankerpunkte definiert sind. Die Rückseite der Segmentierung, die in der ROI liegen kann (Abb. 1(c)), wird ebenfalls fixiert, um ungewünschte Nebeneffekte zu verhindern.

2.3   3D-Ausbreitung

Unser Live-Wire-Werkzeug breitet die schichtbasierte Manipulation des Live-Wire-Algorithmus über das Laplacian Framework aus, so dass eine dreidimensionale Manipulation des Polygonnetzes erfolgt (Abb. 3). Optional kann eine zweite, auf der betrachteten Schicht senkrecht stehende, Dijkstra-Kontur verwendet werden. Diese bezieht Bildinformationen der benachbarten Schichten ein.

2.4   Geführte Navigation

Im Gegensatz zum linearen Scrollen durch die Schichten erfolgen die Schichtwechsel bei der geführten Navigation nach einer binären Suchstrategie. Zu Beginn segmentiert der Mediziner die beiden äußeren Schichten des Zielobjekts und springt im Anschluss immer in die Schichten zentral zwischen zwei bereits bearbeiteten Schichten. Durch die Ausbreitung der anfänglichen Korrekturen reduziert sich der Umfang der nötigen Bearbeitung in späteren Schichten. Die

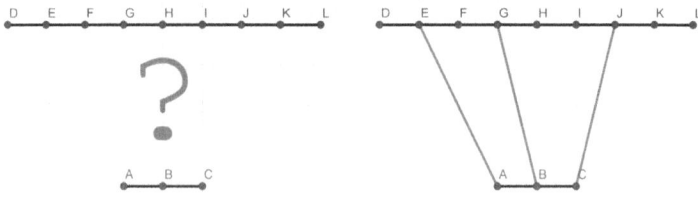

(a) Knotenzuweisungsproblem.   (b) Ergebnis des Algorithmus.

Abb. 2. Knotenzuweisung zwischen zwei unterschiedlich langen Konturen. Die Lösung (b) ordnet Knoten von links nach rechts zu. Die durchschnittliche Lückengröße in der größeren Kontur beträgt für die ersten beiden Knoten 1, anschließend 2.

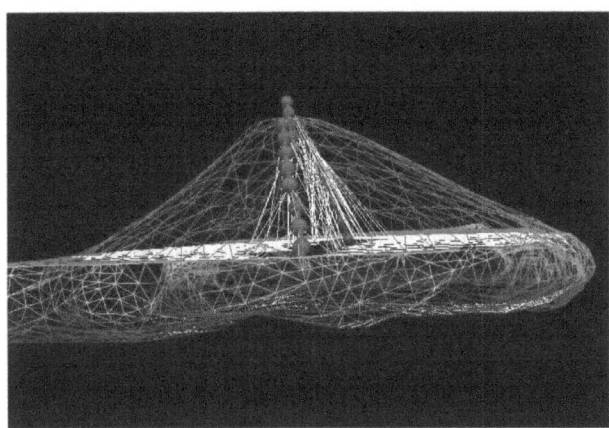

Abb. 3. 3D-Ausbreitung der Live-Wire-Manipulation (rot) durch das Laplacian Framework (grün). Die Punktezuordnung zwischen Dijkstra-Kontur und Polygonnetz ist in Weiß eingezeichnet.

eingesetzte Strategie der Schichtwechsel nutzt diesen Effekt aus um die Effizienz zu steigern. Die Ausbreitung der 3D-Manipulation wird entsprechend des Abstandes zur nächsten bereits bearbeiteten Schicht automatisch begrenzt. Das Segmentierungspolygonnetz wird nach jedem Schichtwechsel dezimiert oder verfeinert um ein präzises und zugleich schnelles Arbeiten zu gewähren.

2.5 Ausbeulwerkzeug

Das Live-Wire-Werkzeug wurde mit einem ursprünglich von Proksch [5] vorgestellten Ausbeulwerkzeug kombiniert. Dieses wurde überarbeitet und um das automatische Einfügen von Knoten erweitert. Wenn der Benutzer in die Kontur greift, arbeitet er mit dem Live-Wire-Werkzeug. Anderenfalls deformiert der Benutzer die Segmentierungskontur freiformend, d.h. ohne Bildinformationen. Dies kann wichtig sein, wenn der Dijkstra-Algorithmus nicht die gewünschte Kontur findet. Ein aufwändiger Wechsel des Werkzeugs ist nicht nötig.

2.6 Implementierung

Das vorgestellte Live-Wire-Werkzeug wurde in dem MITK-Framework umgesetzt. Das Werkzeug ist sowohl in den mitk::toolmanager als auch in das MITK Undo-/Redokonzept eingearbeitet. In einem Model View Controller Ansatz ist die Benutzeroberfläche durch Threads von dem arbeitenden Werkzeug getrennt. Performanceintensive Rechnungen, wie beispielsweise das Lösen des Gleichungssystems im Laplacian Framework, sind zusätzlich parallelisiert und als Kernels auf die GPU ausgelagert.

2.7 Statistische Auswertung

Das Live-Wire-Werkzeug wurde in einer empirischen Diskrepanzanalyse mit den in MITK integrierten klassischen Segmentierungswerkzeugen Add/Substract und

Paint/Wipe verglichen. Eine Konvertierung zwischen binärem Voxelvolumen und Polygonnetz ist fehlerbehaftet. Der Vergleich mit dem Goldstandard wurde daher im Polygonnetzbereich, über die Hausdorff-Distanz und den beidseitigen durchschnittlichen Fehler [6], und im Voxelbereich, über die Überlappungsmaße Dice- und Tanimoto-Koeffizient [7], durchgeführt. Über den Variationskoeffizienten wurde die Reproduzierbarkeit der Segmentierung bestimmt.

Die Messergebnisse gehen aus den Segmentierungen von 11 Probanden hervor. Eine Protokollierungsfunktion hat in fünfsekündigen Abständen Segmentierungszwischenstände abgespeichert, wodurch der Zeitverlauf der erstellten Segmentierungen rekonstruiert werden kann. Über den Student's t-Test, den F-Test und den Welch-Test wurden zudem Rückschlüsse auf die Grundgesamtheit gezogen und die Ergebnisse auf Signifikanz getestet. Die Probanden bewerteten die Segmentierungswerkzeuge mit ganzzahligen Schulnoten (1 (sehr gut) bis 6 (ungenügend)) nach den 5 in Tab. 1 dargestellten Kriterien.

3 Ergebnisse

Der zeitliche gemittelte Verlauf des Dice-Koeffizienten ist stellvertretend für alle angeführten Maße in Abb. 4 (links) gezeigt. Die Auswertung im Polygonnetz- und Voxelbereich kommt zu vergleichbaren Ergebnissen. Das Live-Wire-Werkzeug überzeugt vor allem in den ersten zwei Minuten und erzielt auch nach 180 Sekunden das beste Ergebnis. In begrenzter Zeit (5-161 Sekunden) lässt sich ein signifikant präziseres Ergebnis als beim Add- und Paint-Werkzeug erzielen. Weiterhin haben Segmentierungen mit unserem Werkzeug geringere Varianzen als andere Werkzeuge (Abb. 4, rechts). Die Ergebnisse der Probandenbefragung sind in Tab. 1 dargestellt. Eignung und Effizienz bewerten die Probanden beim neu entwickelten Werkzeug geschlossen besser als bei den klassischen Werkzeugen, die jedoch in Bezug auf die Intuition und Reaktionszeit besser bewertet werden.

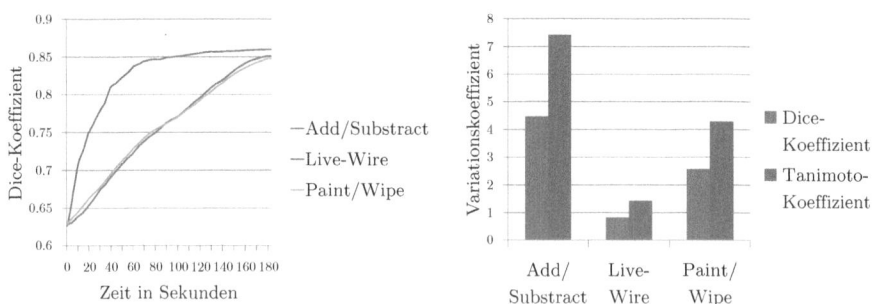

Abb. 4. Zeitlicher Verlauf des Dice-Koeffizienten gemittelt über alle Probanden (links) und Inter-Reader-Variabilität bzw. Reproduzierbarkeit von Segmentierungen (rechts).

Tabelle 1. Ergebnisse der Befragung von 11 Probanden. In jeder Zelle der Tabelle sind der Mittelwert (oben) und die Standardabweichung (unten) der Noten eingetragen.

	Intuition	Reaktionszeit	Präzision	Effizienz	Eignung
Add/Substract	⌀ 1,64	⌀ 1,36	⌀ 2,36	⌀ 2,82	⌀ 2,82
	± 0,809	± 0,6742	± 0,809	± 0,8739	± 0,4045
Paint/Wipe	⌀ 1,09	⌀ 1,00	⌀ 1,73	⌀ 3,36	⌀ 2,73
	± 0,3015	± 0,0000	± 0,7862	± 0,809	± 0,4671
Live-Wire	⌀ 2,09	⌀ 2,73	⌀ 1,82	⌀ 1,18	⌀ 1,64
	± 0,8312	± 1,009	± 0,603	± 0,4045	± 0,5045

4 Diskussion

Die Kombination aus 3D-Live-Wire-Werkzeug, Ausbeulwerkzeug und geführter Navigation hat sich als mächtiges interaktives Segmentierungswerkzeug bewiesen. Dies bestätigt die vorab erwartete Effizienzsteigerung und gute Eignung, die auch in der Probandenbefragung unterstrichen werden. Das Live-Wire-Werkzeug stellt insbesondere eine praktische Alternative für zeitkritische Segmentierungen dar. Im Alltagsbetrieb ist zu erwarten, dass die Intuition ein ähnlich gutes Niveau wie das der klassischen und damit bereits bekannten Werkzeuge erreicht. Die geringeren Variationskoeffizienten zeigen, dass reproduzierbarere Ergebnisse als mit den klassischen Werkzeugen erzielbar sind.

In Zukunft kann ausgehend von den senkrecht aufeinander stehenden Dijkstra -Konturen (Abschnitt 2.3) sukzessive eine sternförmige Dijkstra-Konturanordnung genutzt werden. Alternativ kann ein Gitter aus Live-Wire-Konturen entstehen, das die gesamte ROI füllt. In diesem Spezialfall, kann auf eine Ausbreitung durch das Laplacian Framework verzichtet werden.

Literaturverzeichnis

1. Ochsmann E, Carl T, Brand P, et al. Inter-reader variability in chest radiography and HRCT for the early detection of asbestos-related lung and pleural abnormalities in a cohort of 636 asbestos-exposed subjects. Int Arch Occup Environ Health. 2010;83:39–46.
2. Maleike D, Nolden M, Meinzer HP, et al. Interactive segmentation framework of the medical imaging interaction toolkit. Comput Meth Prog Bio. 2009;96(1):72–83.
3. Dijkstra EW. A note on two problems in connexion with graphs. Numerische Mathematik. 1959;1:269–71.
4. Lipman Y, Sorkine O, Alexa M, et al. Laplacian Framework for Interactive Mesh Editing. Int J Shape Model. 2005;11(1):43–61.
5. Proksch D, Dornheim J, Preim B. Interaktionstechniken zur Korrektur medizinischer 3D-Segmentierung. In: Proc BVM; 2010. p. 420–4.
6. Cignoni P, Rocchini C, Scopigno R. Metro: measuring error on simplified surfaces. Comput Graph Forum. 1998 Juni;17(2):167–74.
7. Heimann T. Optimierung des Segmentierungsvorgangs und Evaluation der Ergebnisse in der medizinischen Bildverarbeitung. Heidelberg: DKFZ; 2003.

MITK-US: Echtzeitverarbeitung von Ultraschallbildern in MITK

Alfred Michael Franz, Keno März, Alexander Seitel, Michael Müller,
Sascha Zelzer, Marco Nodeln, Hans-Peter Meinzer, Lena Maier-Hein

Abteilung für Medizinische und Biologische Informatik, DKFZ Heidelberg
a.franz@dkfz.de

Kurzfassung. Ultraschall (US) als bildgebendes Verfahren in der Medizin ist nicht invasiv, schnell, vielerorts verfügbar, kommt ohne Strahlenbelastung aus und liefert kontinuierlich Daten in Echtzeit. Die Nutzung von US für computerassistierte Interventionen (CAI) stellt jedoch nicht nur extrem hohe Anforderungen an die Methoden zur Bildverarbeitung aufgrund der beschränkten Bildqualität, sondern bedeutet auch einen beträchtlichen Integrationsaufwand wenn die Daten in Echtzeit weiterverarbeitet werden sollen. Mit MITK-US stellen wir in dieser Arbeit ein neues Modul für das Open Source verfügbare Medical Imaging Interaction Toolkit (MITK) vor, welches die einheitliche Einbindung und Weiterverarbeitung von Echtzeitultraschalldaten ermöglicht und somit den Aufwand für die Integration von US in CAI Systeme verringert. Da die Verwendung von Echtzeitdaten insbesondere im Bereich der CAI zahlreiche neue Möglichkeiten bietet, erwarten wir einen hohen Nutzen dieses Moduls für künftige Projekte.

1 Einleitung

Computerassistierte Systeme gewinnen zunehmend an Bedeutung im Bereich der minimalinvasiven Medizin. Während sich derartige Systeme für rigide Strukturen, wie z.b. bei der Neurochirurgie, bereits in der klinischen Praxis etablieren konnten, sind sie für bewegte Strukturen im Weichgewebe weiterhin Gegenstand der Forschung. Offene Probleme sind hierbei unter anderem die durch Atmung und andere Faktoren verursachte Bewegung der Zielstruktur und die Einbindung komplexer Systeme in den klinischen Workflow. Im Verlauf der meisten minimalinvasiven Interventionen im Weichgewebe stehen Echtzeitinformationen wie Ultraschall-, Fluoroskopie- oder Endoskopiebilder zur Verfügung. Während diese Daten in der Vergangenheit häufig erst einige Zeit nach der Bildakquisition zur Diagnosefindung oder Therapieplanung weiterverarbeitet wurden [1, 2], könnten sie bei computerassistierten Interventionen (CAI) neue Möglichkeiten eröffnen, wenn sie in Echtzeit vorliegen und vom System als zusätzliche Information genutzt werden können. Ultraschall (US) hat in diesem Zusammenhang eine besondere Bedeutung, da diese Art der Bildgebung nicht invasiv ist, keine Strahlenbelastung für den Patienten mit sich bringt, sehr schnell durchgeführt werden kann und vielerorts verfügbar ist [3].

H.-P. Meinzer et al. (Hrsg.), *Bildverarbeitung für die Medizin 2013*, Informatik aktuell,
DOI: 10.1007/978-3-642-36480-8_53, © Springer-Verlag Berlin Heidelberg 2013

Die Nutzung von US für CAI stellt jedoch nicht nur extrem hohe Anforderungen an die Methoden zur Bildverarbeitung aufgrund der beschränkten Bildqualität, sondern bedeutet auch einen beträchtlichen Integrationsaufwand wenn die Daten in Echtzeit weiterverarbeitet werden sollen. Daher ist es nötig, einheitliche Schnittstellen für US-Echzeitbildquellen im Bereich der CAI Systeme zu schaffen. In der Vergangenheit vorgestellte Open Source Ansätze für US-Bildverarbeitung, wie zum Beispiel eine von Wang et al. vorgestellte Erweiterung für die Bibliothek ITK[1] [4] oder die Public software Library for UltraSound imaging research (PLUS) [5, 6], konzentrieren sich auf reine US-Bildverarbeitung bzw. Prototyping von US-Navigationsanwendungen. Eine Bereitstellung von weiteren für CAI benötigten Methoden, wenn z.b. Ultraschalldaten mit präoperativen Computertomographiedaten kombiniert werden sollen, gestaltet sich in diesem Fall relativ aufwändig. Das Medical Imaging Interaction Toolkit (MITK) stellt hingegen sowohl Methoden zur medizinischen Bildverarbeitung als auch für CAI zur Verfügung [7, 8] und wurde in der Vergangenheit bereits zur Weiterverarbeitung von US-Bildern eingesetzt [1, 2]. Allerdings war diese Bildquelle innerhalb der Software bisher nicht in Echtzeit verfügbar.

In dieser Arbeit präsentieren wir daher mit MITK-US ein neues Modul für MITK, das die einheitliche Einbindung und Weiterverarbeitung von Echtzeit-Ultraschalldaten ermöglicht.

2 Methoden

Zu Beginn der Entwicklung des Softwaremoduls MITK-US wurden die Anforderungen an dieses Modul wie folgt festgelegt:

- *Anbindung der Hardware:* Hierzu soll es möglich sein, die Geräte sowohl als Videoquelle, als auch über herstellerspezifische Programmierschnittstellen (Application Programming Interface, API) anzubinden.
- *Erweiterbarkeit:* Das Modul soll auf künftige Anwendungsfälle, wie z.B. Echtzeitverarbeitung von 3D-Ultraschall, erweiterbar sein.
- *Flexibilität:* Es soll ein flexibles Konzept zur Echtzeitdatenverarbeitung bereitstehen, das es ermöglicht, einzelne Softwarekomponenten auszutauschen oder Funktionalität hinzuzufügen.
- *Performanz:* Die Bildwiederholrate soll mindestens 20 Bilder pro Sekunde betragen, um einen Echtzeiteinsatz der Software zu ermöglichen.
- *Applikationsweite Unterstützung:* Ultraschallbildquellen sollen auf einfache Weise applikationsweit in MITK zur Verfügung stehen. Die Verwaltung der Bildquellen soll zentral erfolgen.
- *Portabilität:* Die Software soll unter den Plattformen Linux, MacOS und Windows verwendbar sein.
- *Robustheit:* Die Software sollte mit einem geeigneten Software-Prozess entwickelt werden, der auch Tests der Klassen umfasst, um einen robusten Code mit hoher Qualität zu gewährleisten.

---

[1] ITK: Insight Segmentation and Registration Toolkit; http://www.itk.org

Der Software-Prozess für die Entwicklung von MITK-US wurde von MITK übernommen und orientiert sich an dem von Schröder et al. vorgestellten Kitware process für Open Source Software [9]. Um die entwickelte Software möglichst flexibel einsetzbar zu gestalten, wurde die Ultraschallunterstützung in drei Komponenten aufgeteilt: das Modul[2] MITK-US, das Modul MITK-USUI und das MITK-Plugin[3] org.mitk.gui.qt.ultrasound mit Benutzeroberfläche (engl. Graphical User Interface, GUI). Die Einordnung dieser Komponenten im Kontext der gesamten Softwarebibliothek MITK ist in Abb. 1 veranschaulicht.

2.1 Das Modul MITK-US

Dieses Modul stellt die Basisfunktionalität zur Anbindung von Echtzeit-US-Quellen und zur Weiterverarbeitung bereit. MITK-US bietet zur Echtzeitbildverarbeitung ein Pipeline-Konzept an, welches auch in der von MITK verwendeten Bibliothek Insight Segmentation and Registration Toolkit (ITK), Abb. 1, für Bilddaten verwendet wird [10]. Für Quellenklassen und für Filterklassen der Pipeline werden in MITK-US jeweils Oberklassen bereitgestellt. US-Bilddaten werden durch eine Datenklasse abgebildet. Diese Klasse erweitert die Bildklasse von MITK mitk::Image um US-spezifische Metadaten, die Angaben zum verwendeten Gerät und zu den Einstellungen, wie z.b. den Zoomfaktor, enthalten. Die Datenstruktur unterstützt dabei sowohl 2D- als auch 3D-Bilder, daher können die entwickelten Strukturen auch für Echtzeit-3D-Ultraschallquellen verwendet werden. Eine gemeinsame Oberklasse für US-Geräte als Bildquelle ermöglicht auch die Einbindung von herstellerspezifischen APIs. Die meisten US-Geräte bieten als einfache Schnittstelle einen Videoausgang (z.B. S-Video oder HDMI) an. Dieser kann als universelle Lösung bereits von einer im Modul enthaltenen Klasse eingebunden werden.

2.2 Das Modul MITK-USUI

Dieses Modul enthält wiederverwendbare GUI-Komponenten, wozu auf die Softwarebibliothek Qt (http://qt.digia.com) zugegriffen wird. Wie in MITK vorgesehen, wird für GUI-Komponenten das Konzept der Qt-Widgets verwendet, was eine einfache Implementierung und Wiederverwendung ermöglicht. Es stehen dabei bereits folgende Widgets innerhalb von MITK-US zur Verfügung:

– *USDeviceManagerWidget:* Dieses Widget bietet eine GUI zur Verwaltung von angebundenen US-Geräten. Dies beinhaltet die Erstellung neuer Geräteverbindung und das Aktivieren/Deaktivieren dieser Verbindungen.

---

[2] Module sind Programmbibliotheken, die Algorithmen und Datenstrukturen thematisch und funktionell gruppieren. Mittels Modulen können Funktionalitäten wiederverwendbar im Projekt zu Verfügung gestellt werden.

[3] Plugins sind Softwarekomponenten, die über das Plugin-Framework von The Common Toolkit (CTK, http://www.commontk.org) in die MITK Basisanwendung eingebunden werden, Abb. 1. Sie können sowohl funktionale Service-Objekte als auch Oberflächenelemente in den Applikationsrahmen einbringen.

– *USNewVideoDeviceWidget:* Mit diesem Widget wird eine GUI zur Einrichtung von neuen US-Quellen, die an einen Videoeingang des Rechners angeschlossen sind, bereit gestellt.

2.3   Das Plugin org.mitk.gui.qt.ultrasound

Dieses Plugin, das innerhalb des MITK-Anwendungsframeworks geladen werden kann, bietet Funktionalität zum Ansteuern von US-Geräten auf Benutzerebene. Mit dem Plugin eingerichtete Geräte sind nach dem Konzept der Serviceorientierten Architektur (SOA) [11] als Service, in MITK als Micro Service (`http://cppmicroservices.org`) bezeichnet, MITK-weit verfügbar und können somit einfach von anderen Plugins verwendet werden.

3   Ergebnisse

Die Ultraschallunterstützung für MITK wurde gemäß den Anforderungen implementiert und ist Open Source als Teil von MITK (`http://www.mitk.org`)

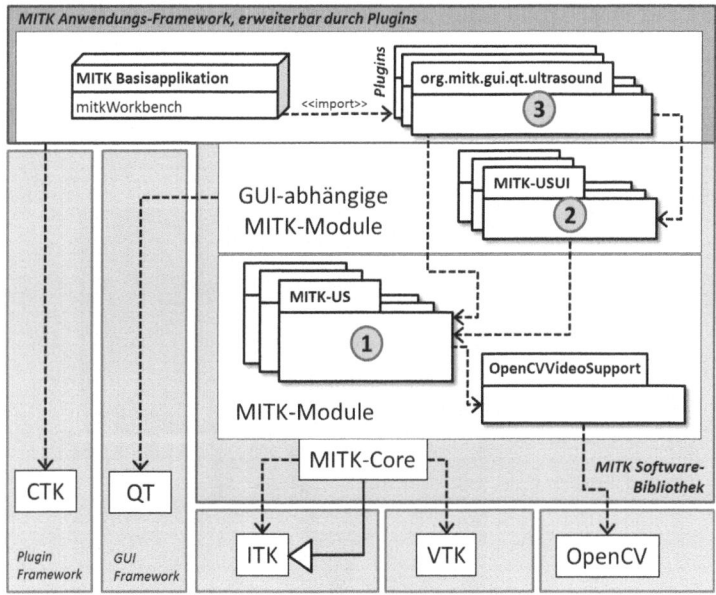

Abb. 1. Überblick über die drei Komponenten zur US-Unterstützung innerhalb der Umgebung MITK. GUI-unabhängige Basisfunktionalität findet sich im Modul MITK-US . Zum Ansprechen der Videoschnittstellen kommt die Bibliothek OpenCV (`http://opencv.org`) zum Einsatz, die über das MITK-Modul OpenCVVideoSupport angesprochen wird. Wiederverwendbare GUI-Elemente werden im Modul MITK-USUI zur Verfügung gestellt. Das Plugin org.mitk.gui.qt.ultrasound bietet eine GUI um Ultraschallgeräte innerhalb der MITK Basisapplikation anzusteuern.

verfügbar. Ein Screenshot der MITK Basisapplikation mit US Plugin ist in Abb. 2 dargestellt. Die Anwendung erreichte bei einer US-Bildquelle mit einer Auflösung von 1920 x 1080 Pixel, die über einen Videoeingang in Form einer Grabberkarte (Unigraf UFG-05 4E, Unigraf Oy, FI-02240 Espoo, Finnland) angeschlossen wurde, eine Updaterate von 21 Bilder pro Sekunde. Für Tests der Software steht außer dem Quellcode auch ein Installer zur Verfügung, der unter http://www.mitk.org/Ultrasound heruntergeladen werden kann. Auf der Konferenz erfolgt des Weiteren eine Softwaredemonstration der Applikation.

4 Diskussion

Im Rahmen dieser Arbeit wurde mit MITK-US eine Erweiterung für MITK präsentiert, welche die Einbindung von Echtzeit-Ultraschallquellen und die Weiterverarbeitung der US-Daten ermöglicht. Portabilität und Robustheit wurden dabei durch den Einsatz des MITK Software-Prozesses erreicht. Die Anbindung neuer Hardware wird durch eine gemeinsame Schnittstelle für Ultraschallgeräte ermöglicht. Flexibilität und Erweiterbarkeit des Moduls werden durch das Piplinekonzept sichergestellt, das eine leichte Austauschbarkeit einzelner Komponenten und Erweiterungen um neue Komponenten ermöglicht. Performanztests bestätigten mit einer Updaterate von 21 Bildern pro Sekunde die Echtzeitfähigkeit der entwickelten Software.

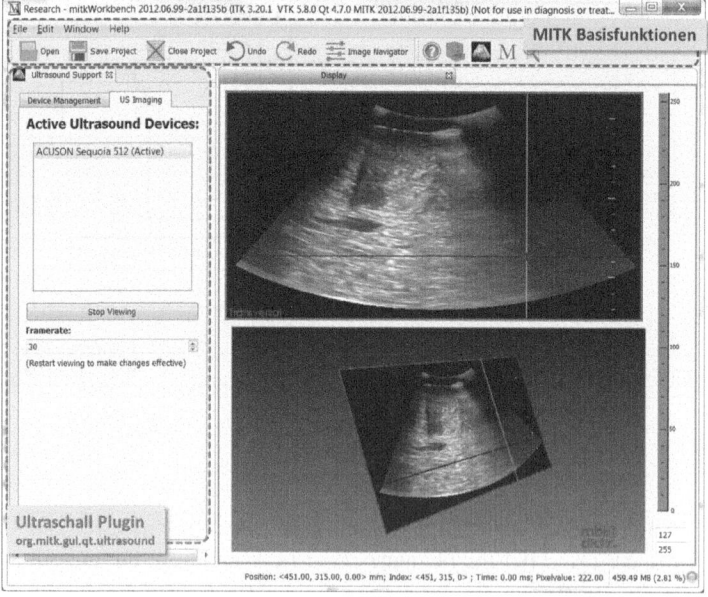

Abb. 2. Screenshot der MITK Basisapplikation mit aktiviertem Ultraschall Plugin. Das Ultraschallgerät kann als Echtzeit-Datenquelle über einen Videoeingang an den Rechner angeschlossen werden.

Im Vergleich zu anderen Open Source Bibliotheken für Ultraschallbildverarbeitung [4, 5, 6] bietet MITK-US über die Basisbibliothek MITK die Möglichkeit, auf einfache Art und Weise auf zahlreiche Softwarekomponenten aus dem gesamten Bereich der medizinischen Bildverarbeitung und CAI zurückzugreifen. So können zum Beispiel in MITK enthaltene Algorithmen der Computertomographie- oder Magnetresonanztomographiebildverarbeitung verwendet werden, wenn ein System entwickelt werden soll, das derartige Informationen mit Ultraschalldaten kombiniert. Mit MITK-IGT [8] steht innerhalb von MITK auch ein Modul zur Verfügung, das bereits viel Funktionalität für CAI bietet.

Abschließend kann gesagt werden, dass mit MITK-US nun ein Modul für die Einbindung von Ultraschallquellen in Echtzeit innerhalb von MITK zur Verfügung steht. Da die Verwendung von Echtzeitdaten insbesondere im Bereich der CAI zahlreiche neue Möglichkeiten bietet, erwarten wir einen hohen Nutzen dieses Moduls für künftige Projekte.

Danksagung. Dieses Projekt wurde im Rahmen des DFG-geförderten Graduiertenkollegs 1126: Intelligente Chirurgie durchgeführt.

Literaturverzeichnis

1. Heimann T, Baumhauer M, Simpfendörfer T, et al. Prostate segmentation from 3D transrectal ultrasound using statistical shape models and various appearance models. Proc SPIE. 2008;6914(1):69141P–69141P8.
2. Graser B, Hien M, Rauch H, et al. Automatic detection of cardiac cycle and measurement of the mitral annulus diameter in 4D TEE images. Proc SPIE. 2012; p. 83140F–83140F7.
3. Khati NJ, Gorodenker J, Hill M. Ultrasound-guided biopsies of the abdomen. Ultrasound Q. 2011;27(4):255–68.
4. Wang DC, Chang W, Stetten GD. Real-time ultrasound image analysis for the insight toolkit. Proc MICCAI. 2005.
5. Boisvert J, Gobbi D, Vikal S, et al. An open-source solution for interactive acquisition, processing and transfer of interventional ultrasound images. Proc MICCAI. 2008.
6. Lasso A, Heffter T, Pinter C, et al. PLUS: An open-source toolkit for developing ultrasound-guided intervention systems. Proc NCIGT. 2011;4:103.
7. Wolf I, Vetter M, Wegner I, et al. The medical imaging interaction toolkit. Med Image Anal. 2005;9(6):594–604.
8. Neuhaus J, Wegner I, Kast J, et al. MITK-IGT: Eine Navigationskomponente für das Medical Imaging Interaction Toolkit. Proc BVM. 2009; p. 454–8.
9. Schroeder WJ, Ibáñez L, Martin KM. Software process: the key to developing robust, reusable and maintainable open-source software. Proc ISBI. 2004; p. 15–8.
10. Ibáñez L, Schroeder W, Ng L, et al. The ITK software guide. 2nd ed. Kitware Inc.; 2005.
11. Josuttis N. Das SOA-Manifest: Kontext, Inhalt, Erläuterung. dpunkt.verlag, Heidelberg; 2010.

Segmentation of Heterochromatin Foci Using a 3D Spherical Harmonics Intensity Model

Simon Eck[1], Stefan Wörz[1], Andreas Biesdorf[1], Katharina Müller-Ott[2],
Karsten Rippe[2], Karl Rohr[1]

[1]Dept. Bioinformatics and Functional Genomics, Biomedical Computer Vision Group
University of Heidelberg, BIOQUANT, IPMB, and DKFZ Heidelberg
[2]Research Group Genome Organization & Function, BIOQUANT and DKFZ
Heidelberg
simon.eck@bioquant.uni-heidelberg.de

Abstract. We introduce a 3D model-based approach for automatic segmentation of 3D fluorescent heterochromatin foci from 3D microscopy images. The approach employs a new 3D parametric intensity model based on a spherical harmonics (SH) expansion and can represent foci of regular and highly irregular shapes. By solving a least-squares optimization problem, the model is directly fitted to the 3D image data, and the model parameters including the SH expansion coefficients are estimated. The approach has been successfully applied to real 3D microscopy image data. A visual comparison and a quantitative evaluation show that the new approach yields better results than previous approaches.

1 Introduction

The analysis of heterochromatin structures and heterochromatin associated proteins from 3D microscopy image data is important to study genome regulation and cell function. Using confocal light microscopy, these structures can be visualized as *fluorescent foci*. Since biological studies often involve large amounts of 3D microscopy image data, manual image analysis is not feasible. Moreover, the size, 3D shape, and signal intensity of the foci can vary significantly (see Fig. 1). Hence, a robust automatic image analysis approach is required which can cope well with *highly irregular shapes* even in the case of high noise.

Previous approaches for segmentation of heterochromatin structures from microscopy images often rely on global intensity thresholds (e.g., [1]). In [2], segmentation is performed by energy minimization within image regions. However, the aforementioned approaches are bound to the pixel raster and do not obtain an analytic representation of the foci. In contrast, model-based approaches, e.g., based on parametric intensity models, are not bound to the pixel raster and allow determining an analytic representation. 3D parametric intensity models have successfully been used for 3D segmentation of subcellular structures from microscopy images (e.g., [3, 4]) and for heterochromatin analysis [5]. However, there only regularly shaped models (e.g., ellipsoids) were used.

H.-P. Meinzer et al. (Hrsg.), *Bildverarbeitung für die Medizin 2013*, Informatik aktuell,
DOI: 10.1007/978-3-642-36480-8_54, © Springer-Verlag Berlin Heidelberg 2013

In this work, we propose an automatic approach for 3D model-based segmentation of fluorescent foci from heterochromatin microscopy images. We introduce a new 3D parametric intensity model based on *spherical harmonics* (SH), which in comparison to [3, 4, 5] copes well with highly irregular foci shapes. SH form a complete orthogonal set of basis functions, enabling spherical functions to be expanded into a series of SH [6, 7]. In biomedical image analysis, SH were previously used, e.g., for shape characterization [8], shape registration [9], and surface smoothing. However, only few approaches *directly* employ SH for model-based *segmentation* [6, 10]. So far, such approaches were not used for microscopy images and they require training data [6] or manual initialization [10]. In our approach, training data is not necessary and the proposed 3D SH intensity model is initialized fully automatically. By solving a least-squares optimization problem, the model is directly fitted to the image data. The new approach has been successfully applied to real 3D microscopy images.

2   Materials and methods

2.1   Spherical harmonics expansion

In our approach, we analytically describe the 3D shape of fluorescent foci using a *spherical harmonics* (SH) expansion. SH form a complete set of basis functions defined on the sphere, enabling spherical functions to be expanded into a series of weighted SH [6, 7]. The real-valued SH of *degree l* and *order m* are defined by

$$Y_l^m(\theta, \varphi) = \begin{cases} \sqrt{2} N_l^m P_l^m(\cos\theta)\cos(m\varphi) & m > 0 \\ N_l^0 P_l^0(\cos\theta) & m = 0 \\ \sqrt{2} N_l^{|m|} P_l^{|m|}(\cos\theta)\sin(|m|\varphi) & m < 0 \end{cases} \tag{1}$$

where P_l^m is an associated Legendre polynomial. The normalization coefficients $N_l^m = \sqrt{\frac{2l+1}{4\pi}\frac{(l-m)!}{(l+m)!}}$ are chosen such that Y_l^m are orthonormal [7]. To describe

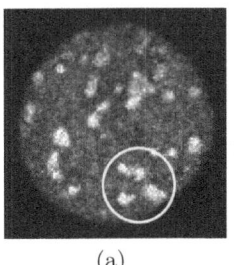
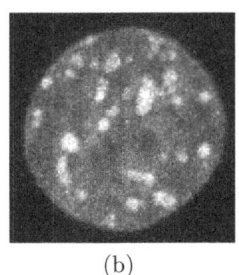
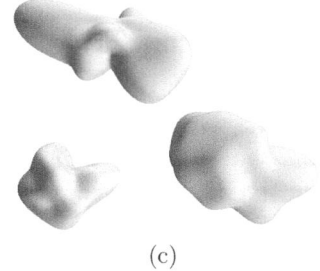

(a)   (b)   (c)

Fig. 1. Maximum intensity projections (MIPs) of a cell nucleus in a 3D two-channel fluorescence microscopy image: Heterochromatin protein 1α (a) and heterochromatin (b). (c) 3D segmentation results of the irregularly shaped foci marked in (a).

the shape of fluorescent foci using a series of SH, we assume the foci to be star-shaped. Let F denote the 3D region of a fluorescent focus, then F is said to be *star-shaped*, if a point $\mathbf{q} \in F$ exists such that each ray originating from $\mathbf{q}$ intersects the surface of F exactly once. If $\mathbf{q}$ is the origin of a spherical coordinate system, then the surface of F can be represented by a 3D radius function $r(\theta, \varphi)$, where $\theta \in [0, \pi]$ and $\varphi \in [0, 2\pi)$ are the inclination and azimuth angles, respectively. Based on (1), the real-valued SH expansion for approximation of $r(\theta, \varphi)$ can be stated as

$$r_{\mathrm{SH}} = \sum_{l=0}^{l_{\max}} \left[a_l^0 N_l^0 P_l^0(\cos\theta) + \sum_{m=1}^{l} \left[a_l^m \cos(m\varphi) + b_l^m \sin(m\varphi) \right] \sqrt{2} N_l^m P_l^m(\cos\theta) \right] \quad (2)$$

where $l_{\max}$ denotes the *series degree* which controls the accuracy of the approximation, and $\mathbf{a} = (a_0^0, ..., a_{l_{\max}}^{l_{\max}})^T$ and $\mathbf{b} = (b_1^1, ..., b_{l_{\max}}^{l_{\max}})^T$ denote the expansion coefficient vectors. A specific 3D shape can be described by adjusting $\mathbf{a}$ and $\mathbf{b}$.

2.2   3D parametric intensity model

To model the imaging process and to incorporate the effect of the point spread function (PSF) into (2), we use a convolution by a Gaussian kernel. The 3D SH intensity model is then given by

$$g_{\mathrm{SH}}(\mathbf{x}) = \Phi_\sigma(r + r_{\mathrm{SH}}(\pi - \theta, \varphi + \pi)) - \Phi_\sigma(r - r_{\mathrm{SH}}(\theta, \varphi)) \quad (3)$$

where Φ_σ is the Gaussian error function with standard deviation σ. To evaluate the model at position $\mathbf{x} = (x, y, z)^T$ in Cartesian coordinates, the spherical parameters r, θ, and φ are computed by $r(\mathbf{x}) = \sqrt{x^2 + y^2 + z^2}$, $\theta(\mathbf{x}) = \cos^{-1}\left(\frac{z}{r(\mathbf{x})}\right)$, and $\varphi(\mathbf{x}) = \tan^{-1}(\frac{y}{x})$. We further include a 3D rigid transform $\mathcal{R}(\mathbf{x}, \mathbf{x_0}, \boldsymbol{\alpha})$ with translation $\mathbf{x_0} = (x_0, y_0, z_0)^T$ and rotation $\boldsymbol{\alpha} = (\alpha, \beta, \gamma)^T$ as well as background and foreground intensity levels a_0 and a_1 to obtain the final 3D SH intensity model

$$g_{\mathrm{M,SH}}(\mathbf{x}, \mathbf{p}) = a_0 + (a_1 - a_0)g_{\mathrm{SH}}(\mathcal{R}(\mathbf{x}, \mathbf{x_0}, \boldsymbol{\alpha})) \quad (4)$$

where $\mathbf{p} = (\mathbf{a}, \mathbf{b}, a_0, a_1, \sigma, \boldsymbol{\alpha}, \mathbf{x_0})^T$ denotes the model parameter vector.

2.3   Automatic 3D foci segmentation

For automatic segmentation of 3D fluorescent foci, we propose a two-step approach. In the first step, initial center positions of different foci are determined using a 3D Gaussian filter for noise reduction followed by background suppression and 3D local maxima search for each individual cell nucleus. In the second step, the 3D SH intensity model (4) is applied to the 3D position of each local maximum. To fit the model to the 3D image data, a least-squares intensity-based optimization is performed within a spherical region of interest. For the optimization, we use the method of Levenberg and Marquardt which incorporates first order partial derivatives of $g_{\mathrm{M,SH}}$ w.r.t. the model parameters. Note that all partial derivatives of $g_{\mathrm{M,SH}}$ can be derived analytically.

3   Results

We have successfully applied our approach to 33 3D confocal microscopy images of mouse fibroblast cells (130 × 130 × 41 or 250 × 250 × 64 voxels). For comparison, we also applied two previous approaches: An approach based on a 3D Gaussian intensity model [4] and a 3D combined approach based on region-adaptive segmentation and a 3D Gaussian intensity model [5]. As an example, Fig. 2 shows 3D foci segmentation results of the heterochromatin protein 1α (HP1α). It can be seen that for small foci the previous approach based on the

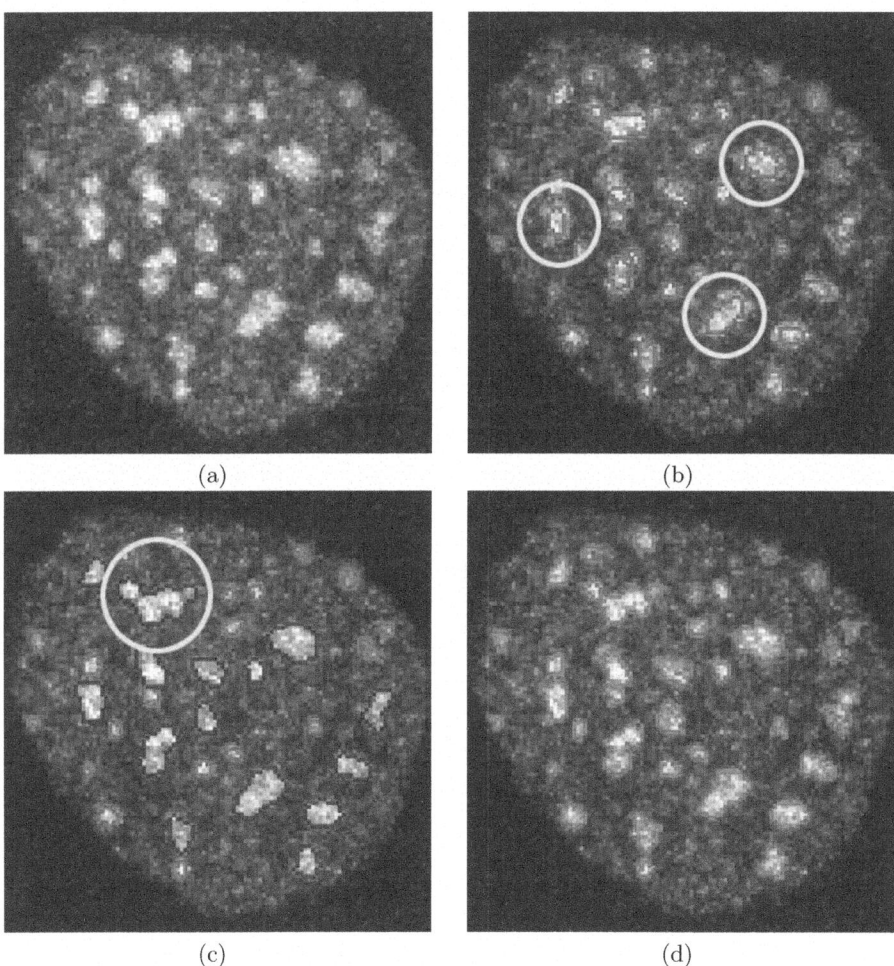

(a)

(b)

(c)

(d)

Fig. 2. MIP of (a) a cell nucleus in a 3D microscopy image and 3D foci segmentation results: (b) 3D Gaussian intensity model (red), (c) 3D combined approach based on region-adaptive segmentation (blue) and a 3D Gaussian intensity model (red), and (d) 3D SH intensity model (magenta).

Table 1. Quantitative results for real 3D microscopy image data: Mean value $\overline{D}$ and standard deviation σ_D of the Dice coefficient for manual segmentation and automatic segmentation based on a 3D Gaussian intensity model, a 3D combined approach based on region-adaptive segmentation and a 3D Gaussian intensity model, and the 3D SH intensity model.

	Manual	3D Gaussian	3D combined	3D SH
$\overline{D}$	**0.694**	0.651	0.682	**0.714**
σ_D	0.054	0.111	0.105	0.098

3D Gaussian model yields relatively good results, however, it fails to accurately segment large foci of irregular shape (see the yellow circles in Fig. 2b). The 3D combined approach generally yields a good result, however, for large foci of irregular shape with other foci in close proximity, undersegmentation occurs (see the yellow circle in Fig. 2c). In comparison, the new approach yields a better result (e.g., undersegmentation does not occur) and the approach can cope well with foci of different size and highly irregular shape (Fig. 2d). 3D visualizations of the segmentation result for several foci are shown in Fig. 1c.

To quantify the segmentation accuracy, we computed the Dice coefficient D between the 3D segmentation results and 3D ground truth data. Ground truth was provided manually by an expert observer for 3D foci in seven 3D microscopy images (7 cell nuclei, 75 foci in total). To determine the interobserver variability, a second observer manually performed 3D segmentation. For the automatic approaches, all foci were segmented using a fixed set of parameters. Table 1 shows the mean value $\overline{D}$ and standard deviation σ_D of the Dice coefficient for the different approaches for all 75 foci. It can be seen, that the new approach outperforms the two previous approaches. In addition, it turns out that the results of the new approach is comparable to manual segmentation (see the bold numbers in Table 1).

4   Discussion

We introduced a 3D model-based approach for automatic segmentation of 3D fluorescent heterochromatin foci. Our approach is based on a new 3D parametric intensity model using spherical harmonics (SH) and yields an analytic description of the segmented foci. Experiments using real 3D microscopy images show that the approach can cope well with foci of highly irregular shape and yields better results than two previous approaches. In future, we plan to apply our approach to a larger number of 3D images.

Acknowledgement. This work has been funded by the BMBF (SysTec) project EpiSys. We thank Dr. Qin Zhang (DKFZ Heidelberg, BIOQUANT, Division of Theoretical Systems Biology) for providing ground truth data.

References

1. Ivashkevich AN, Martin OA, Smith AJ, et al. H2AX foci as a measure of DNA damage: a computational approach to automatic analysis. Mutat Res. 2011;711(1-2):49–60.
2. Dzyubachyk O, Essers J, van Cappellen WA, et al. Automated analysis of time-lapse fluorescence microscopy images: from live cell images to intracellular foci. Bioinformatics. 2010;26(19):2424–30.
3. Thomann D, Rines DR, Sorger PK, et al. Automatic fluorescent tag detection in 3D with super-resolution: application to the analysis of chromosome movement. J Microscopy. 2002;208:49–64.
4. Wörz S, Sander P, Pfannmöller M, et al. 3D geometry-based quantification of colocalizations in multichannel 3D microscopy images of human soft tissue tumors. IEEE Trans Med Imaging. 2010;29(8):1474–84.
5. Eck S, Rohr K, Müller-Ott K, et al. Combined model-based and region-adaptive 3D segmentation and 3D co-localization analysis of heterochromatin foci. Proc BVM. 2012; p. 9–14.
6. Székely G, Kelemen A, Brechbühler C, et al. Segmentation of 2-D and 3-D objects from MRI volume data using constrained elastic deformations of flexible Fourier contour and surface models. Med Image Anal. 1996;1(1):19–34.
7. Arfken GB, Weber HJ, Harris FE. Mathematical Methods for Physicists. Sixth ed. Academic Press; 2005.
8. El-Baz A, Nitzken M, Khalifa F, et al. 3D shape analysis for early diagnosis of malignant lung nodules. Lect Notes Comput Sci. 2011;6801:772–83.
9. Shen L, Firpi HA, Saykin AJ, et al. Parametric surface modeling and registration for comparison of manual and automated segmentation of the hippocampus. Hippocampus. 2009;19(6):588–95.
10. Baust M, Navab N. A spherical harmonics shape model for level set segmentation. Lect Notes Comput Sci. 2010;6313:580–93.

Automatic Detection of Osteolytic Lesions in Rat Femur With Bone Metastases

Andrea Fränzle[1], Maren Bretschi[2], Tobias Bäuerle[2], Rolf Bendl[1,3]

[1]Division of Medical Physics in Radiation Oncology, DKFZ Heidelberg
[2]Division of Medical Physics in Radiology, DKFZ Heidelberg
[3]Department of Medical Informatics, Heilbronn University
a.fraenzle@dkfz-heidelberg.de

Abstract. A method for the automatic detection of osteolytic lesions caused by bone metastases is presented. Osteolytic means that bone mass is lost and these lesions are visible as holes in the bone structure. For the analysis of the process of metastases and their response to therapies the measurement of these lesions is neccessary. As manual segmentation of all lesions is too complex for a larger study, automatic tools are needed. The challenging task of measuring missing structures is solved here by comparison of a modified bone with a healthy model. The algorithm is tested on rat femur bones. First tests have shown that the presented algorithm can be used for the global identification of osteolytic regions.

1 Introduction

For a better understanding of bone metastases and their response to different therapies in case of mamma carcinoma, rat models with site specific metastases are analyzed [1]. In addition to a tumor part, bone metastases can have both osteolytic (bone mass is destroyed) and osteoblastic (new bone mass is built) effects on bone. Fig. 1 shows an example for the progress of osteolytic lesions in the hind leg bones of a rat from day 30 to day 55 after tumor cell inoculation. At the beginning of the process, bone mass is dissolved, which results in small caves in the cortical bone (Fig. 1(a), 1(b)). As the metastasis inside the bone grows larger, the remaining bone mass is pushed aside by the tumor mass, so that the bone and bone fragments are spread (Fig. 1(d)).

For the quantitative analysis of bone deformation the volume of the bone lesions has to be determined. Therefore an exact segmentation of the bone lesion is needed. In a larger study manual segmentation of all bone lesions is too complex and too time consuming. The challenge for developing automated tools for the segmentation of osteolytic lesions is the segmentation of missing structures. Here an approach for the automatic detection of osteolytic lesions in a rat femur by comparison with a healthy model is presented.

2 Material and methods

Since the whole hind anatomy of the animal is visible, that means the field of view is not limited to a specific region, a global approach for detecting osteolytic regions is needed. The basic idea to find osteolytic lesions is to compare the modified bone structure with a healthy model. An example for a model based approach for detecting bone lesions is presented by [2]. As in [1] described, vessel clips are used in this rat model to lead the tumor cells, therefore metastases can only occur in the right hind leg. That means that in this case under these controlled conditions an unaffected body side exists. We assume that the left and right limbs develop symmetrically and therefore we can simulate the healthy right body side by mirroring the healthy left body side. First, the healthy femur is segmented and the femur segmentation is then mirrored along the median plane. The mirrored segmentation is registered to the affected body side. Finally, a gray value based decision is performed for each voxel. The following sections describe the data material and the single steps of the algorithm.

2.1 Experimental rat model data

The algorithm is developed on 3D CT data that shows the hind part of the anatomy. The field of view is not limited to a specific leg region, the whole anatomy of the hind part of the animal is visible. A transversal slice has 512 x 512 voxels, a data cube has about 200 slices. The voxel size is 0.17mm x 0.17mm x 0.20mm. Image data is acquired for each animal on day 30, 35, 45, and 55 after tumor cell inoculation.

2.2 Healthy model segmentation

For the healthy femur segmentation a statistical shape model [3] is used. The advantage of using shape models for segmenting single bones is that they already include appearance information and can cope with diffuse edge information in the joints contrary to a segmentation with a simple thresholding. The shape model is constructed by using 10 manually segmented femur bones. The initial positioning of the shape model is done automatically by using bone marrow caves, that have similar properties concerning position and orientation as the bone itself. The process of using bone marrow caves for shape model initialization, including bone marrow cave segmentation and finding the according bone structure with

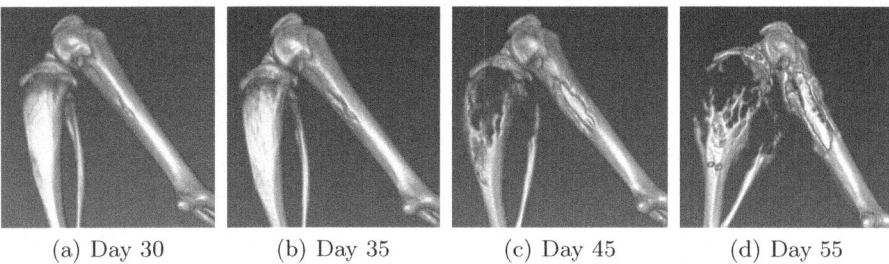

(a) Day 30   (b) Day 35   (c) Day 45   (d) Day 55

Fig. 1. Right leg bones of a rat with osteolytic lesions on day 30, 35, 45 and 55 after tumor cell inoculation.

pattern recognition is described for human bone structures in [4] and transferred to long bones in rats. A masked image of the femur segmentation is created with original values within the segmented contours and zero in the background and then mirrored along the median plane.

2.3   Registration of healthy model and modified bone

The mirrored segmentation mask is registered rigidly to the original skeleton by maximizing mutual information [5]. A rigid transformation is used here to prevent deformation of the healthy model in regions with osteolytic lesions since this would make a comparison between healthy model and modified bone worthless. Mutual information is used because it does not demand additional user interaction, e.g. setting landmarks.

2.4   Gray value based decision

After registration of the model with the right femur, each voxel v enclosed by the model contour is checked, if it is within an osteolytic lesion. The decision for each voxel v to be an osteolytic lesion based on its gray value $g_{\text{healthy}}(v)$ in the registered healthy model image and its gray value $g_{\text{modified}}(v)$ in the modified bone and using a threshold t_{bone} for cortical bone is as follows: if

$$(g_{\text{healthy}}(v) \geq t_{\text{bone}}) \wedge (g_{\text{modified}}(v) < t_{\text{bone}})$$

v is considered to be located in an osteolytic region.

3   Results

A prototype of the presented algorithm is tested for an osteolytic lesion in the femur in 3 rats on day 35 and day 45. These timepoints were selected because an osteolytic lesion is clearly visible then and the bone structure of the femur is still in such a condition the algorithm can deal with. Day 55 was excluded, since the bone loss and the bone deformation is so large, that the healthy model cannot be positioned reliably. Fig. 2 shows all objects in the femur recognized as osteolytic lesion by the algorithm, including false posititive results. The additionally found false positive regions also meet the criteria for an osteolytic lesion according to the voxel based decision but result from a non-perfect fit of the healthy model.

Fig. 3 shows the results of the automatic segmentation of an selected osteolytic lesion in the femur in 3 rats on day 35 (Fig. 3(d)- 3(f)) and on day 45 (Fig. 3(j)- 3(l)).

4   Discussion

The presented algorithm is able to detect osteolytic lesions automatically in a rat femur with bone metastases at an early stage. It completes a bone structure with missing parts by using a healthy model which makes a segmentation and measurement of the missing bone mass possible. The accuracy of the example segmentations (Fig. 3) delivered by the presented algorithm for lesions at an early stage, except for the segmentation of rat no. 3 on day 45 (Fig. 3(l)), is sufficient for a radiologist.

An obvious limitation is given if the metastasis grows too large (Fig. 1(d)), so that the bone is not only destroyed in some well bounded regions but spread and has therefore a totally modified shape. In this case, the actual size of the osteolytic region cannot be determined with this algorithm, because the healthy model does not adapt to this new shape. In clinical cases in patients with metastases osteolytic lesions with such large bone deformations are rather unlikely. In the present rat experiment, such large osteolytic lesions occur in rats in a control group without a therapy. A patient would be diagnosed with metastases at an earlier stage and get a therapy to stop the process. That means, this limitation of the algorithm is rather irrelevant for clinical data.

The presented algorithm is based on the assumption that the contralateral healthy side of the skeleton can be used as a model. We do not use a shape model directly for segmentation of the right femur, since those models would tend to adapt to the already deformed osteolytic bone boundaries.

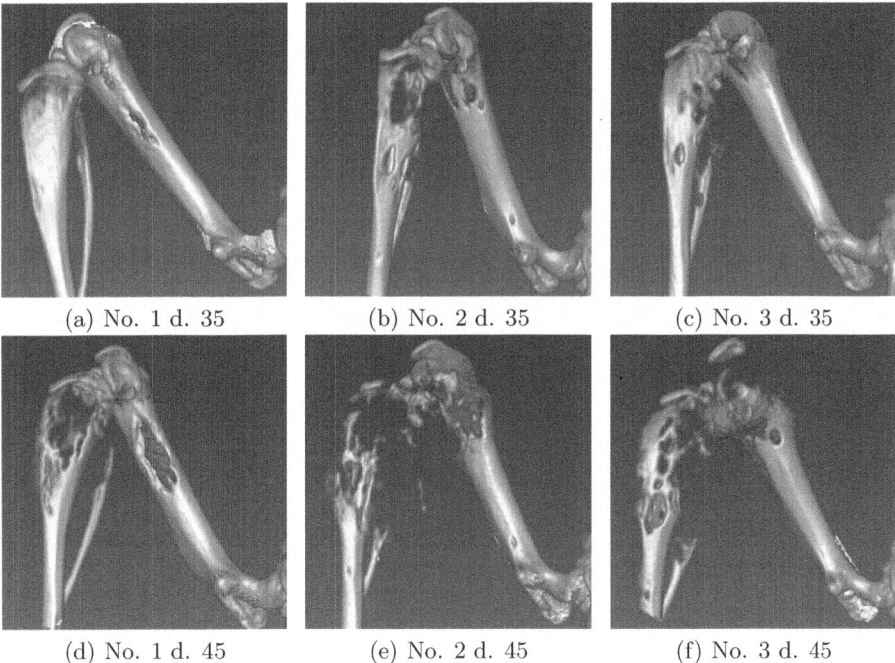

(a) No. 1 d. 35   (b) No. 2 d. 35   (c) No. 3 d. 35

(d) No. 1 d. 45   (e) No. 2 d. 45   (f) No. 3 d. 45

Fig. 2. All automatically found segmentations in 3 rats on day 35 and day 45. Red: correctly recognized osteolytic lesion. Yellow: false positive segmentations.

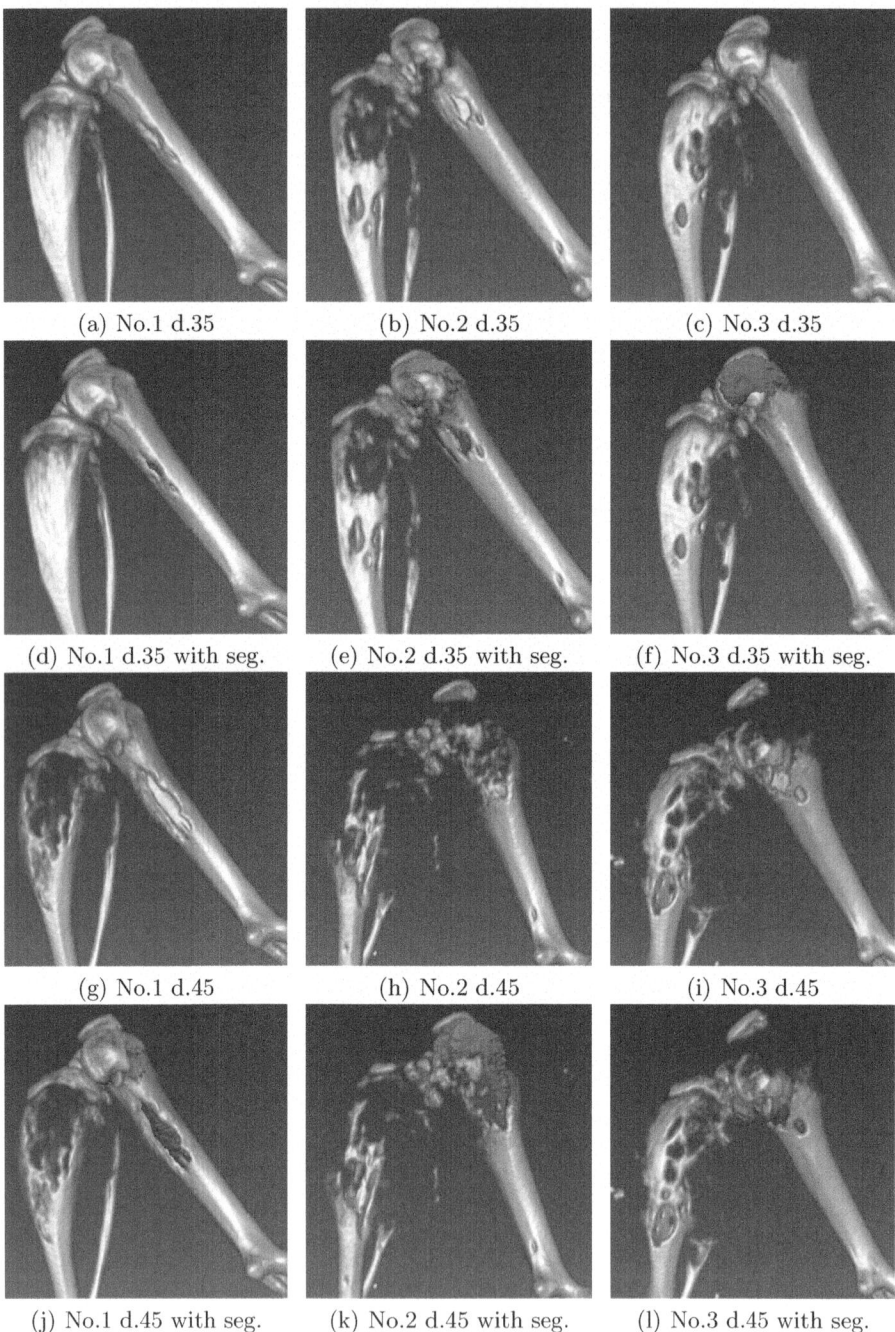

(a) No.1 d.35   (b) No.2 d.35   (c) No.3 d.35

(d) No.1 d.35 with seg.   (e) No.2 d.35 with seg.   (f) No.3 d.35 with seg.

(g) No.1 d.45   (h) No.2 d.45   (i) No.3 d.45

(j) No.1 d.45 with seg.   (k) No.2 d.45 with seg.   (l) No.3 d.45 with seg.

Fig. 3. Osteolytic lesions in 3 rats on day 35 and day 45. Red: result of the automatic segmentation of the osteolytic lesion in the femur.

This way they would not allow to determine the deformed parts precisely. By using the healthy body side we have a model that has not to be deformed.

So far, the algorithm is still detecting a number of false positives (Fig. 2), which are caused by a non-perfect fit of the healthy model. Currently we work on an implementation of some volume completion algorithms [6], [7] to overcome this limitation. These algorithms are able to detect cavities in objects. Their results can build the base of classifying found regions as osteolytic cavities and also improve the found boundaries. So the presented algorithm could be used as a global approach to identify regions of interest and locally applied volume completion might refine the results.

References

1. Bäuerle T, Adwan H, Kiessling F, et al. Characterization of a rat model with site-specific bone metastasis induced by MDA-MB-231 breast cancer cells and its application to the effects of an antibody against bone sialoprotein. Int J Cancer. 2005;115(2):177–86.
2. Malizos KN, Siafakas MS, Fotiadis DI, et al. An MRI-based semiautomated volumetric quantification of hip osteonecrosis. Skeletal Radiol. 2001;30(12):686–93.
3. Heimann T, Meinzer HP. Statistical shape models for 3D medical image segmentation: a review. Med Image Anal. 2009;13(4):543–63.
4. Fränzle A, Bendl R. Automatische Segmentierung und Klassifizierung von Knochenmarkhöhlen für die Positionierung von Formmodellen. Procs BVM. 2012; p. 280–5.
5. Maes F, Collignon A, V D, et al. Multimodality image registration by maximization of mutual information. IEEE Trans Med Imaging. 1997;16:187–98.
6. Janaszewski M, Couprie M, Babout L. Hole filling in 3D volumetric objects. Pattern Recognit. 2010;43:3548–59.
7. Sharf A, Alexa M, Cohen-Or D. Context-based surface completion. ACM Trans Graph. 2004;23(3):878–87.

A Generic Approach to Organ Detection Using 3D Haar-Like Features

Florian Jung[1], Matthias Kirschner[2], Stefan Wesarg[1]

[1]Cognitive Computing & Medical Imaging, Fraunhofer IGD, Darmstadt, Germany
[2]Graphisch-Interaktive Systeme, TU Darmstadt, Darmstadt, Germany
`florian.jung@igd.fraunhofer.de`

Abstract. Automatic segmentation of medical images requires accurate detection of the desired organ as a first step. In contrast to application-specific approaches, learning-based object detection algorithms are easily adaptable to new applications. We present a learning-based object detection approach based on the Viola-Jones algorithm. We propose several extensions to the original approach, including a new 3D feature type and a multi-organ detection scheme. The algorithm is used to detect six different organs in CT scans as well as the prostate in MRI data. Our evaluation shows that the algorithm provides fast and reliable detection results in all cases.

1 Introduction

The segmentation of organs is one of the major tasks in medical imaging. Common segmentation algorithms operate locally, that is why a preceding detection of the organ is needed to approximate its position. Many segmentation algorithms still need a manual placement of a seed point in order to successfully segment the desired structure. In order to achieve a fully automatic organ segmentation, the detection task has to be automated as well. Many object detection methods are tailored to a specific application. As an example, Kainmüller et al. [1] detect the liver by searching for the right lung lobe, which can be relatively easily detected by thresholding and voxel counting. The problem of such approaches is that they do not generalize to other structures or image modalities. Learning-based approaches such as Discriminative Generalized Hough transform [2] and Marginal Space Learning (MSL) [3, 4] are more general and can be adapted to a wide variety of detection tasks by simply exchanging the training data.

In this paper, we propose a learning-based organ detection approach for 3D medical images based on the Viola-Jones object detection algorithm [5]. We use a bootstrapping approach to automatically select important training data. Moreover, we propose several extensions to the original approach tailored to medical images, namely a new pure-intensity feature type, and a multi-organ detection that exploits spatial coherence in medical data. Finally, we provide a detailed evaluation of the algorithm by detecting six different organs in CT data sets as well as the prostate in T2-weighted MRI scans. Hereby, we show that our algorithm can successfully detect these seven different structures.

H.-P. Meinzer et al. (Hrsg.), *Bildverarbeitung für die Medizin 2013*, Informatik aktuell,
DOI: 10.1007/978-3-642-36480-8_56, © Springer-Verlag Berlin Heidelberg 2013

2   Methods

The basis of this algorithm is the Viola-Jones face detection [5] which builds a strong classifier based on Haar-like features. We use AdaBoost to train this classifier and to select a subset of 3D Haar-like features [4] within an iterative training process. We made several modifications to the algorithm in order to be able to use it in 3D.

2.1   Bootstrapped learning process

The number of subregions per image is huge and the time needed to train a classifier using all the regions is not negligible. Therefore we extract only a subset of subregions from the training images. In order to extract regions with high information value for the training process we implemented a bootstrapped process which trains a classifier and then starts a detection on the training images. All resulting false positives are added as additional negative samples to the already existing examples. Finally a new training process is executed. With the use of these additional samples, we expect that the classifier can better discriminate regions that are hard to classify.

2.2   Adjusting the ROI

In most cases, we use the organ's bounding box as positive training example. As the tissue within an organ is relatively homogeneous and 3D Haar features describe the intensity contrast between adjacent regions, 3D Haar features are usually more discriminative when they cover tissue of both the organ and its surroundings. In cases where the bounding box alone does not provide sufficiently discriminative features, the ROI can be enlarged by a constant factor to include additional tissue. After detection, the detected bounding box can be easily reconstructed by downsizing the enlarged ROI.

2.3   New feature type

A Haar-like feature consists of two (or more) rectangular areas which are summed up and subtracted from each other. The difference between these area-sums is the resulting Haar-like feature value. A Haar-like feature is defined by its type, its size and its position inside the current window.

In order to account for regions with approximately constant image intensities that are often observed in CT images we create a new feature type that only sums up all pixels within its area without doing any subtraction. Therefore we expect the feature we added to be an enrichment for our algorithm and improve the detection results.

Fig. 1. Illustration of the eight 3D Haar-like feature types we are using for our organ detection algorithm.

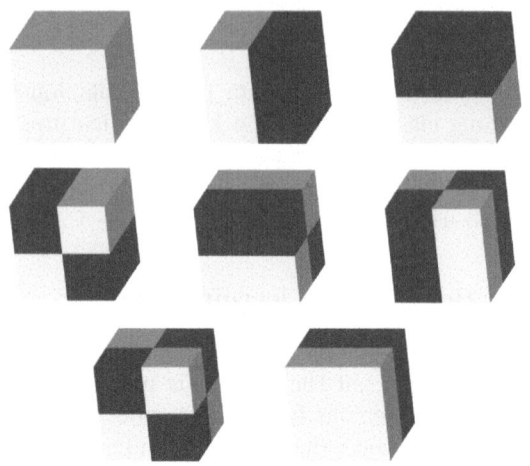

2.4 Detection

The organ detection is done using the sliding window. At each window position all feature values for the selected subset of 3D Haar-like features are calculated, multiplied with the weight that was stored during the training process and finally summed up. If this value exceeds the threshold defined during the training phase, it is assumed that the region contains the relevant structure. The detection is done using 5 different sliding window sizes. Starting with the mean size of the organ the window is downsized twice and upsized twice according to observed organ size variations. In contrast to face detection, where every image can potentially contain many faces, or no face at all, we can safely assume that there is exactly one organ per image. Therefore, the final detection result is the sub window with the highest signed distance to the decision threshold.

Fig. 2. Illustration of the relationship model between different organs. The usage of this model improves the detection results significantly.

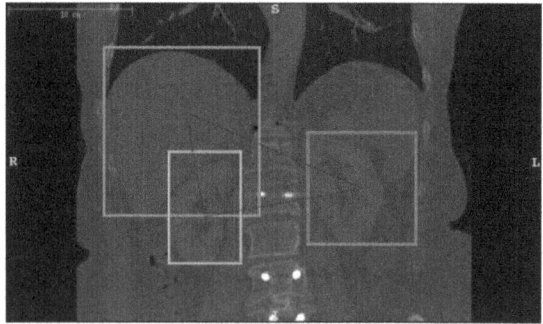

2.5   Multi-organ detection

In order to further improve the detection results and to be able to detect organs which could not be detected with the default detection approach, we implemented a multi-organ detection. For this purpose, we use a PCA (principal component analysis) and train a model consisting of the organs of interest and their relative positions to each other using the center of gravity. During the detection phase we analyze the positions of the detected organs and compare them with the trained PCA model. A probability function returns us the likelihood of a valid organ model. We create a ranking of the 30 best results for each organ and than calculate a detection score for each possible permutation considering the probability as an additional weight.

2.6   Experimental setup

For tests on contrast enhanced CT data, we used 210 images to train the classifier and 10 images to evaluate the results. The images contained the following organs: liver, heart, bladder, kidneys and the spleen. The spacing of the images varies between: x: 0.57, y: 0.57, z: 1 and x: 0.97, y: 0.97, z: 5. The detected ROIs are compared with the ground truth bounding boxes of the images using the Dice Coefficient. We trained more than 250 classifiers for different organs and with varying window size. Performing some tests we found out that an Dice overlap of 60-70 % for the detection is enough to accomplish a good segmentation.

For tests on MR data, we detected the prostate on T2-weighted MRI scans. The data was obtained from the MICCAI Grand Challenge: Prostate MR Image Segmentation 2012. For training the detector, we used the 50 training images, and then performed tests on the 30 test images. As the ground truth of the 30 test scans is not available to us, the results were assessed by visual inspection only. Because in contrast to CT images, MRI data has non-standardized image intensities, all images were pre-processed. Intensity inhomogeneities within a single a image, the so-called bias-field, was removed with Coherent Local Intensity Clustering [6]). Afterwards, image intensities are normalized using robust statistics and rescaled to the interval $[0, 1000]$.

Adjusting the ROI on MRI. Because the tissue within the prostate's bounding box is very inhomogeneous, we adjusted the ROI around the prostate (see Section 2.2) in x and y-direction by 40 % in order to achieve more robust detection results.

Multi-organ detection. The multi-organ detection was applied to the task of simultaneously detecting liver and both kidneys, because the latter are difficult to detect. As test images we choose images in which the detection of at least one organ failed.

3   Results

Fig. 3 shows quantitative results obtained on the CT data with a detection window size of 10^3. We achieve a median Dice coefficient with the ground truth bounding box of 0.71-0.87, depending on the data set. Only for the kidneys, we observed misdetections.

The size of the sliding window has major impact on the training time. A training run with a resolution of 5^3 can be accomplished within 5 minutes, while a classifier trained with a resolution of 15^3 needs two and a half days. However, we observed that the classifiers trained with a resolution of 5^3 already yield some usable detection results. Here, the median Dice coefficient is between 0.62 and 0.78.

On 30 MRI test scans, visual inspection showed that the detection results were sufficient for segmentation. Indeed, in a subsequent Active Shape Model segmentation, we achieved a median Dice coefficient of 0.86 [7].

The detection itself is very fast. Although it depends on the image size, the size of the sliding window and some other factors, it takes less than one second in the majority of cases.

3.1   New feature type

The new feature type we created is used in 15 per cent of cases for an average classifier and was thereby the second most used classifier. Considering that the boosting algorithm chooses the feature that can distinguish best between the samples, it can be said that the inclusion of the new feature type turns out to be an enrichment for the algorithm.

Fig. 3.   Illustration of the overlaps of six different organs. Comparison was done between the ground-truth bounding-box and the detected bounding box. All results are located between 0.6 and 0.95 %(except for three kidney results), what turned out to be enough to do a proper segmentation of the organ.

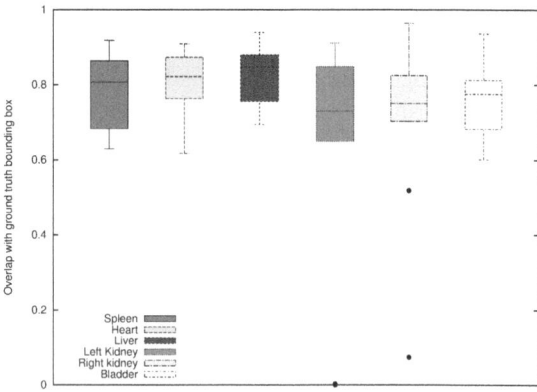

Multi-organ detection. The use of the multi-organ detection improves the detection results for organs that are more difficult to detect (like the kidneys)

significantly. In 75% of the cases the missclassified organ was detected due to the usage of the multi-organ detection. Additionally the average overlap of the three detected organs increased by 20% thanks to this approach.

4 Discussion

We proposed several extensions to the Viola-Jones face detection algorithm and applied them to the detection of organs in 3D medical images. Our approach achieves good detection results on seven different organs, including six CT and one MRI data set. This shows the broad applicability of our approach in contrast to methods tailored to specific applications. In cases where the detection is difficult, for example for the kidneys, the use of the multi-organ detection improves the results and enables use to locate organs that can not be robustly detected with a single detector. Alternatively, it might be possible to improve the results by enlarging the ROI, as it was done for the prostate.

In contrast to MSL, we do not estimate the orientation of the organ. This estimation is, in most cases, not necessary because of the scanning protocol. For example, patients are always oriented upright in CT images. We also use a simple learning algorithm, namely boosting instead of the probabilistic boosting tree used in MSL. However, our results show that this simpler algorithm provides sufficient results in practice, and is applicable to a large variety of different organs.

References

1. Kainmüller D, Lange T, Lamecker H. Shape constrained automatic segmentation of the liver based on a heuristic intensity model. Proc MICCAI Grand Challenge: 3D Segmentation in the Clinic. 2007; p. 109–16.
2. Ruppertshofen H, Lorenz C, Schmidt S, et al. Discriminative generalized hough transform for localization of joints in the lower extremities. CSRD. 2011;26:97–105.
3. Ling H, Zhou SK, Zheng Y, et al. Hierarchical, learning-based automatic liver segmentation. Proc IEEE CVPR. 2008; p. 1–8.
4. Zheng Y, Barbu A, Georgescu B, et al. Four-chamber heart modeling and automatic segmentation for 3-D cardiac CT volumes using marginal space learning and steerable features. IEEE Trans Med Imaging. 2008;27(11):1668–81.
5. Viola P, Jones M. Rapid object detection using a boosted cascade of simple features. Proc CVPR. 2001;1:511–18.
6. Li C, Xu C, Anderson A, et al. MRI tissue classification and bias field estimation based on coherent local intensity clustering: A unified energy minimization framework. IPMI. 2009; p. 288–99.
7. Kirschner M, Jung F, Wesarg S. Automatic prostate segmentation in MR images with a probabilistic active shape model. Proc MICCAI Grand Challenge: Prostate MR Image Segmentation. 2012.

Mobile Detektion viraler Pathogene durch echtzeitfähige GPGPU-Fuzzy-Segmentierung

Pascal Libuschewski[1,2], Dominic Siedhoff[1], Constantin Timm[2], Frank Weichert[1]

[1]Lehrstuhl für Graphische Systeme, Technische Universität Dortmund
[2]Lehrstuhl für Eingebettete Systeme, Technische Universität Dortmund
pascal.libuschewski@tu-dortmund.de

Kurzfassung. Die vorliegende Arbeit stellt einen neuartigen Fuzzy-Logik-basierten Segmentierungsalgorithmus zur Detektion von biologischen Viren in stark Artefakt-behafteten Bildsequenzen vor, der konform ist zu den differenzierten Ressourcenbeschränkungen mobiler Endgeräte. Als Sensor kommt der neuartige PAMONO-Biosensor zum indirekten Nachweis von Viren mittels optischer Mikroskopie zum Einsatz. Die Segmentierungen weisen eine hohe positive Übereinstimmung bei idealisierten synthetischen Segmentierungen auf, die durch den Fuzzy-Ansatz insbesondere bei kleinen Viren/schlechtem Signal-Rausch-Verhältnis nochmals verbessert wird. Ferner wird gezeigt, dass eine GPU-gestützte Datenanalyse die Detektion viraler Strukturen in Echtzeit auf mobilen Endgeräten ermöglicht, und im Vergleich zur CPU den Energieverbrauch im Durchschnitt um Faktor 3.7 senkt.

1 Einleitung

Um das Ausbreitungsverhalten von Virus-Epidemien zu verstehen und Präventivmaßnahmen zu ergreifen, ist es erforderlich, Diagnosen viraler Infektionen schnell, verlässlich und vor Ort durchführen zu können. Das vorgestellte PAMONO-Verfahren (Plasmon-Assisted Microscopy of Nano-Objects) [1] erfüllt diese Eigenschaften. Es ist ein modifiziertes Oberflächen-Plasmonen-Resonanz-Verfahren (SPR-Verfahren), das im Vergleich zu konventionellem SPR jede Virus-Anhaftung einzeln nachweisen kann. Im Unterschied zu Methoden wie ELISA und PCR [2] kann der Nachweis in Echtzeit, während die Viren durch eine Flusszelle auf den Sensor geleitet werden, geschehen. Die Funktionsweise des Biosensors wird zu Beginn von Abschnitt 2 kurz zusammengefasst.

Der Fokus des neuartigen Ansatzes liegt in der Detektion viraler Strukturen in stark Artefakt-innervierten Bilddatenfolgen unter Einsatz unscharfer Bewertungsregeln. Eine besondere Herausforderung besteht in den Ressourcenlimitierungen, da der Sensor und die Verarbeitungseinheit als tragbares, kostengünstiges Gerät realisiert werden sollen. Der Stand der Technik lässt sich ausgehend von diesen Anforderungen in modell- oder trackingbasierte Ansätze, Verfahren der künstlichen Intelligenz, Mustererkennung oder neuronalen Netzwerken differenzieren. Eine Übersicht findet sich in [3]. Bei der medizinischen Bildverarbeitung

H.-P. Meinzer et al. (Hrsg.), *Bildverarbeitung für die Medizin 2013*, Informatik aktuell,
DOI: 10.1007/978-3-642-36480-8_57, © Springer-Verlag Berlin Heidelberg 2013

stellen Ultraschallaufnahmen vergleichbare Herausforderungen an die Segmentierung und Klassifikation wie die hier vorgestellte Technik – eine Übersicht zu aktuellen Methoden beschreibt z.B. [4]. Im Gegensatz zur bisherigen Datenanalysemethodik [5] kommen ortszeitliche Fuzzy-Regeln (Abschnitt 2.1) zum Einsatz. Der experimentelle Aufbau wird in Abschnitt 2.2 beschrieben. Die Resultate werden schließlich in Abschnitt 3 dargestellt und in Abschnitt 4 diskutiert.

2   Material und Methoden

Ausgangsbasis der Analysealgorithmen bilden die Daten des PAMONO-Sensors (Plasmon-Assisted Microscopy of Nano-Objects), welcher es erlaubt, Objekte im Nanometer-Bereich mittels optischer Mikroskopie nachzuweisen [1]. Hierbei wird eine dünne, mit Antikörpern beschichtete Goldschicht unter Zuhilfenahme eines Lasers bestrahlt (Abb. 1(a)), wobei Viren innerhalb einer Pufferlösung über die Antikörper mittels einer Pumpe geleitet werden. Wenn ein Virus an einen Antikörper gebunden wird, ändern sich die Oberflächen-Plasmonen-Resonanz-Eigenschaften in einer Mikrometer-großen Umgebung um das Virus. Resultierend reflektiert dieser Bereich mehr Licht als umgebende Bereiche – der Nachweis des Intensitätsanstiegs geschieht dabei mittels optischer Mikroskopie. Neben der markierungsfreien Viren-Detektion kann der Sensor auch zur Diagnose der Funktionsfähigkeit von Antikörpern, sowie zum Nachweis anderer Nano-Teilchen, wie etwa von Feinstaub-Partikeln, verwendet werden.

Eine 12-Bit CCD Kamera zeichnet 30 Bilder der Oberflächenreflektion pro Sekunde auf, bei einer Auflösung von 1024×256 Pixeln. Ein anhaftendes Virus zeichnet sich in diesen Daten als sprunghaft auftauchender, schwacher Fleck ab. Für ein Pixel innerhalb dieses Flecks bedeutet dies einen Sprung in der am Pixel gemessenen Zeitreihe, Abb. 1(b), wodurch sich Virus-Kandidaten-Pixel von Hintergrund-Pixeln unterscheiden lassen [1].

2.1   Fuzzy-Detektor

Dieser Abschnitt skizziert, ausgehend von der existierenden Methodik zur Datenanalyse [5], den neuen Stream-basierten Ansatz unter Verwendung von Fuzzy Lo-

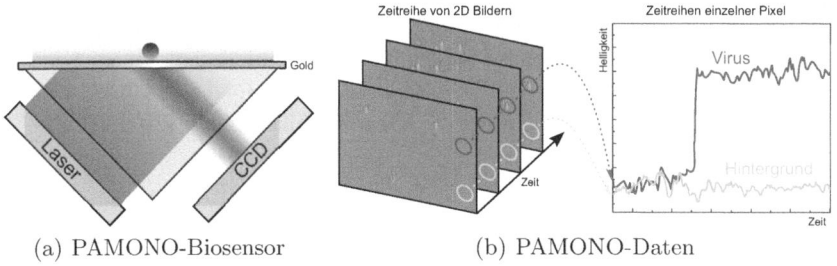

(a) PAMONO-Biosensor   (b) PAMONO-Daten

Abb. 1. a) Schematischer Aufbau des PAMONO-Biosensors und b) exemplarische Darstellung zur Zeitreihenanalyse für ein Virus- und Hintergrund-Pixel.

gik. Im initialen Vorverarbeitungsschritt erfolgt ein Denoising der Daten mittels Wavelets [6]. Eine Mustererkennung bestimmt ein Ähnlichkeitsmaß D der akquirierten Zeitreihen zu idealen Modellzeitreihen für Virus-Pixel, welche bei einem vorliegenden hohen Ähnlichkeitsmaß über einen Marching-Squares Algorithmus zu Polygonen aggregiert werden. Im letzten Schritt erfolgt eine Klassifikation der Polygone mit Methoden des Maschinellen Lernens anhand von Formfaktoren, um echte Viren von Falschdetektionen aufgrund von Artefakten im Signal zu unterscheiden. Mit Blick auf die Echtzeit-Anforderungen wurden diese Methoden unter Verwendung von Grafikprozessoren, implementiert („General-purpose computing on graphics processing units"(GPGPU)).

Der hier vorgestellte Fuzzy-Detektor setzt zwischen der Mustererkennung und dem Marching-Squares Algorithmus an und verarbeitet das Ähnlichkeitsmaß D. Anstatt eines harten Schwellwerts zur Binarisierung von D werden Fuzzy-Regeln genutzt, die zusätzliches Wissen einfließen lassen. Sei $D(x, y, t)$ das Ähnlichkeitsmaß der Mustererkennung mit Ortskoordinate x, y an Zeitpunkt t (im Kontext von PAMONO dient die normalisierte Kreuzkorrelation als D). Sei ferner $N^{x,y,t}_{b \times h \times l}$ die Multimenge der Werte, die D in einem $b \times h \times l$ Fenster mit x, y, t im Zentrum annimmt. Der Fuzzy-Detektor ordnet der Koordinate x, y, t auf Basis von $D(x, y, t)$ und der Nachbarschafts-Information $N^{x,y,t}_{b \times h \times l}$ die Klassen "Virus„oder "Hintergrund„zu. Dies geschieht zunächst unscharf über Fuzzy-Regeln, die einer Koordinate Zugehörigkeitgrade zu Fuzzy-Mengen zuweisen. Diese Grade liegen in [0,1] und können sich zu Werten größer eins summieren. Der beschriebene Ansatz erweitert das in [7] zur Rauschreduktion vorgestellte Pixelklassifikations-Verfahren zu einem Segmentierungs-Verfahren und parallelisiert es auf der GPU.

Der erste Schritt des Verfahrens ist die Fuzzyfizierung, die jedem Wert $d :=$ $D(x, y, t)$ eine Zugehörigkeit zur Fuzzy-Menge $\mu_{\text{Sprung}} \in [0, 1]$ zuweist, welche die Ähnlichkeit d zu eine Sprung-Funktion mittels zweier unscharfer Schwellwerte $0 \leq \pi_1 < \pi_2$ normiert

$$\mu^{\pi_1, \pi_2}_{\text{Sprung}}(d) = \begin{cases} 1 & \text{für } d \geq \pi_2 \\ \frac{d - \pi_1}{\pi_2 - \pi_1} & \text{für } \pi_1 < d < \pi_2 \\ 0 & \text{sonst} \end{cases} \tag{1}$$

Diese Regel charakterisiert Virus-Pixel durch hohe Werte. Über ergänzende Regeln wird zudem differenziertes Anwendungswissen über die Struktur von Virus-Anhaftungen und das Hintergrundsignal in deren Klassifikation integriert – dies wird im Folgenden an zwei exemplarischen Regeln aufgezeigt. Hierbei bezeichnet $r(k, S)$ das k-größte Element der Menge S. Die folgende Regel dient der Erkennung von Pixeln, die am Rand von Virus-Anhaftungen liegen

$$\mu^{\pi_1, \pi_2}_{\text{Rand}}(d) = d > \pi_1 \text{ AND } \mu^{\pi_1, \pi_2}_{\text{Sprung}}(r(15, N^{x,y,t}_{7 \times 7 \times 3})) \tag{2}$$

Der Fuzzy-Operator a AND b ist hierbei als $\min(a, b)$ definiert. Diese Regel trägt der Tatsache Rechnung, dass die Amplitude des Resonanzeffekts in den Randbereichen abnimmt, sodass ein schlechtes Signal-Rausch-Verhältnis die korrekte Klassifizierung des Sprungs mittels eines einzelnen scharfen Schwellwerts verhindert. Liegt d jedoch im Trägerintervall der unscharfen Funktion aus Gleichung (1), so wird die Nachbarschaft des Pixels betrachtet und das Pixel anhand der Anzahl und Stärke der benachbarten Virus-Pixel klassifiziert, was eine korrekte Klassifizierung des Randbereichs ermöglicht. Die zweite Regel dient der Synchronisierung multipler zeitlicher Instanzen der selben Virus-Anhaftung

$$\mu_{\text{Synch}}^{\pi_1,\pi_2}(d) = d > \pi_1 \text{ AND } \mu_{\text{Sprung}}^{\pi_1,\pi_2}(r(1,N_{1\times1\times5}^{x,y,t})) \tag{3}$$

Resultierend steht eine Regelbasis zur Charakterisierung der Klasse der Virus-Pixel zur Verfügung, welche u.a. aus den Gleichungen (1)–(3) besteht. Ferner existieren Regelgruppen zur Differenzierung der Hintergrund-Klasse, sowie signalspezifischer Artefakte. Die Zugehörigkeitsfunktionen werden in einem abschließenden Schritt defuzzyfiziert, wodurch die Pixel zur Weiterverarbeitung mittels Marching-Squares klassifiziert werden.

2.2 Experimenteller Aufbau und Mobile Echtzeit-Analyse

Die Qualitätssteigerung durch den Fuzzy-Detektor wurde durch Vergleich mit einer scharfen Schwellwert-Methode mit genetisch optimiertem Schwellwert gemessen. Per datengetriebener Synthese wurden echte Daten zu synthetischen Daten mit bekannter idealer Segmentierung und Klassifikation transformiert. Nach dieser Methode wurden sechs verschiedene Ausprägungen von Datensätzen mit jeweils 2000 Bildern erzeugt. Ein Typus von erzeugten Daten nutzt einen synthetisch Poisson-verrauschten Hintergrund, der andere Typus nutzt reale Sensordaten ohne Viren als Hintergrund, was neben Poisson-Rauschen weitere Signaldegradationen bedingt, die etwa von Staub und Luftblasen in der Pufferlösung herrühren. Pro Typus wurden drei Datensätze mit den simulierten Virusgrößen 200 nm, 150 nm und 100 nm erzeugt. Die Fragestellung hierbei war, ob die Erkennung der Viren durch nicht-scharfe Schwellwerte und Fuzzy-Anwendungswissen verbessert werden kann.

Als Gütemaß diente die positive Übereinstimmung [8] zwischen idealer synthetischer Segmentierung und Detektionsergebnis, sodass sowohl falsch positive als auch falsch negative Detektionen berücksichtigt wurden. Die negative Übereinstimmung wurde nicht gemessen, da der Begriff der wahren negativen Detektion in diesem Kontext nicht definiert ist.

Für das mobile Szenario war die Fragestellung, ob die dort beschränkten Ressourcen „Rechenzeit"und „Energie"für die vorgestellte Echtzeit Datenanalyse-Methodik ausreichen. Der Versuchsaufbau war wie folgt: Es wurde für verschiedene Systeme gemessen, wie viele Bilder pro Sekunde analysiert werden können. Die Größe der analysierten Bilder und die Anzahl der enthaltenen Viren wurde graduell erhöht, indem eine 64×64 Pixel große Kachel wiederholt wurde, um Datensätze der Größen $1024 \times \{128, 256, 512, 1024\}$ Pixel pro Bild zu erzeugen. Die erreichten Bildraten wurden für eine mobile GPU (Nvidia Quadro NVS 3100M 256MB) gemessen, sowie zum Vergleich für eine mobile CPU (Intel Core i7 620M) und eine Desktop-CPU (Intel Core i7 2600). Für die beiden mobilen Plattformen wurde der Energieverbrauch über die Batterie-Status-Information innerhalb von `sysfs` unter Linux gemessen und verglichen.

3 Ergebnisse

Der vorgestellte Fuzzy-Detektor erhöht die positive Übereinstimmung für alle Datensätze (Abb. 2(a)). Bei synthetischem Poisson-Rauschen und größeren Partikeln ist der Unterschied weniger stark, weil das Signal-zu-Rausch-Verhältnis hoch genug für einen scharfen Schwellwert ist – geringere simulierte Virus-Größe und Datensätze mit realem Sensorrauschen verdeutlichen die Verbesserung signifikant. Bei Sensorrauschen kann die Übereinstimmung im Durchschnitt um sieben Prozentpunkte gesteigert werden, wobei die relative Verbesserung bei sinkender simulierter Virus-Größe steigt. Folglich ermöglicht der Fuzzy-Detektor eine verbesserte Erkennung insbesondere kleinerer Viren.

Für die Evaluation der Echtzeitfähigkeit wurde die Anzahl der verarbeiteten Bilder pro Sekunde erfasst (Abb. 2(b)), unterschieden nach Ausführungsplattform und Größe der Datensätze. Um Echtzeitfähigkeit im Kontext von PAMONO zu gewährleisten, müssen mindestens 30 Bilder pro Sekunde bei einer Auflösung von 1024 × 256 Pixeln analysiert werden können. Dieses Ziel wird weder von der mobilen, noch von der Desktop CPU erreicht, jedoch von der mobilen GPU. Der durchschnittliche Geschwindigkeitszuwachs von der mobilen CPU zur GPU beläuft sich auf den Faktor 3.6. Gleichzeitig sinkt der Energieverbrauch des Gesamtsystems durchschnittlich um einen Faktor 3.7 für das mobile Gerät: Die Verarbeitung eines Bildes der Auflösung 1024 × 256 verbraucht unter Verwendung der CPU 5.84 J, hingegen 1.56 J bei der GPU (1024 × 512: 10.52 J (CPU) und 2.76 J (GPU); 1024 × 128: 3.26 J (CPU) und 0.93 J (GPU)) – für weitere Methoden zur Senkung des GPU-Energieverbrauchs sei auf [9] verwiesen.

4 Diskussion

Ausgehend von der Herausforderung, eine konzeptionelle und algorithmische Basis für eine Echtzeit-konforme und portable Analyseeinheit zur Erkennung viraler

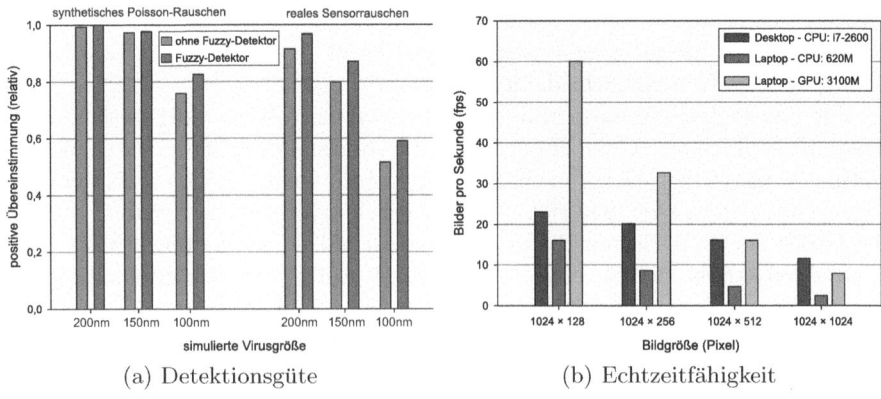

(a) Detektionsgüte   (b) Echtzeitfähigkeit

Abb. 2. a) Evaluation der Detektionsgüte für unterschiedliches Rauschen und Signalstärke und b) der Echtzeitfähigkeit für verschiedene Bildgrößen und Systeme.

Strukturen unter dem zusätzlichem Gesichtspunkt der Kosteneffizienz zu entwickeln, konnte aufgezeigt werden, dass der vorgestellte Fuzzy-Detektor diesen Anforderungen entspricht und zudem eine hohe Detektionsgüte aufweist. Die positive Übereinstimmung zwischen idealen synthetischen Daten und Detektionsergebnis wurde in allen untersuchten Fällen verbessert. Die Verbesserung zeigt sich insbesondere bei kleineren Viren und dem damit verbundenen schlechteren Signal-zu-Rausch-Verhältnis. Ferner wurde dargelegt, dass die vorgestellte Datenanalyse in Echtzeit auf einem mobilen Endgerät durchgeführt werden kann. Hierbei erwies sich die Verwendung der GPU als notwendig, da selbst aktuelle Desktop CPUs keine Echtzeit-Analyse gewährleisten. Die Verwendung der GPU ist außerdem, mit Blick auf den mobilen Einsatz, deutlich energiesparender.

Damit ist der aktuelle Prototyp der PAMONO-Analyseeinheit ein effizientes und mobiles Gerät mit hoher Detektionsrate für virale Strukturen. Der Prototyp besteht aus einem handelsüblichen Laptop-Computer und dem tragbaren Sensoraufbau in ähnlicher Größe. Da Viren durch die Echtzeit-Datenanalyse bereits kurz nach dem Einleiten der Probe in den Flüssigkeitskreislauf des Sensors erkannt werden können, lassen sich Diagnosen im Vergleich zu ELISA und PCR stark beschleunigen. Mit Blick auf einen ubiquitären Einsatz wird eine weitere Miniaturisierung des Sensor-Aufbaus angestrebt. Ferner sollen GPUs von Tablet-Computern und Smartphones als Analyseplattform untersucht werden. Neben Messungen zum Nachweis von Feinstaub ist ein Fernziel die Untersuchung von Netzwerken aus PAMONO Sensorknoten, die der Messung des großräumigen Ausbreitungsverhaltens von Nanopartikeln in der Umwelt dienen.

Danksagung. Teile dieser Arbeit wurden von der Deutsche Forschungsgemeinschaft (DFG) im Sonderforschungsbereich SFB 876 „Verfügbarkeit von Information durch Analyse unter Ressourcenbeschränkung", Projekt B2, unterstützt.

Literaturverzeichnis

1. Zybin A, et al. Real-time detection of single immobilized nanoparticles by surface plasmon resonance imaging. Plasmonics. 2010;5:31–5.
2. Karlovsky P. Moderne Diagnosemethoden und Nachweisverfahren. Schriftenreihe der Deutschen Phytomedizinischen Gesellschaft. 2006; p. 104–18.
3. Zhang YJ. Advances in image and video segmentation. IRM Press; 2006.
4. Noble JA, Boukerroui D. Ultrasound image segmentation: A survey. IEEE Trans Med Imaging. 2006;25(8):987–1010.
5. Siedhoff D, et al. Detection and classification of nano-objects in biosensor data. Microscop Image Anal Appl Biol. 2011; p. 1–6.
6. Mittermayr CR, et al. Wavelet denoising of Gaussian peaks: a comparative study. Chemometrics Intell Labor Syst. 1996;34:187–202.
7. Mélange T, et al. Fuzzy random impulse noise removal from color image squences. IEEE Trans Image Process. 2011;20:959–70.
8. Cicchetti DV, Feinstein AR. High agreement but low kappa: II. Resolving the paradoxes. J Clin Epidemiol. 1990;43:551–8.
9. Timm C, et al. Design space exploration towards a realtime and energy-aware GPGPU-based analysis of biosensor data. Comput Sci Res Dev. 2011; p. 1–9.

Towards Deformable Shape Modeling of the Left Atrium Using Non-Rigid Coherent Point Drift Registration

Martin Koch[1], Sebastian Bauer[1], Joachim Hornegger[1,2], Norbert Strobel[3]

[1]Pattern Recognition Lab, Friedrich-Alexander-Universität Erlangen-Nürnberg
[2]Erlangen Graduate School in Advanced Optical Technologies (SAOT),
Friedrich-Alexander-Universität Erlangen-Nürnberg
[3]Siemens AG, Healthcare Sector, Forchheim
martin.koch@cs.fau.de

Abstract. Modeling the deformable shape of the left atrium is of strong interest for many applications in cardiac diagnosis and intervention. In this paper, we propose a method for left atrium shape modeling using non-rigid point cloud registration. In particular, we build upon the concept of Coherent Point Drift (CPD) registration that considers the alignment as a probability density estimation problem. Based on the set of non-rigidly registered point clouds, we perform a principle component analysis to establish a deformable shape model. In an experimental study on ten clinical data sets, we evaluated the registration accuracy in terms of average mesh-to-mesh distance, as well as on anatomical landmarks on the left atrium. With the proposed method, we achieved registration results with an average mesh-to-mesh error of 3.4 mm. The average landmark offset was 8.5 mm.

1 Introduction

Statistical shape models are widely used today in different fields of medical image processing. A common application is the use as prior information for segmentation of 3-D medical image data [1]. The left atrium is a challenging structure, as it shows a large amount of variation in surface topology and shape across different patients. Examples of 3-D mesh models for different atria are shown in Fig. 1. In addition to the anatomical differences among subjects, there is the aspect of cardiac motion which leads to deformations of the left atrium in different heart phases. In electrophysiology ablation procedures, a model of the underlying anatomical structure could be used for planning of the intervention as, e.g., suggested by Keustermans et al. using patient specific 3-D data sets for planning of atrial fibrillation treatment [2].

In this paper, we propose a method for left atrium shape modeling using non-rigid point cloud registration. In our approach, we generate the shape model from 3-D magnetic resonance imaging (MRI) volume data sets. We exclusively used data sets of left atria with four pulmonary veins, which reflects the most common anatomic configuration [3]. First, the relevant structure was segmented and represented as a triangle mesh. Then we used the Coherent Point Drift (CPD) algorithm [4] to pairwise align meshes via non-rigid point cloud registration. Basically, CPD registration is performed based on a Gaussian Mixture Model (GMM) framework and a regularization of the displacement field. Benefits of the CPD algorithm are the generation of smooth deformation fields while being robust against noise and outliers [4].

2   Materials and methods

Left atrium mesh models of ten subjects were extracted from contrast enhanced 3-D MRI volume data sets. The MRI data sets were acquired with a resolution of $256 \times 256 \times 68$ voxels. The in-plane pixel spacing was $1.23 \times 1.23\,\mathrm{mm}$ and the slice thickness $1.5\,\mathrm{mm}$. The left atrium was segmented from MRI voxel data sets using a semi-automatic segmentation software (syngo InSpace EP, Siemens AG, Forchheim, Germany). The segmentation process is initialized by manually selecting a point inside the left atrium. Based on this seed point, the complete left atrium is segmented automatically. The segmentation results are represented

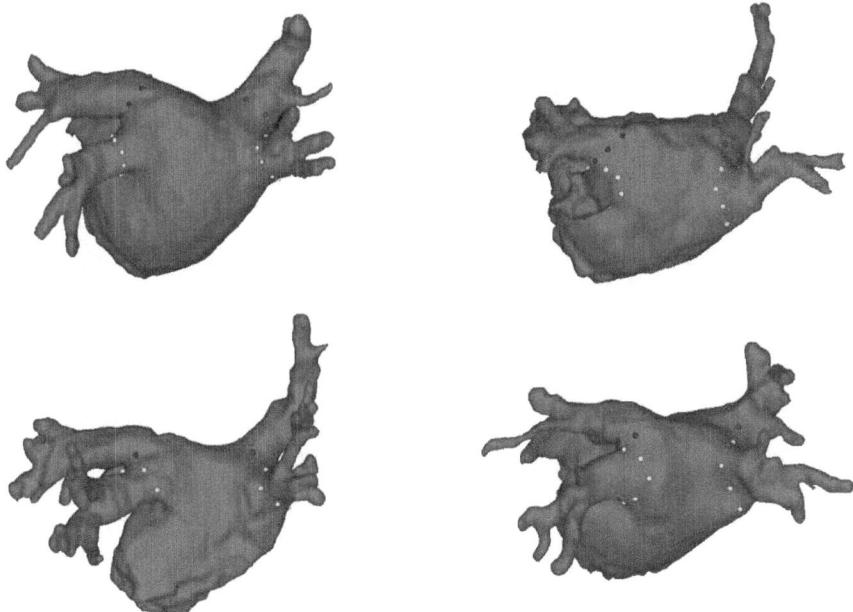

Fig. 1. Mesh models of the left atrium segmented from 3-D MRI volumes from four subjects. The colored spheres depict the anatomic position of the pulmonary vein ostia and were labeled by an expert: right superior (dark green), right inferior (light green), left superior (dark blue) and left inferior (light blue).

as triangle meshes. Fig. 1 depicts models of the left atrium from four different subjects.

For registration, let us consider the mesh as a point cloud $\mathcal{M}$ consisting of N points $x_i \in \mathbb{R}^3$

$$\mathcal{M} \equiv \boldsymbol{m} = \left[\boldsymbol{x}_1^\top, \ldots, \boldsymbol{x}_N^\top\right]^\top \in \mathbb{R}^{3N} \tag{1}$$

In a first step, we selected one left atrium mesh model as a reference mesh. The reference mesh was chosen based on visual inspection to clearly express the LA anatomy. The reference mesh $\boldsymbol{m}_{\mathrm{Ref}}$ is then registered to a set of sample meshes $\{\boldsymbol{m}_t\}_{t=1}^{T}$, with $T = 9$, using the CPD algorithm. All meshes have the same anatomical orientation, and are zero centered before applying the registration.

2.1 Non-rigid point cloud registration using CPD

We used the coherent point drift algorithm to register the reference mesh to the set of sample meshes. CPD follows a probabilistic approach by considering the alignment of the two point sets as a probability density estimation problem. The basic idea is to fit the GMM centroids, represented by the points of the reference mesh $\boldsymbol{m}_{\mathrm{Ref}}$, to the sample mesh $\boldsymbol{m}_t$, by maximizing the likelihood. This optimization is performed with the expectation maximization algorithm. During the optimization process, the GMM centroids are forced to move coherently as a group, to ensure preservation of the topological structure of the point set.

The displacement function v for the reference mesh is defined as

$$\hat{\boldsymbol{m}}_{\mathrm{Ref}} = \boldsymbol{m}_{\mathrm{Ref}} + v(\boldsymbol{m}_{\mathrm{Ref}}) \tag{2}$$

with $\boldsymbol{m}_{\mathrm{Ref}}$ as the initial centroid positions. $\hat{\boldsymbol{m}}_{\mathrm{Ref}}$ and v, respectively, are obtained by minimizing the following energy function [5]

$$E\left(\hat{\boldsymbol{m}}_{\mathrm{Ref}}\right) = -\sum_{n=1}^{N} \log \sum_{m=1}^{M} e^{-\frac{1}{2}\left\|\frac{x_n - y_m}{\sigma}\right\|^2} + \frac{\lambda}{2}\phi\left(v\right) \tag{3}$$

where $\phi(v)$ is a regularization to ensure the displacement field to be smooth. $\boldsymbol{x}_n$ denotes a point of the mesh $\boldsymbol{m}_t$, $\boldsymbol{y}_m$ a point of the transformed mesh $\hat{\boldsymbol{m}}_{\mathrm{Ref}}$, respectively. N and M refer to the number of points within the respective mesh. The parameter λ determines the trade-off between data fitting and smoothness of the deformation field. We empirically determined a suitable value for this parameter ($\lambda = 2.0$).

2.2 Deformable shape model generation

The reference mesh $\boldsymbol{m}_{\mathrm{Ref}}$ is registered to every sample mesh $\boldsymbol{m}_t$. The transformed mesh $\hat{\boldsymbol{m}}_{\mathrm{Ref}}$ is labeled $\boldsymbol{v}_t$ for ease of use. The training set is defined as $\mathcal{V} = \{\boldsymbol{m}_{\mathrm{Ref}}, \boldsymbol{v}_1, \ldots, \boldsymbol{v}_T\}$. We used a Principle Component Analysis (PCA) approach [6] to compute the modes of variation. Applying PCA to the covariance matrix of the centered version of $\mathcal{V}$ yields a set of eigenvectors $\boldsymbol{e}_i$ describing the principle modes of variation in the training data set. The eigenvectors are ordered in descending order based on the value of their corresponding eigenvalue. The P largest eigenvectors are stored in the matrix $\boldsymbol{\Phi} = [\boldsymbol{e}_1, \ldots, \boldsymbol{e}_P] \in \mathbb{R}^{3N \times P}$. A linear combination of the P principal modes of variation, with $\boldsymbol{b} \in \mathbb{R}^P$ as weighting factors, spans a subset of linearized mesh models composed of the given modes of variation

$$\boldsymbol{m}^* = \bar{\boldsymbol{v}} + \boldsymbol{\Phi}\boldsymbol{b} \tag{4}$$

The mean shape $\bar{\boldsymbol{v}}$ is defined as

$$\bar{\boldsymbol{v}} = \frac{1}{T+1}\left(\boldsymbol{m}_{\mathrm{Ref}} + \sum_{t=1}^{T} \boldsymbol{v}_{\mathrm{t}}\right) \tag{5}$$

For quantitative evaluation of the proposed framework, we used ten clinical data sets with manually annotated pulmonary vein (PV) ostia. These landmarks are labeled RSPV (Right Superior Pulmonary Veins), RIPV (Right Inferior Pulmonary Veins), LSPV (Left Superior Pulmonary Veins), and LIPV (Left Inferior Pulmonary Veins). The quality of the registration is measured based on residual landmark distances and mesh-to-mesh distance. The residual landmark error is defined as the Euclidean distance of the center of corresponding PV ostia and measured after non-rigid CPD registration.

3 Results

Fig. 2 shows the average mesh-to-mesh distance, as well as the initial and residual landmark offset per data set. The initial and residual offsets per landmark are shown in Fig. 3. The average mesh-to-mesh distance is between 2.5 and 5.1 mm, the average landmark offset is between 2.9 and 13.9 mm. Fig. 4 depicts the residual registration error for data set 4, which shows the highest mesh-to-mesh error. The highest mesh-to-mesh distance occurs at the end of the pulmonary veins. In this case especially on the right inferior PV.

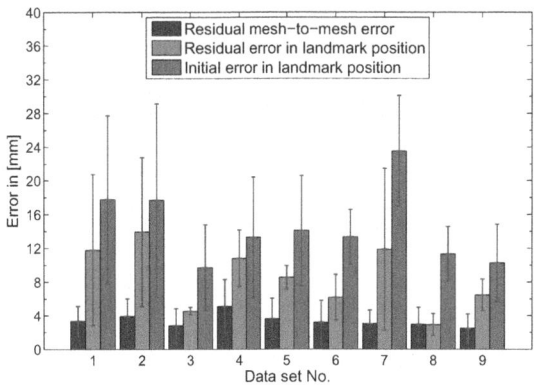

Fig. 2. Evaluation per data set. Mean and standard deviation of the residual mesh-to-mesh error, landmark error after registration, and initial landmark error are shown per data set.

Fig. 3. Evaluation per landmark. Mean and standard deviation of the initial and residual landmark error.

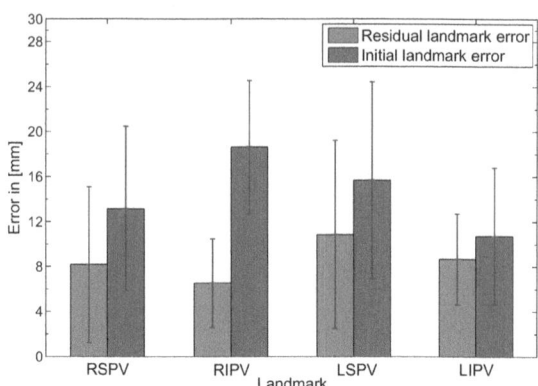

4 Discussion

We described a method for left atrium shape modeling using non-rigid point cloud registration. The overall performance of the mesh registration shows a mean mesh-to-mesh error of 3.4 mm over all data sets. The coherent point drift algorithm was capable of dealing with high variations in anatomy. The highest residual mesh-to-mesh distance results from different extents of the pulmonary veins. The average landmark offset was 8.5 mm. Landmarks on the right side of the left atrium, namely RSPV and RIPV, show a lower residual error compared to left sided landmarks LSPV and LIPV. This might be due to the additional pouch on the left side of the left atrium, the left atrial appendage, which is anterior to the PV ostia.

The mesh models of the left atrium also contained a large part of the connected pulmonary veins. Removing or trimming these extensions might improve

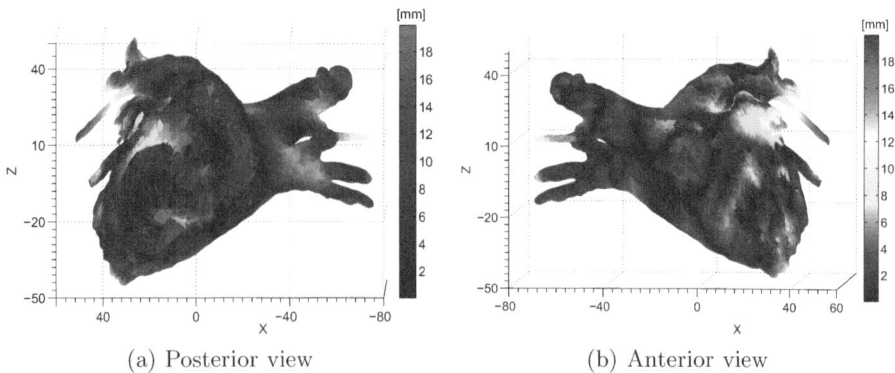

(a) Posterior view   (b) Anterior view

Fig. 4. Residual mesh-to-mesh error color coded on one example mesh. The error is measured as Euclidean distance in [mm]. The highest mesh-to-mesh distance occurs at the end of the pulmonary veins. In this case especially on the right inferior PV.

the accuracy, since these structures show a high variation in shape and size. For the modeling of the atrium, short pulmonary vein ostia would be sufficient. This work is a first step towards our goal of automatic planning of ablation regions for atrial fibrillation procedures. Planning structures could be transfered to augmented fluoroscopy systems used to guide the procedure and overlaid to the X-ray images.

Acknowledgement. This work was supported by the German Federal Ministry of Education and Research (BMBF) in the context of the initiative Spitzencluster Medical Valley - Europäische Metropolregion Nürnberg, project grant Nos. 01EX1012A and 01EX1012E, respectively. Additional funding was provided by Siemens AG, Healthcare Sector. S. Bauer acknowledges support by the Graduate School of Information Science in Health (GSISH) and TUM Graduate School.

References

1. Heimann T, Meinzer HP. Statistical shape models for 3D medical image segmentation: a review. Med Image Anal. 2009;13(4):543–63.
2. Keustermans J, De Buck S, Heidbuechel H, et al. Automated planning of ablation targets in atrial fibrillation treatment. Proc SPIE. 2011;7962:796207.
3. Kautzner J, Micochova H, Peichl P. Anatomy of the left atrium and pulmonary veins–lessons learned from novel imaging techniques. Eur Cardiol. 2006;2(1):89–90.
4. Myronenko A, Song X. Point set registration: Coherent Point Drift. IEEE Trans Pattern Anal Mach Intell. 2010;32(12):2262–75.
5. Myronenko A, Song X, Carreira-Perpinan M. Non-rigid point set registration: Coherent Point Drift. Adv Neural Inf Process Syst. 2007;19:1009–16.
6. Jolliffe I. Principal Component Analysis. Wiley Online Library; 2005.

Convolution-Based Truncation Correction for C-Arm CT Using Scattered Radiation

Bastian Bier[1], Chris Schwemmer[1,2], Andreas Maier[1,3], Hannes G. Hofmann[1],
Yan Xia[1], Joachim Hornegger[1,2], Tobias Struffert[4]

[1] Pattern Recognition Lab, Universität Erlangen-Nürnberg
[2] Erlangen Graduate School in Advanced Optical Technologies (SAOT)
[3] Siemens AG, Healthcare Sector, Forchheim, Germany
[4] Department of Neuroradiology, Universitätsklinikum Erlangen
bastian.bier@medtech.stud.uni-erlangen.de

Abstract. Patient dose reduction in C-arm computed tomography by volume-of-interest (VOI) imaging is becoming an interesting topic for many clinical applications. One limitation of VOI imaging that remains is the truncation artifact in the reconstructed 3-D volume. This artifact can either be a cupping effect towards the boundaries of the field-of-view (FOV) or an offset in the Hounsfield values of the reconstructed voxels. A new method for the correction of truncation artifacts in a collimated scan is introduced in this work. Scattered radiation still reaches the detector and is detected outside of the FOV, even if axial or lateral collimation is used. By reading out the complete detector area, we can use the scatter signal to estimate the truncated parts of the object: The scattered radiation outside the FOV is modeled as a convolution with a scatter kernel. This new approach is called scatter correction. The reconstruction results using Scatter convolution are at least as good or better than the results with a state-of-the-art method. Our results show that the use of scattered radiation outside the FOV improves image quality by 1.8 %.

1 Introduction

In many clinical applications, intra-procedural imaging is required. This is often done with fluoroscopy. Sometimes the information out of these 2-D images is not enough. Then a 3-D reconstruction is desirable, e.g. for a fluoroscopic overlay [1]. In order to reduce the patient dose, the X-rays are collimated so that only a small part of the detector size is used.

Collimated projection data leads to a problem when using filtered backprojection for 3-D reconstruction. Strong truncation artifacts appear at the boundary of the FOV, due to the ramp filtering of the projection data. The collimation introduces a sharp boundary into the projection data, which is amplified during the filtering step. These artificially high frequencies are backprojected into the volume and generate the truncation artifacts [2].

Due to the collimation, the scan does not cover the full spatial extent of the object. For an exact reconstruction, the full extent of the object has to be known

H.-P. Meinzer et al. (Hrsg.), *Bildverarbeitung für die Medizin 2013*, Informatik aktuell,
DOI: 10.1007/978-3-642-36480-8_59, © Springer-Verlag Berlin Heidelberg 2013

from a prior scan [3], or a small part of the object has to be known [4]. If no prior knowledge is available, heuristic methods have to be applied. These methods are often called truncation correction in the literature. The better the heuristic fits the truncated object, the better the resulting reconstruction is. Some methods model the outside of the FOV, which was not measured [4, 5]. Others require extrapolation only implicitly [6, 7]. With respect to image quality, these heuristic methods provide acceptable results. In [8], an approach is presented that uses a filter to attenuate the radiation outside the FOV to a minimal dose. In a post-processing step, this information is then used to solve the truncation problem. The approach presented here is similar to [8] as we also used a small amount of radiation outside the regular FOV. In contrast to [8], no additional dose has to be applied to the patient, as we employ the scattered radiation that is caused by the collimator edges and the object itself. This information is always present in a truncated FOV scenario but usually not measured.

Fig. 1 shows projection images of the skull of one patient. In Fig. 1(a), the full projection and in Fig. 1(b), the collimated projection are shown with the same grayscale window. Fig. 1(c) shows the same projection as in Fig. 1(b), but with a narrow windowing. It can be seen that the attenuated signal caused by the scattered radiation clearly depicts the shadow of the skull (cf. arrow).

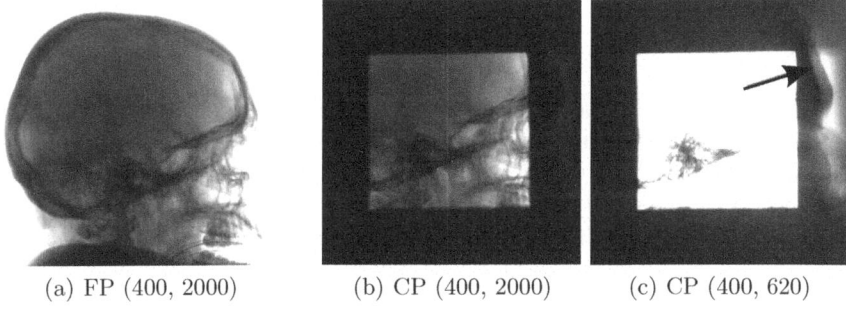

    (a) FP (400, 2000)   (b) CP (400, 2000)   (c) CP (400, 620)

Fig. 1. Projection images. FP = full projection; CP = collimated projection; The numbers determine the grayscale window.

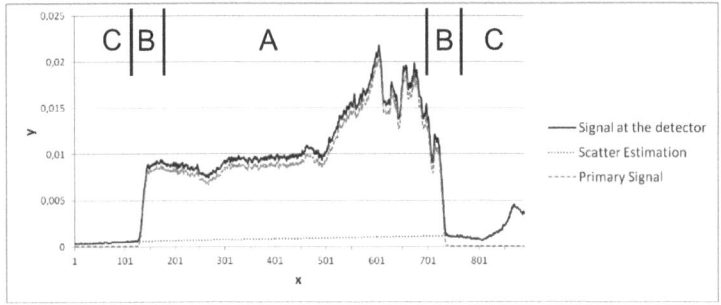

Fig. 2. Scatter estimation.

This information can be used to improve the image quality of the reconstruction inside the FOV.

2   Materials and methods

In Fig. 2, an intensity profile through a collimated projection is plotted. The projection is divided into three parts: the FOV (area A), the area outside the FOV (area C), and the shadow of the collimator edge (area B).

2.1   Edge detection

First, the edges of the collimator have to be detected. An edge is modeled as two lines that describe the beginning and the end of the collimator shadow (Fig. 2). Since the truncation correction is applied in row direction, only the vertical collimator edges need to be detected.

For the initial detection, the Hough transformation (HT) is applied. After that, the collimator edge is approximated with a sigmoid curve in each row. On this sigmoid curve, the beginning and the end points of the collimator edge are calculated. RANSAC is used to fit continuous lines through the corresponding points of the four edges in each projection.

2.2   Scatter convolution

A scatter model must be assumed before a correction is possible. There are different approaches for scatter estimation. They are either based on measurements, mathematical-physical models, or a combination of both ([9] gives an overview). One possibility is the beam-scatter-kernel superposition approach, a measurement-based method: The primary signal ϕ is convolved with a spatially invariant scatter kernel to estimate the scatter effect. ϕ is the primary signal without scatter and measured in the intensity domain I/I_0. Note that all the following calculations are done in the intensity domain instead of the line integral domain, because scatter is always additive to the intensity measured at the detector. The scatter estimation can be written as

$$\phi_{\text{scatter}} = \phi * G \qquad (1)$$

where G is a scatter kernel and ϕ_{scatter} is the resulting scatter estimate.

Another measurement-based method presented in [10] is called collimator-shadow continuation method. This method is only possible if collimation is applied. The scattered radiation outside the FOV is measured. It is assumed that the scatter distribution in the FOV can be obtained by an interpolation between the measured boundary data. An example for this estimation is shown in Fig. 2. The dotted line represents the scatter estimate. Inside the FOV (area A), this estimate is linearly interpolated using areas B and C. The signal at the detector is defined as

$$\phi_T = \phi + S_c \tag{2}$$

ϕ_T is the intensity measured at the detector. ϕ is the primary signal and S_c is the scatter estimate using linear interpolation and measured data. Both scatter estimation models are used in the following.

Next, a suitable scatter correction method is needed. In [9], several are presented. For this approach, a projection-based deterministic scatter compensation approach is used. The initial equation is

$$\phi_T = \phi + H(\phi) \tag{3}$$

$H(\phi) = T \cdot (\phi * G)$ transforms the primary signal to the estimated scatter. By rearranging, the following fixed-point equation is found

$$\phi = \phi_T - H(\phi) \tag{4}$$

Let the fixed-point be $\phi = \phi_c$. If ϕ_c is the primary signal, then $H(\phi)$ is the correct scatter. After subtracting $H(\phi)$ from ϕ_T, the primary signal is gained. Both ϕ and $H(\phi)$ are non-negative, since they represent intensities. Out of this equation, an iterative subtractive algorithm with relaxation can be derived [9]

$$\phi^{(n+1)} = \phi^{(n)} + \lambda^{(n)}(\phi_T - (\phi^{(n)} + H(\phi^{(n)}))) \tag{5}$$

λ is the step size of the iteration and n the current iteration number. This equation is reformulated by inserting $\phi_T = \phi + S_c$, where S_c is the initial scatter estimate from (2)

$$\phi^{(n+1)} = \phi^{(n)} + \lambda^{(n)}(S_c - H(\phi^{(n)})) \tag{6}$$

$$\text{with: } H(\phi^{(n)}) = T \cdot (\phi^{(n)} * G) \tag{7}$$

T is a scaling factor to adjust the estimated scatter to the initial scatter estimate S_c. G is assumed to be a Gaussian kernel here. The results presented were calculated with two different Gaussians. The first kernel has a size of 150 pixels with $\sigma = 10$, the second kernel has a size of 300 pixels and $\sigma = 30$. Convolution is done row-wise.

$\phi^{(0)} = S_c - \phi_T$. Sometimes this value can be negative. To avoid this, only a small constant scatter is subtracted from the total signal. This constant is the minimum of the first and last pixel of the area C of the initial scatter estimate. Areas B and C of ϕ^0 are extrapolated with the common water cylinder correction for the initial estimate.

Convolution is done in frequency domain. 40 iterations are performed with a constant step size of 0.1. After each iteration, the area A of $\phi^{(n+1)}$ is replaced with the initial $\phi^{(0)}$. When a pixel in $\phi^{(n+1)}$ gets negative, the value from $\phi^{(n)}$ is taken.

3   Results

We used two different datasets for evaluation. Both datasets were reconstructed using the new scatter correction approach and the water cylinder correction. Quantitative measurements use the correlation coefficient (CC) and the structural similarity (SSIM) index, since a reference dataset without collimation exists.

The results for dataset 1 and 2 are shown in Fig. 3 and 4 and Tab. 1. Scatter convolution shows no cupping artifact. In the water cylinder correction, an intensity increase towards the boundary of the FOV is visible (cf arrows). At the boundary of the FOV, scatter correction retains more details than the water cylinder correction. Quantitatively, scatter correction also performs better than water cylinder correction.

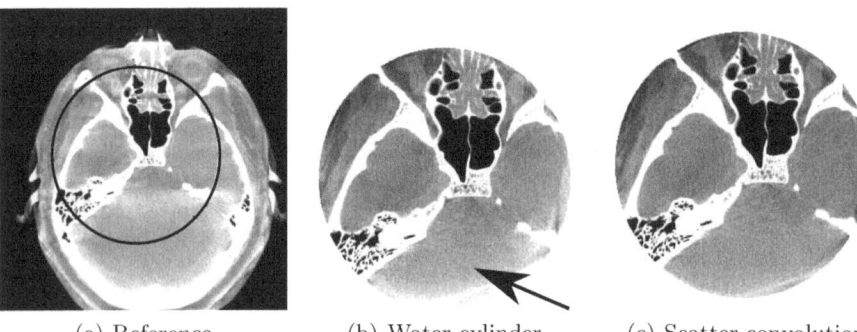

(a) Reference   (b) Water cylinder   (c) Scatter convolution

Fig. 3. Results of dataset 1. Corrected reconstructions shown for FOV denoted by circle in reference. Grayscale window (600, 1400).

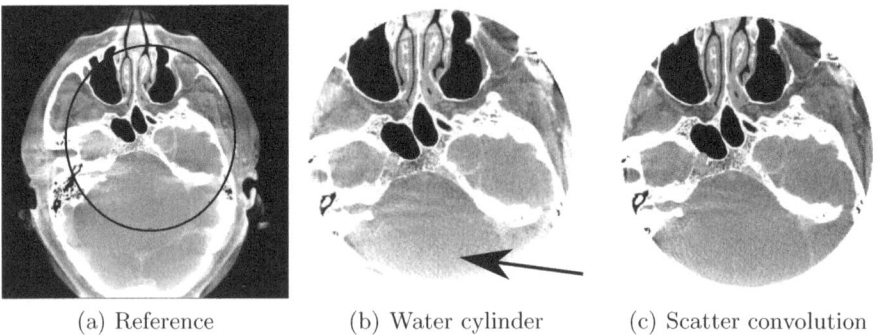

(a) Reference   (b) Water cylinder   (c) Scatter convolution

Fig. 4. Results of dataset 2. Corrected reconstructions shown for FOV denoted by circle in reference. Grayscale window (600, 1400).

Table 1. Error measurements.

	CC	SSIM
Dataset 1 Water cylinder correction	0.9461	0.9444
Scatter convolution (kernel size 150, $\sigma = 10$)	0.9589	0.9527
Scatter convolution (kernel size 300, $\sigma = 30$)	0.9593	0.9533
Dataset 2 Water cylinder correction	0.9228	0.9224
Scatter convolution (kernel size 150, $\sigma = 10$)	0.9403	0.9368
Scatter convolution (kernel size 300, $\sigma = 30$)	0.9401	0.9367

4 Discussion

The method scatter convolution does not work when no scattered radiation is measured. This can however be detected, and only the normal water cylinder correction can be applied. Thus, the method performs at least as good as the water cylinder correction. Further improvements could come from a refined physical model. Here, only simple scatter estimation and correction methods were used, which already lead to good reconstruction results.

References

1. Chintalapani G, Chinnadurai P, Maier A, et al. The value of volume of interest (VOI) C-arm CT imaging in the endovascular treatment of intracranial aneurysms: a feasibility study. Procs ASNR. 2012;12-O-1509-ASNR.
2. Zeng L. Medical Image Reconstruction. 1st ed. Heidelberg: Springer Verlag; 2010.
3. Kolditz D, Kyriakou Y, Kalender WA. Volume-of-interest (VOI) imaging in C-arm flat-detector CT for high image quality at reduced dose. Med Phys. 2010;37(6):2719–30.
4. Kudo H, Courdurier M, Noo F, et al. Tiny a priori knowledge solves the interior problem in computed tomography. Phys Med Biol. 2008;53(9):2207–31.
5. Hsieh J, Chao E, Thibault J, et al. A novel algorithm to extend the CT scan field-of-view. Med Phys. 2004;31(9):2385–91.
6. Dennerlein F, Maier A. Region-of-interest reconstruction on medical c-arms with the ATRACT algorithm. Medical Imaging 2012: Physics of Medical Imaging. 2012;8313:83131B–83131B–9.
7. Xia Y, Maier A, Dennerlein F, et al. Efficient 2D filtering for cone-beam VOI reconstruction. IEEE MIC. 2012;P. to appear.
8. Chityala R, Hoffmann KR, Bednarek DR, et al. Region of interest (ROI) computed tomography. Proc Soc Photo Opt Instrum Eng. 2004;5745(1):534–41.
9. Rührnschopf EP, Klingenbeck K. A general framework and review of scatter correction methods in x-ray cone-beam computerized tomography. Part 1+2. Med Phys. 2011;38(7):4296–311, 5186–99.
10. Siewerdsen JH, Daly MJ, Bakhtiar B, et al. A simple direct method for x-ray scatter estimation and correction in digital radiography and cone-beam CT. Med Phys. 2006;33(1):187–97.

Hyperelastic Susceptibility Artifact Correction of DTI in SPM

Lars Ruthotto[1], Siawoosh Mohammadi[2], Constantin Heck[1], Jan Modersitzki[1], Nikolaus Weiskopf[2]

[1]Institute of Mathematics and Image Computing, Universität zu Lübeck
[2]Wellcome Trust Center for Neuroimaging, University College London
lars.ruthotto@mic.uni-luebeck.de

Abstract. Echo Planar Imaging (EPI) is a MRI acquisition technique that is the backbone of widely used investigation techniques in neuroscience like, e.g., Diffusion Tensor Imaging (DTI). While EPI offers considerable reduction of the acquisition time one major drawback is its high sensitivity to susceptibility artifacts. Susceptibility differences between soft tissue, bone and air cause geometrical distortions and intensity modulations of the EPI data. These susceptibility artifacts severely complicate the fusion of micro-structural information acquired with EPI and conventionally acquired structural information. In this paper, we introduce a new tool for hyperelastic susceptibility correction of DTI data (HySCO) that is integrated into the Statistical Parametric Mapping (SPM) software as a toolbox. Our new correction pipeline is based on two datasets acquired with reversed phase encoding gradients. For the correction, we integrated the variational image registration approach by Ruthotto et al. 2007 into the SPM batch mode. We briefly review the model, discuss involved parameter settings and exemplarily demonstrate the effectiveness of HySCO on a human brain DTI dataset.

1 Introduction

Echo planar imaging (EPI) is a commonly available ultrafast MRI acquisition technique [1]. It is routinely used for key investigation techniques in modern neuroscience like, e.g., diffusion tensor imaging (DTI) [2] or functional MRI.

While offering a considerable reduction of acquisition time, a drawback of EPI is the low bandwidth in phase-encoding direction. Therefore, EPI is highly sensitive to inhomogeneities in the magnetic field. In practice, the MRI scanner's almost perfectly homogeneous magnetic field is perturbed by the different magnetic susceptibilities of soft tissue, bone and air associated with the subject. Field inhomogeneities cause geometrical distortions and intensity modulations, the so-called susceptibility artifacts in EPI. Susceptibility artifacts considerably complicate the fusion of functional and micro-structural information acquired using EPI with conventionally acquired anatomical image data, for which susceptibility artifacts are almost negligible [3].

H.-P. Meinzer et al. (Hrsg.), *Bildverarbeitung für die Medizin 2013*, Informatik aktuell, 344
DOI: 10.1007/978-3-642-36480-8_60, © Springer-Verlag Berlin Heidelberg 2013

A number of approaches have been proposed to reduce susceptibility artifacts in EPI. For instance, fieldmap methods measure the inhomogeneities by a reference scan and subsequently correct the data [4]. An alternative is the reversed gradient method presented by [5]. It requires the acquisition of an image pair, acquired using phase encoding gradients of positive and negative polarity, which results in oppositely distorted data. Subsequently, the data are corrected for susceptibility artifacts using modified image registration approaches [5, 6, 7, 3].

In this work, we present a novel hyperelastic susceptibility correction pipeline termed HySCO, which is integrated as a batch tool into the Statistical Parametric Mapping (SPM) toolbox (http://www.fil.ion.ucl.ac.uk/spm/). The backbone of HySCO is a reversed gradient method and the freely available toolbox FAIR [8] that features also the code underlying [3]. The key feature of the scheme [3] is a tailored regularization functional inspired by hyperelasticity that ensures invertibility of the geometric transformations. We integrated the new pipeline into SPM to allow convenient susceptibility artifact correction of large datasets. We exemplify the effectiveness of the method on a human brain DTI dataset. HySCO will be made freely available after publication.

2   Materials and methods

2.1   Data acquisition

One healthy, male volunteer was scanned on a TIM Trio 3T scanner (Siemens Healthcare, Erlangen, Germany) with written informed consent. The acquisition protocol provides two DTI datasets: 66 images with positive phase encoding $\mathcal{I}_1^k$ and 66 images with negative phase encoding $\mathcal{I}_2^k$, where $k = 1, \ldots, 66$. Each DTI dataset was acquired using the following parameters: 6 non-diffusion-weighted (DW) images (image number: $k = 1, \ldots, 6$), 60 DW images with spherically distributed diffusion-gradient directions (image number: $k = 7, \ldots, 66$), matrix 96×96, 60 slices, 2.3mm isotropic resolution, 5/8 Partial Fourier in PE direction using zero filling reconstruction, TE=86ms, volume TR=10.5ms. Note that for each pair of images, $\mathcal{I}_1^k$ and $\mathcal{I}_2^k$, the diffusion direction and diffusion-weighting was the same in both datasets. We thus assumed that differences in $\mathcal{I}_1^k$ and $\mathcal{I}_2^k$ were mostly due to field inhomogeneities.

2.2   Hyperelastic susceptibility correction of echo-planar MRI

We briefly summarize the numerical implementation of the reversed gradient method in [3]. Given are two oppositely distorted images $\mathcal{I}_1$ and $\mathcal{I}_2$. Based on the physical distortion model derived in [5], the goal is to estimate the field inhomogeneity $B : \Omega \to \mathbb{R}$ by minimizing the distance functional

$$\mathcal{D}[B] = \frac{1}{2} \int_\Omega \left(\mathcal{I}_1(x + B(x)v)\,(1 + \partial_v B(x)) - \mathcal{I}_2(x - B(x)v)\,(1 - \partial_v B(x)) \right)^2 dx,$$

$$(1)$$

where v denotes the phase-encoding direction, typically $v = (0, 1, 0)^T \in \mathbb{R}^3$ is the second unit vector. The transformations applied to the images have two components: A displacement that is restricted along v and an intensity modulation given by the Jacobian determinant of the geometrical transformation [5]. Note the opposite signs of the displacement and intensity modulations for $\mathcal{I}_1$ and $\mathcal{I}_2$. Following [3], the field inhomogeneity is estimated numerically by solving

$$\min_{B} \mathcal{J}[B] := \mathcal{D}[B] + \alpha \mathcal{S}^{\mathrm{diff}}[B] + \beta \mathcal{S}^{\mathrm{jac}}[B], \tag{2}$$

where $\mathcal{S}^{\mathrm{diff}}$ is a diffusion-, and $\mathcal{S}^{\mathrm{jac}}$ is a nonlinear regularization term that ensures $-1 < \partial_v B < 1$, which translates to invertible geometrical transformations and positive intensity modulations. The parameters $\alpha, \beta > 0$ balance between minimization of the distance and the regularization functionals.

Problem (2) is solved using the publicly available registration framework FAIR [8] in Matlab. More precisely, a regularized cubic B-spline interpolation is used as image model, where a regularization parameter $\theta \geq 0$ can be used to improve robustness against noise [8]. Problem (2) is discretized on a coarse to fine hierarchy of discretization levels and solved on each level using a Gauss Newton optimization scheme. The coarse grid solution is used as a starting guess for the optimization on the fine grid [8].

2.3   Susceptibility artifact correction pipeline for DTI in the SPM batch mode

Before tensor estimation two pre-processing steps were applied. First, the non-DW and DW images were corrected for motion and eddy current effects using the ECMOCO toolbox [9]. Second, each image was corrected for susceptibility artifacts using three different methods: (a) none, (b) the fieldmap toolbox ([4] following the pipeline described in [9]), and (c) the HySCO toolbox. The diffusion tensors and the root-mean square of the tensor-fit error ($\mathrm{rms}(\epsilon)$) were estimated for the DTI datasets $\mathcal{I}_1$ and $\mathcal{I}_2$ using ordinary least squares as in [9].

In the first step of the HySCO method we solved Problem (2) for the non-diffusion weighted images $\mathcal{I}_1^1$ and $\mathcal{I}_2^1$ Tab. 1. To this end, we used the above outlined multilevel strategy with three discretization levels $24 \times 24 \times 15$, $48 \times 48 \times 30$, and $96 \times 96 \times 60$. Thereby, we obtained an estimate of the field inhomogeneity denoted by B^1. Subsequently, we solved (2) for $\mathcal{I}_1^k$ and $\mathcal{I}_2^k$ on the finest discretization level with the starting guess B^1 and obtained B^k for $k = 2, \ldots, 66$. These correction steps account for small variations in the field inhomogeneity arising from other effects like residual eddy currents [10]. Finally, the corrected images are obtained by applying the transformations in (1) for B^k on $\mathcal{I}_1^k$ and $\mathcal{I}_2^k$.

For convenient access to the correction scheme, we designed a graphical user interface in the batch mode of SPM. The user can control the regularization parameters (default: $\alpha = 50, \beta = 10$), the resolutions of the levels in the multilevel strategy, and the smoothing parameter (default: $\theta = 0.01$).

Table 1. Effect of 3D susceptibility artifact correction. We visualize axial (left) and sagittal (right) projections of the images $\mathcal{I}_1^1$ and $\mathcal{I}_2^1$, acquired without diffusion weighting. The oppositely distorted images and their absolute difference are depicted using equally scaled intensities. Considerable susceptibility artifacts manifest in the original data; compare image pairs in first row. Using the SPM fieldmap toolbox improved the similarity of $\mathcal{I}_1^1$ and $\mathcal{I}_2^1$, however, structures in the difference image remained; second row. Superior correction results were obtained using the proposed `HySCO` method; third row.

	axial			sagittal		
	$\mathcal{I}_1^1$	$\mathcal{I}_2^1$	$\lvert\mathcal{I}_1^1 - \mathcal{I}_2^1\rvert$	$\mathcal{I}_1^1$	$\mathcal{I}_2^1$	$\lvert\mathcal{I}_1^1 - \mathcal{I}_2^1\rvert$
data						
fieldmap						
`HySCO`						

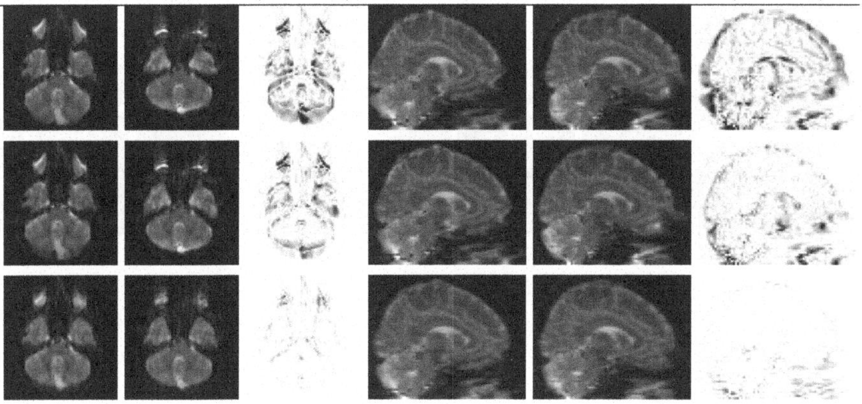

2.4 Comparison of susceptibility artifact correction methods

We compared the correction results of the fieldmap correction and HySCO based on two criteria. As a first step, we compared the similarity of the first image pair acquired without diffusion weighting, i.e.,$k = 1$. To this end, we used visual assessment of uncorrected, fieldmap corrected, and HySCO corrected image pairs, as well as their respective difference images given by (1). In a second step, we compared the impact of the correction pipeline on the diffusion tensor reconstruction using visual inspection of the rms(ϵ) maps as well as quantification of the rms(ϵ) over the whole brain.

3 Results

In Tab. 1 we visualize axial and sagittal slices of the original 3D data, fieldmap corrected data, and results of HySCO. Severe distortions manifest in the original data, especially at the transition between bone and air; compare images in first row and difference images. Similarity between both images was increased by the fieldmap correction indicated by a reduction of the distance functional in (2) from 100% to 52.91%; second row in Tab. 1. A considerable improvement was achieved by HySCO, which relies on the correction scheme [3]. The image pairs were visually almost indistinguishable; third row in Tab. 1. The superiority

Table 2. Impact of susceptibility correction methods on tensor-fit error rms(ϵ) (axial and sagittal slices). The root-mean square of rms(ϵ) (3rd and 6th column) and the non-diffusion weighted images $\mathcal{I}_1^1$ and $\mathcal{I}_2^1$ (1st, 2nd, 4th, and 5th column) are visualized. The tensor-fit error is larger in regions, where the effect of susceptibility artifacts has been insufficiently corrected, e.g. bright spots at the sinuses and frontal areas, highlighted by arrows. Over the whole brain HySCO yielded a considerably smaller average tensor-fit error as compared to the fieldmap correction; 0.1 mm^2/s vs. 0.15 mm^2/s.

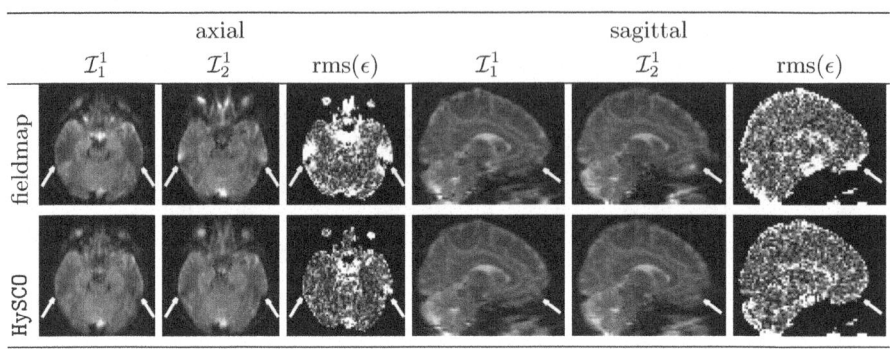

manifests also in the reduction of the distance functional to 8.8%. The multi-level correction required about 20 seconds on a current standard computer.

The distance between the image pairs $\mathcal{I}_1^k$ and $\mathcal{I}_2^k$, where $k = 2, \ldots, 66$, was on average reduced from 100% to 50% for the fieldmap correction. By applying the transformation model described in (1) with the inhomogeneity estimate B^1 from the first problem the image distance was on average reduced to 38.4%. Best results were obtained by performing correction steps on the finest resolution with an average distance reduction to 18.1%. All intensity modulations were positive and overall in a range between 0.03 and 1.97. The average runtime for the correction steps was around 12 seconds on a current standard computer.

Tab. 2 shows axial and sagittal slices of the fieldmap and HySCO corrected non-diffusion-weighted images and tensor-fit error maps. Using the HySCO method resulted in a smaller tensor-fit error than when using the fieldmap method; see, eg., bright spots in the sinuses and frontal areas highlighted by arrows. The mean tensor fit error over the whole brain was 0.15 mm^2/s for the fieldmap approach and 0.1 mm^2/s for HySCO.

4   Discussion

We introduced HySCO, a novel pipeline for susceptibility artifact correction of DTI data. Our pipeline requires two DTI datasets, acquired with reversed phase encoding gradients and thus opposite distortion effects. The backbone of our pipeline is the susceptibility correction scheme presented in [3]. HySCO is integrated as a toolbox into the Statistical Parametric Mapping (SPM) software in Matlab. To enable convenient processing of large datasets, a graphical user interface was designed and integrated into the batch mode of SPM.

In our pipeline, the first image pair, acquired without diffusion weighting, is corrected for susceptibility artifacts using a multi-level strategy. Based on this starting guess correction steps are performed for the diffusion weighted images. This leads to a considerable reduction of computation times, which is desirable for the correction of DTI datasets with many diffusion measurements.

The proposed pipeline requires the acquisition of two DTI datasets and thus doubles scan time, which might not always be feasible. As our results indicate, however, even solving the correction problem once for non-diffusion weighted images and applying the transformation to the remaining image volumes can considerably reduce susceptibility artifacts. In this case, only one image needs to be acquired with reversed phase encoding gradients. This case is also covered by our HySCO implementation.

Preliminary results indicate that HySCO gives superior correction results compared to fieldmap approaches [4], with respect to image similarity and tensor fit error. Extensive evaluations will be a main focus of future work. Further, combinations with other correction techniques like [9] will be investigated.

References

1. Stehling M, Turner R, Mansfield P. Echo-planar imaging: magnetic resonance imaging in a fraction of a second. Science. 1991;254(5028):43–50.
2. Le Bihan D, Mangin J, Poupon C. Diffusion tensor imaging: concepts and applications. J Magn Reson Imaging. 2001;13:534–46.
3. Ruthotto L, Kugel H, Olesch J, et al. Diffeomorphic susceptibility artefact correction of diffusion-weighted magnetic resonance images. Phys Med Biol. 2012;57:5715–31.
4. Hutton C, Bork A, Josephs O, et al. Image distortion correction in fMRI: a quantitative evaluation. Neuroimage. 2002;16(1):217–40.
5. Chang H, Fitzpatrick JM. A technique for accurate magnetic resonance imaging in the presence of field inhomogeneities. IEEE Trans Med Imaging. 1992;11(3):319–29.
6. Andersson J, Skare S, Ashburner J. How to correct susceptibility distortions in spin-echo echo-planar images: application to diffusion tensor imaging. Neuroimage. 2003;20(2):870–88.
7. Holland D, Kuperman JM, Dale AM. Efficient correction of inhomogeneous static magnetic field-induced distortion in echo planar imaging. Neuroimage. 2010;50(1):175–83.
8. Modersitzki J. FAIR: flexible algorithms for image registration. SIAM Rev Soc Ind Appl Math; 2009.
9. Mohammadi S, Nagy Z, Hutton C, et al. Correction of vibration artifacts in DTI using phase-encoding reversal (COVIPER). Magn Reson Med. 2012;68(3):882–9.
10. Jezzard P, Barnett A, Pierpaoli C. Characterization of and correction for eddy current artifacts in echo planar diffusion imaging. Magn Reson Med. 2005;39(5):801–12.

Simulation und Evaluation tiefenbildgebender Verfahren zur Prädiktion atmungsbedingter Organ- und Tumorbewegungen

Maximilian Blendowski, Matthias Wilms, René Werner, Heinz Handels

Institut für Medizinische Informatik, Universität zu Lübeck
blendows@informatik.uni-luebeck.de

Kurzfassung. Lokalisationsunsicherheiten von Tumoren und umliegender Risikostrukturen durch Atembewegungen stellen ein zentrales Problem bei der Bestrahlung von abdominalen und thorakalen Tumoren dar. Moderne Ansätze zur Kompensation der Atembewegung werden in der Regel durch externe Atemsignale gesteuert, die ein Surrogat der inneren Tumor- und Organbewegung darstellen. Unter der Annahme eines Wirkungszusammenhangs zwischen Surrogatsignal und interner Bewegung lassen sich patientenspezifische Korrespondenzmodelle trainieren, um die internen Bewegungen zu prädiktieren. In diesem Beitrag wird der Einfluss der Dimensionalität des Surrogats auf die Genauigkeit der Prädiktion von Organ- und Tumorbewegungen mit Hilfe eines multivariaten linearen Modells untersucht. Hierzu wird die externe Verfolgung der Brustwandbewegung durch tiefenbildgebende Verfahren simuliert und das resultierende Signal als mehrdimensionales Surrogat aufgefasst. Resultate auf der Basis von 10 Lungentumorpatienten zeigen, dass durch den Einsatz von mehrdimensionalen externen Atemsignalen (Linien- und Regionenabtastungen) im Vergleich zu eindimensionalen Signalen eine signifikante Verbesserung der Prädiktionsgenauigkeit erreicht wird.

1 Einleitung

Atmungsbedingte Bewegungen stellen eines der Hauptprobleme bei der Strahlentherapie abdominaler und thorakaler Tumoren dar. Moderne Ansätze zur Kompensation der Atembewegung (z.B. Gating und Tumortracking) werden in der Regel durch externe Atemsignale gesteuert [1]. Unter der Annahme einer Korrelation lassen sich patientenspezifische Korrespondenzmodelle zwischen extern beobachtetem Atemsignal (Surrogat) und der internen Organ- und Tumorbewegungen trainieren, die zur Bewegungsprädiktion eingesetzt werden können. Die Bewegungen des Tumors und umliegender Risikoorgane sind durch ihre Dreidimensionalität und ggf. lokal auftretende Deformationen komplexer Natur. Daher stellt sich die Frage, ob die Nutzung einfacher eindimensionaler Surrogate (z.B. Spirometer-Daten oder Bauchgurtmessungen) sinnvoll ist oder ob mehrdimensionale Signale, die beispielsweise durch tiefenbildgebende Sensorsysteme erfasst werden können [2], präzisere Bewegungsvorhersagen für die relevanten internen Strukturen ermöglichen.

H.-P. Meinzer et al. (Hrsg.), *Bildverarbeitung für die Medizin 2013*, Informatik aktuell,
DOI: 10.1007/978-3-642-36480-8_61, © Springer-Verlag Berlin Heidelberg 2013

In diesem Beitrag wird deshalb der Einfluss der Dimensionalität des Surrogats auf die Genauigkeit der Prädiktion von Organ- und Tumorbewegungen im Kontext der Strahlentherapie von Lungentumorpatienten untersucht.

2 Material und Methoden

Die externe Verfolgung der Brustwandbewegung wird durch tiefenbildgebende Verfahren (z.b. Linienscanner und Time-of-Flight-Kameras) anhand von 4D-CT-Datensätzen simuliert und als mehrdimensionales Atemverlaufssignal aufgefasst. Um den Zusammenhang zwischen den komplexen internen Bewegungsmustern und dem Surrogat mathematisch zu beschreiben, wird – durch die Korrelationsbetrachtungen in [3] motiviert und von uns in [4] vorgeschlagen – ein (multi-) lineares Korrespondenzmodell eingesetzt, dessen Parameter mit Hilfe einer multivariaten linearen Regression (MLR) geschätzt werden. Die Repräsentation der internen Bewegungen erfolgt hierbei durch nicht-lineare, diffeomorphe Transformationen, um die Topologie der anatomischen und pathologischen Strukturen zu erhalten. Der Einfluss von verschiedenen Abtastmustern (einzelne Punkte, Linien und Regionen) und -positionen der Brustwandbewegung auf die Präzision der surrogatbasierten Bewegungsprädiktion wird anhand von 10 4D-CT-Datensätzen untersucht.

2.1 Framework zur surrogatbasierten Bewegungsvorhersage

Es seien $(I_j)_{j \in \{1,...,n_{ph}\}}$ 3D-CT-Bilddaten $I_j : \Omega \to \mathbb{R}$ $(\Omega \subset \mathbb{R}^3)$ eines aus n_{ph} Phasen bestehenden 4D-CT-Datensatzes gegeben, wobei j die Atemphase bezeichne. Zusätzlich liegen jeweils die phasenweise korrespondierenden n_{sur}-dimensionalen externen Atemsurrogate $(\xi_j)_{\in \{1,...,n_{ph}\}}$ mit $\xi_j \in \mathbb{R}^{n_{sur}}$ vor. Durch Anwendung eines diffeomorphen Registrierungsverfahrens [5] liegen die Informationen über die Bewegungen der einzelnen Punkte interner Strukturen zwischen einer Referenzatemphase I_{ref} und der Phase I_j in Form nicht-linearer Transformationen $\varphi_j : \Omega \to \Omega$ vor, die auf Basis des Log-Euclidean-Frameworks durch stationäre Geschwindigkeitsfelder v_j mit $\varphi_j = exp(v_j)$ beschrieben werden.

Sowohl die Geschwindigkeitsfelder v_j als auch die korrespondierenden Atemsurrogatsmessungen ξ_j werden als Zufallsvariablen $\mathbf{V}_j \in \mathbb{R}^{3m}$ (mit m als Anzahl der Bildvoxel) bzw. $\mathbf{Z}_j \equiv \xi_j$ aufgefasst. Diese werden in den Matrizen $\mathbf{V} = (\mathbf{V}_1^c, ..., \mathbf{V}_{n_{ph}}^c)$ bzw. $\mathbf{Z} = (\mathbf{Z}_1^c, ..., \mathbf{Z}_{n_{ph}}^c)$ zusammengefasst, wobei $\mathbf{V}_j^c = \mathbf{V}_j - \bar{\mathbf{V}}$ bzw. $\mathbf{Z}_j^c = \mathbf{Z}_j - \bar{\mathbf{Z}}$ mittelwertzentriert sind.

$$\hat{\mathbf{V}} = \bar{\mathbf{V}} + \mathbf{B}(\hat{\mathbf{Z}} - \bar{\mathbf{Z}}) \qquad (1)$$

gibt an, wie sich das vorherzusagende Geschwindigkeitsfeld $\hat{\mathbf{V}}$ (Regressand) aus einer Messung des Surrogatsignals $\hat{\mathbf{Z}} \equiv \hat{\xi}$ (Regressor) linear berechnet. Die Koeffizienten der Schätzmatrix $\mathbf{B}$ ergeben sich unter Verwendung des Kleinste-Quadrate-Ansatz beim Training des Korrespondenzmodells durch

$$\mathbf{B} = \arg\min_{\mathbf{B}'} \text{tr} \left[(\mathbf{V} - \mathbf{B}'\mathbf{Z})(\mathbf{V} - \mathbf{B}'\mathbf{Z})^T \right] = \mathbf{V}\mathbf{Z}^T (\mathbf{Z}\mathbf{Z}^T)^{-1} \qquad (2)$$

Nahezu unvermeidbare lineare Abhängigkeiten innerhalb des multidimensionalen Atemsignals bereiten Probleme beim Invertieren der Matrix $\mathbf{ZZ}^T$, da diese
fast nie vollen Rang besitzt. Um die Invertierbarkeit zu gewährleisten, wird eine
Tikhonov-Regularisierung angewandt, d.h. $\mathbf{ZZ}^T$ wird durch $\mathbf{ZZ}^T + \gamma\mathbf{I}$ approximiert (Regularisierungsparameter $\gamma > 0$ heuristisch gewählt).

2.2 Simulation der Tiefenbildgebung

Da für diesen Beitrag keine realen Tiefenbildgebungsdaten vorlagen, wurden
punkt-, linien- und regionenweise Abtastungen der sich hebenden und senken-
den Brustwand aus den 4D-CT-Daten der Patienten simuliert. Im Falle der Regionenabtastung werden von einer gegebenen Sensormatrixposition oberhalb des
Patienten in anterior-posteriorer Richtung für jede Atemphase j Strahlverfolgun-
gen durchgeführt, bis subvoxelgenau der Luft-Gewebe-Übergang (Schwellwert:
-500 HU) für die äquidistant verteilten Abtastpunkte innerhalb einer zwischen
den Patienten anatomisch vergleichbaren Region of Interest (ROI) bestimmt ist
(Abb. 1a). Auf die Daten der Matrix wird ebenfalls zur Abtastung cranio-caudal-
verlaufender Linien und einzelner Punkte zurückgegriffen (Abb. 1b,c).

2.3 Bilddaten und Experimente

Für die Evaluation des Einflusses der Dimensionalität der als Surrogat genutzten Brustwandbewegung und der Position des Abtastmusters auf die Vorhersagegenauigkeit des linearen Korrespondenzmodells stehen 10 thorakale 4D-CT-
Datensätze von Lungenkrebspatienten zur Verfügung (10-14 Atemphasen, durchschnittliche Auflösung 512×512×270 Voxel, Voxelgröße von ca. $1{\times}1{\times}1.5$ mm^3).
Ausgehend von der endinspiratorischen Atemphase (EI) als Referenz soll die interne Bewegung zwischen EI und der endexpiratorische Phase (EE) vorhergesagt
werden. Hierzu werden verschiedene Modelle generiert, die sich durch das simulierte Surrogatsignal und die internen Bewegungsinformationen unterscheiden.

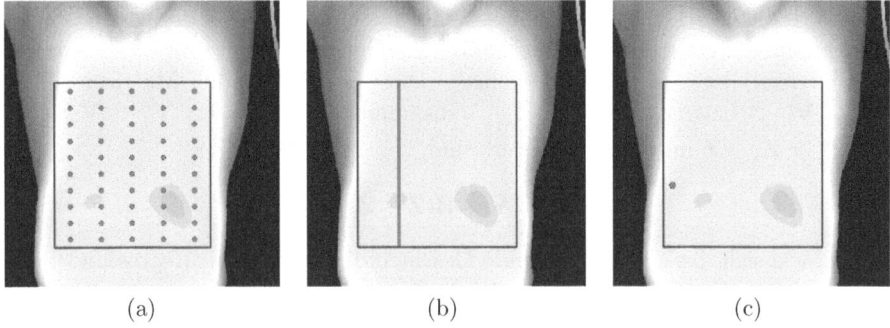

(a)   (b)   (c)

Abb. 1. Illustration der Simulation der verschiedenen Abtastmuster der Brustwandbewegung: (a) Regionenabtastung (b) Linienabtastung (c) Punktabtastung. Die blaue
Box veranschaulicht die genutzte ROI.

Tabelle 1. Prädiktionsergebnisse der verschiedenen Surrogate für die Tumorschwerpunktsbewegung (COM-D) und die gesamte Lunge (TRE), siehe Text für Erläuterungen. Die Ergebnisse sind gemittelt über alle Patienten angegeben als $\mu \pm \sigma$. Zum Vergleich enthält die Tabelle zusätzlich die Abweichungen ohne Bewegungsschätzung und der Intrapatienten-Registrierung zwischen der Referenzphase EI und der vorherzusagenden Phase EE.

Bewegungsschätzung	COM-D [mm]	TRE [mm]
ohne Bewegungsschätzung	6.93 ± 6.06	6.80 ± 1.80
Intrapatienten-Registrierung	0.90 ± 0.50	1.37 ± 0.16
Surrogatbasierte Bewegungsprädiktion; Surrogat =		
$\zeta^{\text{sternum,point}}$	3.83 ± 5.04	4.21 ± 1.87
$\zeta^{\text{opt,point}}$	3.89 ± 4.05	4.00 ± 1.60
$\zeta^{\text{sternum,line}}$	1.59 ± 1.24	1.81 ± 0.25
$\zeta^{\text{opt,line}}$	1.36 ± 1.00	1.73 ± 0.20
$\zeta^{\text{ROI,50}}$	1.36 ± 1.24	1.81 ± 0.26
$\zeta^{\text{ROI,100}}$	1.32 ± 1.16	1.77 ± 0.24
$\zeta^{\text{ROI,150}}$	1.37 ± 1.26	1.75 ± 0.22

Für das Training der Modelle werden die Informationen der EE-Phase sowie ihre beiden benachbarten Phasen nicht berücksichtigt (Leave-Out-Test). Als vorherzusagende interne Bewegungsinformation (Regressand) wird sowohl die komplette Lungenbewegung (inkl. Tumor) als auch der Tumorschwerpunkt betrachtet. Auf Seiten des Atemverlaufssignals (Regressor) werden flächenweise Abtastungen mit 50/100/150 Samplingpunkten generiert ($\zeta^{\text{ROI},50/100/150} \in \mathbb{R}^{50/100/150}$). Die maximale Anzahl der Abtastpunkte wird hier auf 150 beschränkt, um die Berechnung von **B** im Speicher des genutzten Testsystems zu gewährleisten (Intel W3520, 2.67GHz, 24GB RAM). Weiterhin werden neben manuell über dem Sternum platzierten Punkt- und Linienabtastungen ($\zeta^{\text{sternum, point}} \in \mathbb{R}$ bzw. $\zeta^{\text{sternum,line}} \in \mathbb{R}^{75}$) auch vorausgewählte Punkte und Linien genutzt, für die die Residuen zum Training der Matrix **B** nach Gleichung (2) minimiert werden ($\zeta^{\text{opt,point}} \in \mathbb{R}$ bzw. $\zeta^{\text{opt,line}} \in \mathbb{R}^{75}$). Insgesamt ergeben sich so für jeden Patienten 14 Modellkonfigurationen. Zur Beurteilung der Prädiktionsergebnisse der gesamten Lungenbewegung wird der Target-Registration-Error (TRE) basierend auf manuellen Landmarkenkorrespondenzen ermittelt (70 manuell gesetzte Landmarken pro Patient und Phase). Im Fall der Tumorschwerpunkte werden die Abweichungen anhand des euklidischen Abstandes der prädiktierten von der realen Punktposition ausgewertet (COM-D).

3 Ergebnisse

Die Ergebnisse der Experimente sind in Tab. 1 und in Abb. 2 dargestellt. Bezüglich des Einflusses der Dimensionalität liefern mehrdimensionale Surrogate für beide Regressanden präzisere Bewegungsvorhersagen als eindimensionale. Im Gegensatz zur Tumorschwerpunktsbewegung als Regressand sind die Unterschiede bei der Bewegungsvorhersage für die gesamte Lunge zwischen dem Einsatz ein- und mehrdimensionaler Atemverlaufssignalen signifikant (zweiseitiger, gepaarter t-Test; $p < 0.05$). Rein quantitativ wird für die Tumorschwerpunktsbewegung durch ein flächenbasiertes Atemverlaufssignal mit 100 Samplingpunkten die genauste Vorhersage erzielt ($\xi^{\mathrm{ROI},100}$). Eine weitere Dimensionserhöhung auf 150 Samplingpunkte verringert jedoch im Mittel die Vorhersagegenauigkeit wieder (Unterschied nicht signifikant; $p = 0.65$). Im Fall der gesamten Lunge als Regressand wird die mittlere Genauigkeit der flächenbasierten Abtastungen knapp durch eine Linienabtastung unter Vorauswahl ($\xi^{\mathrm{opt},\mathrm{line}}$) übertroffen. Zusammenfassend lässt sich hier allerdings kein signifikanter Einfluss der verschiedenen mehrdimensionalen Abtastmuster auf die Präzision der Bewegungsvorhersagen feststellen (z.B. TRE: $\xi^{\mathrm{opt},\mathrm{line}} \leftrightarrow \xi^{\mathrm{ROI},150}; p = 0.54$). Weiterhin ergibt sich bei beiden Versuchsreihen (COM-D und TRE) keine signifikante Verbesserung der Genauigkeit durch eine zeitintensive Vorauswahl der Punkt- oder Linienposition gegenüber der patientenindividuell festen Sternumsposition. Die Rechenzeit für die Prädiktion liegt im Maximum ($\xi^{\mathrm{ROI},150}$) bei circa 1 Sekunde, wobei die Implementierung bislang nicht laufzeitoptimiert ist.

4 Diskussion

In diesem Beitrag wurde der Einsatz von tiefenbildgebenden Verfahren zur surrogatbasierten Prädiktion von atmungsbedingten Organ- und Tumorbewegungen untersucht und der Einfluss der Dimensionalität (Punkte, Linien und Regionen)

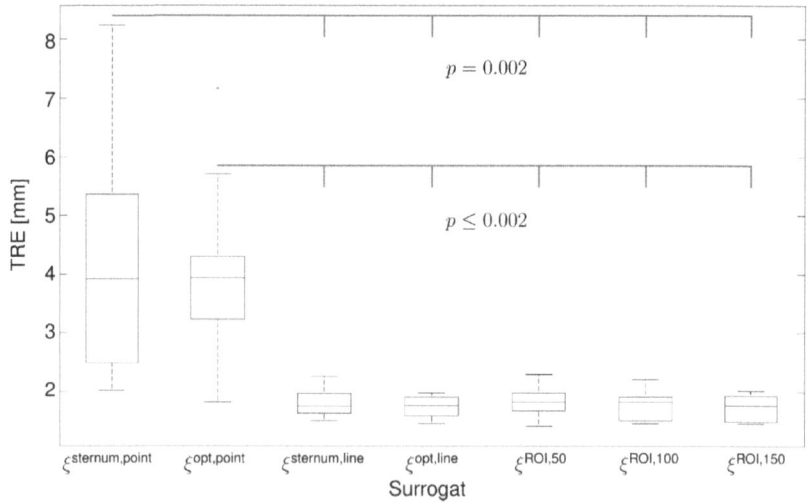

Abb. 2. Darstellung der TRE-Werte der verschiedenen Atemsurrogate bei Betrachtung der gesamten Lunge als Regressand. Es ergaben sich die aufgeführten, signifikanten Unterschiede zwischen den ein- und mehrdimensionalen Signalen.

sowie der Position des Abtastmusters der Brustwandbewegung auf die Präzision der Bewegungsprädiktion evaluiert. Die Resultate zeigen, dass durch den Einsatz von mehrdimensionalen, externen Atemsignalen im Vergleich zu eindimensionalen Signalen eine signifikante Verbesserung der Prädiktionsgenauigkeit erreicht werden kann. Es lässt sich jedoch kein signifikanter Unterschied zwischen der Nutzung eines Linienscanners und der Abtastung der kompletten Brustwand feststellen. Weitere Dimensionserhöhungen gehen nicht beliebig mit einer stetigen Verbesserung der Vorhersagegenauigkeit einher, sondern erhöhen vor allem den Speicherbedarf. So ergibt die Erhöhung der Dimensionalität des abgetasteten Signals zwar prinzipiell mehr Freiheitsgrade beim linearen Korrespondenzmodell, führt aber durch die lineare Abhängigkeit der Bewegung der einzelnen Oberflächenpunkte eher zur Zunahme von redundanten Informationen. Eine Dimensionsreduktion z.B. per Hauptkomponentenanalyse könnte daher Gegenstand zukünftiger Betrachtungen im Rahmen des vorgestellten Frameworks sein. Weiterhin zeigt sich, dass die berechnungsintensive Vorauswahl der Abtastpositionen nicht in einer signifikant verbesserten Prädiktion der internen Strukturen resultiert.

Die Ergebnisse dieses Beitrags illustrieren das Potential der Bewegunsgprädiktion anhand von zeitlichen Oberflächenabtastungen der Brustwand in Kombination mit einem linearen Korrespondenzmodell. Für weitere Aussagen über die Prädiktionsgenauigkeit sind allerdings noch umfangreiche Studien mit realen Daten notwendig, insbesondere im Hinblick auf die intra- und interfraktionelle Variabilität der Bewegungsmuster.

Danksagung. Die präsentierte Arbeit wurde von der Deutschen Forschungsgemeinschaft gefördert (DFG, HA-2355/9-2).

Literaturverzeichnis

1. Keall P, Mageras G, Balter J, et al. The management of respiratory motion in radiation oncology report of AAPM TG 76. Med Phys. 2006 Oct;33(10):3874–900.
2. Schaller C, Penne J, Hornegger J. Time-of-flight sensor for respiratory motion gating. Med Phys. 2008 Jul;35(7):3090–3.
3. Fayad H, Pan T, Clement JF, et al. Technical Note: Correlation of respiratory motion between external patient surface and internal anatomical landmarks. Med Phys. 2011 Jun;38(6):3157–65.
4. Werner R, Wilms M, Ehrhardt J, et al. A diffeomorphic MLR framework for surrogate-based motion estimation and situation-adapted dose accumulation. In: Image-Guidance and Multimodal Dose Planning in Radiation Therapy, a MICCAI Workshop - MICCAI 2012; 2012. p. 42–9.
5. Schmidt-Richberg A, Ehrhardt J, Werner R, et al. Diffeomorphic diffusion registration of lung CT images. In: Workshop Medical Image Analysis for the Clinic: A Grand Challenge - MICCAI 2010; 2010. p. 55–62.

Total Variation Regularization in Digital Breast Tomosynthesis

Sascha Fränkel[1,2], Katrin Wunder[1], Ulrich Heil[2], Daniel Groß[2], Ralf Schulze[3], Ulrich Schwanecke[4], Christoph Düber[1], Elmar Schömer[2], Oliver Weinheimer[1]

[1]Department of Radiology, University Medical Center (UMC) of the Johannes Gutenberg-University Mainz (JGU), Germany
[2]Institute for Computer Science, JGU
[3]Department of Oral Surgery (and Oral Radiology), UMC of the JGU
[4]Department of Design, Computer Science and Media, RheinMain University of Applied Sciences, Wiesbaden
`sasfraen@students.uni-mainz.de`

Abstract. We developed an iterative algebraic algorithm for the reconstruction of 3D volumes from limited-angle breast projection images. Algebraic reconstruction is accelerated using the graphics processing unit. We varied a total variation (TV)-norm parameter in order to verify the influence of TV regularization on the representation of small structures in the reconstructions. The Barzilai-Borwein algorithm is used to solve the inverse reconstruction problem. The quality of our reconstructions was evaluated with the Quart Mam/Digi Phantom, which features so-called Landolt ring structures to verify perceptibility limits. The evaluation of the reconstructions was done with an automatic LR detection algorithm. The LR feature of the Quart Mam/Digi Phantom is well suited for the evaluation of DBT algorithms with respect to the visibility of small structures. TV regularization is not the technique of choice to improve the representation of small structures in DBT. The BB solver provides good results after just 4 iterations.

1 Introduction

Breast cancer remains a significant threat to women's health with almost 60000 newly diagnosed cases per year in Germany. Early detection of breast cancer is important for good healing prognoses. The 2D mammography is still the standard method for detecting suspicious lesions but in certain cases, especially in dense breasts, lesions are sometimes not visible [1]. Driven by now available fast detectors and fast computers the old tomography technique has been revitalized in breast diagnostics to overcome the typical limitations of 2D mammography: superimposing tissue. The generated 3D information in digital breast tomosynthesis (DBT) should improve lesion detection through reduction of superimposition. The results in [2] indicate that there may also be a substantial advantage in using total variation (TV) regularization for microcalcification imaging.

In the DBT technique, a 3D volume, respectively a stack of 2D slices, is computed by the use of a few projected X-ray images. Different algorithms like

H.-P. Meinzer et al. (Hrsg.), *Bildverarbeitung für die Medizin 2013*, Informatik aktuell, DOI: 10.1007/978-3-642-36480-8_62, © Springer-Verlag Berlin Heidelberg 2013

filtered back-projection (FBP), shift-and-add (SAA) or algebraic reconstruction techniques (ART) are employed to produce the 3D volume. Improvements for DBT algorithms are needed especially to enhance resolution and minimize radiation exposure [3]. In this paper, we investigate iterative image-reconstruction in DBT based on ART and TV.

ART formulates the projection of a volume to images as the system of linear equations $\mathbf{Ax} = \mathbf{y}$, where $\mathbf{x} \in \mathbb{R}^n$ is an unknown 3D volume composed of n voxels written in a plain 1D vector, $\mathbf{y} \in \mathbb{R}^{pm}$ is the set of p 2D images, each consisting of m pixels and $\mathbf{A}$ is the Radon transform operator. To solve this equation means to reconstruct the volume. Other groups have shown, that a regularization of total variation leads to a better signal to noise ratio and to a reduction of streaking artifacts [4, 5], but one may ask, whether small structures are better recognizable. With the regularization of total variation the linear equation becomes a convex optimization problem of the form

$$\min_{\mathbf{x}} f(\mathbf{x}) := \|\mathbf{Ax} - \mathbf{y}\|_2^2 + \lambda TV(\mathbf{x}) \tag{1}$$

$$TV(\mathbf{x}) := \sum_{ijk} \sqrt{(x_{i-1,j,k} - x_{i,j,k})^2 + (x_{i,j-1,k} - x_{i,j,k})^2 + (x_{i,j,k-1} - x_{i,j,k})^2}$$

where the $TV(\mathbf{x})$ denotes the total variation and the indices i, j and k refer the position in the 3D volume. In [6] the iterative Barzilai-Borwein (BB) solver was successfully used for reconstruction of low-dose cone-beam computed tomography (CBCT) images, delivering good results after just a few (12-30) iterations.

2   Materials and methods

We scanned the Quart Mam/Digi Phantom with a Hologic Selenia Dimensions system at exposures between 3 mAs and 120 mAs (31 kVp). 3 mAs was the minimal, 120 mAs the maximal adjustable value and 59 mAs was given by the automatic exposure control (AEC) function of the device. One scan consists of 15 projection views (pixel size: $0.117 \times 0.117 \, \text{mm}^2$, image matrix: $\approx 1800 \times 2500$), acquired by the X-ray tube moving over the phantom in a 15° arc. Since we have no access to the raw projection data, we used the 15 projections marked as „for presentation" by the device for our reconstruction process – Hologic uses the 15 raw projections for reconstruction. To evaluate the quality of our reconstructions we used the so-called Landolt ring structures of the Quart Mam/Digi Phantom. The more LRs are detected correctly in the reconstructions, the better the image quality is. For a fast and objective evaluation we implemented an automatic LR detection algorithm (section 2.2).

2.1   Reconstruction method

We define a 3D Volume $\mathbf{x}$ with a voxel size of $0.117 \times 0.117 \times 1 \, \text{mm}^3$ and use the iterative BB solver for minimizing f in Eq. (2). The BB algorithm is based on a Quasi-Newton-Method, so an iteration step has the form

$$\mathbf{x}_{n+1} = \mathbf{x}_n - \mathbf{H}_n^{-1} \nabla f(\mathbf{x}_n) \tag{2}$$

where $\mathbf{H}_n$ is an approximation to the Hessian of $f(\mathbf{x})$. Barzilai and Borwein set $\mathbf{H}_n = \alpha_n \mathbf{I}$ where and α_n minimizes $\|(\mathbf{x}_k - \mathbf{x}_{k-1}) - \alpha_n(\nabla f(\mathbf{x}_n) - \nabla f(x_{n-1}))\|$ and is hence assigned to

$$\alpha_n = \frac{(\mathbf{x}_n - \mathbf{x}_{n-1})^T(\nabla f(\mathbf{x}_n) - \nabla f((\mathbf{x}_{n-1})))}{(\mathbf{x}_n - \mathbf{x}_{n-1})^T(\mathbf{x}_n - \mathbf{x}_{n-1})} \tag{3}$$

We start with $\mathbf{x}_0 = 0$. The influence of TV on the reconstruction process can be managed by the regularization constant λ in Eq. (2). To speed up the reconstruction process forward and back projection are written as shaders running on the graphics processing unit (GPU) [7]. To keep the size of the volume as small as possible we separate the region of the phantom from the air in every projection and define all voxels, which are projected only in phantom regions, as our volume.

2.2   Automatic Landolt ring detection

Fig. 1(a) shows a projection image of the Quart Mam/Digi Phantom. The phantom has 12 steps with increasing densities and each step contains a group of six LRs with diameters from $800\,\mu m$ down to $260\,\mu m$ (Fig. 1(b)). These LRs consist of a ring that has a gap at one of the four positions: left, right, bottom or top. The Hologic tomosynthesis system did not display Step 11 and Step 12.

Fig. 2(a) shows the layout of a LR. Three features are calculated for the description of a LR (Fig. 2(b)):

1. Contrast c, based on the gray value v_1 at the center, the mean value v_2 of the ring values on a path inside the ring and the mean value v_3 on the circle-path outside: $c = ((v_1 - v_2) + (v_3 - v_2))/2$.
2. Standard deviation sd of the ring values.
3. Difference d between mean gap value and mean ring value.

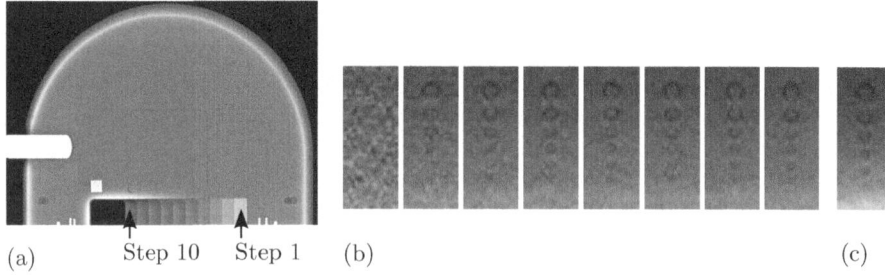

(a)   Step 10   Step 1   (b)   (c)

Fig. 1. 2D projection of the Quart Mam/Digi Phantom (a). Step 11 and 12 are not displayed. Six LRs at Step 7, BB reconstruction, TV $\lambda = 0.0$, iteration 4. Exposures (l.t.r.): 3 mAs, 24 mAs, 45 mAs, 59 mAs, 63 mAs, 84 mAs, 99 mAs, 120 mAs (b). Hologic reconstruction, Step 7, 99 mAs (c).

The calculations are performed with sub-pixel accuracy using bi-linear interpolation. The positions of the 12 groups of LRs in the phantom are fix. In order to ensure a more flexible usability of the detection method, offset jumps from an automatically detected landmark to the LR groups are used. Caused by small inaccuracies in the landmark detection, a small search window of $0.5{\times}0.5{\times}1.0\,\mathrm{mm}^3$ for searching the center of the first LR of a group is used - this ensures that the first ring of a group can be determined correctly. A ring is marked at the position where the sum

$$D = \omega_1 c + \omega_2 sd + \omega_3 d, \text{ with } \boldsymbol{\omega} = (\omega_1, \omega_2, \omega_3) = (3, -1, 1) \tag{4}$$

is maximized, varying the center of the LR and the position of the gap. $\boldsymbol{\omega}$ was heuristically defined. A ring is counted as detected if the detection sum D is greater than a threshold and the gap is correctly detected – the correct gap positions are known for all LRs of the phantom.

3   Results

The rings on Step 1 to Step 10 were analyzed, altogether 60 LRs. We assigned 0.0, 0.5 and 1.0 to the regularization constant λ and compared the reconstructions using 1 to 12 iteration steps. Fig. 3(a)-(c) shows the results for assigned λ values for the different mAs settings. In the following we consider the maximum number of LRs recognized by the automatic detection algorithm over all iterations for a single mAs setting. Then the reconstructions with $\lambda = 0.0$ delivered the best results (228 rings summed up over all mAs settings, 218 for $\lambda = 0.5$, 205 for $\lambda = 1.0$). Summing up TV regularization with $\lambda \neq 0$ did not lead to higher LR counts by the automatic detection method. Fig. 3(d) compares the results of our method with the DBT images provided by the manufacturer of the device (223 rings). Fig. 3(e) shows the ring detection value D (Eq. (4)) for the first LR on Step 8. This value is increasing over the number of iterations, the same applies to the underlying features contrast c, standard deviation sd and difference d (Fig. 3(f)-(h)). The computer used for reconstruction has an Intel Core i7

(a)   (b)   (c)   (d)   (e)

Fig. 2. LR with gap on the right side (a). Marked features (b): center of ring (dot), path inside the ring (line), path in the gap (dotted line) and circle-path outside (line). LRs on Step 7, Exposure 99 mAs, Barzilai Borwein reconstruction, TV $\lambda = 0.5$ (c). Visual output of the automatic LR detection for the first Ring in (c): center, ring and gap are marked correctly (d). Values on the circle-path through the ring and the gap: the highest peak belongs to the gap (e).

CPU with 2.97 GHz clock speed and 12 GB RAM. We use a 64-bit Windows 7 OS, the GPU is a NVIDIA GeForce GTX 280. The reconstruction program is compiled as an 32-bit application. Interim reconstruction volumes needed in the reconstruction process had to be stored on the hard disk, while they were not needed because of the large size of the Quart Mam/Digi Phantom. The runtime for 1 iteration was approx. 2 minutes.

4   Discussion

We showed in this paper that the LR feature of the phantom is an adequate tool for the evaluation of DBT algorithms with respect to the representation of small

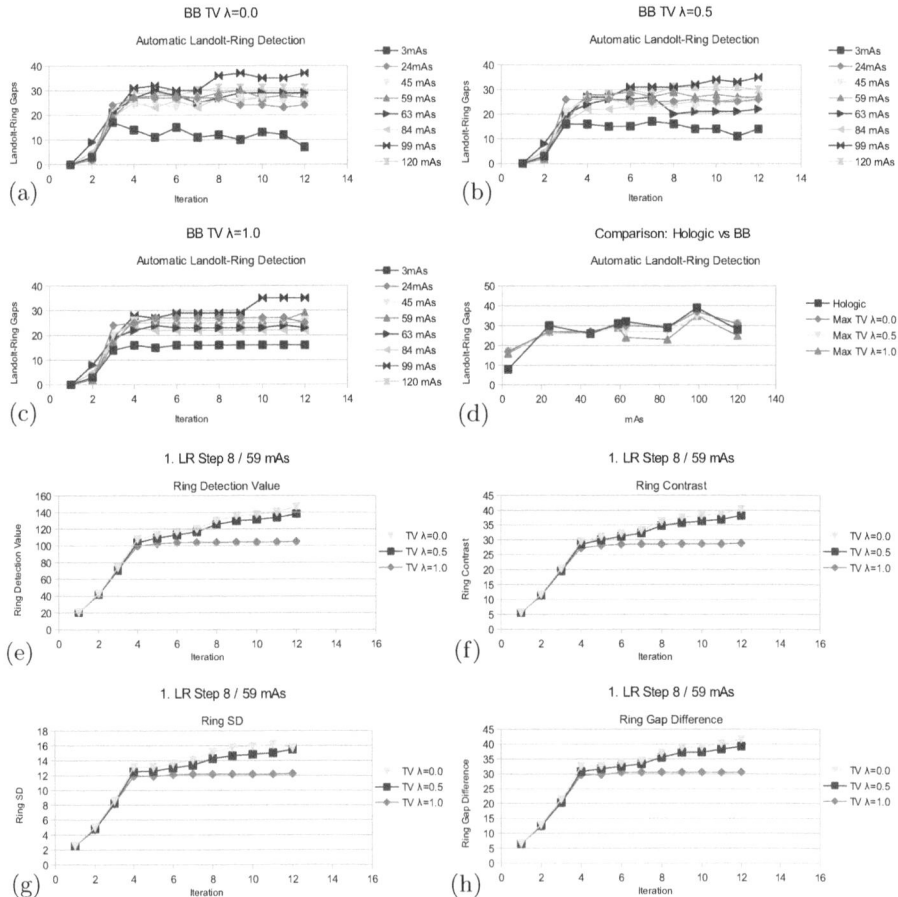

Fig. 3. LR counts for TV reconstructions with different λ values (a)–(c). Comparison of BB and Hologic output (d). Exemplary inspection of the LR detection and feature values for the first LR on Step 8 ((e)–(f).

structures. TV regularization did not lead to better perceptibility of the LRs contained in the Quart Mam/Digi Phantom. TV regularization is therefore not the technique of choice to improve the representation of small structures in DBT. The BB solver provides after just 4 iterations good results. Our reconstructions without TV ($\lambda = 0.0$) are comparable with the DBT images provided by the manufacture with respect to the LR visibility. It is likely that we can (slightly) improve our results by simply feeding our reconstruction program with the true raw projection images. Even though the ring detection value D increases with the iteration number for the example given in the results section, no more rings will be detected for more than 4 iterations. A possible explanation for this is the simultaneously increasing standard deviation sd of the values on the ring – we get more contrast, but also more noise. Different steps are planed for the future. We will compare the results of the automatic LR detection with the reading of radiologists to evaluate reconstruction quality in a clinical context. Our software should be compilable as 64-bit application to overcome the mentioned memory problems. Also we will systematically evaluate our reconstructions for more than 12 iterations. Reconstructing with projections of other DBT systems should be possible in the near future. Investigation and possibly modification of other regularization methods are planed. With ongoing improvement of our reconstruction algorithm the minimal needed radiation dose could possibly be further reduced.

Acknowledgement. Many thanks to the companies Hologic and Quart for giving us the opportunity to work with the preprocessed projection images and with the phantom.

References

1. Helvie MA. Digital mammography imaging: breast tomosynthesis and advanced applications. Rad Clin North Am. 2010;48(5):917–29.
2. Sidky EY, Pan X, Reiser IS, et al. Enhanced imaging of microcalcifications in digital breast tomosynthesis through improved image-reconstruction algorithms. Med Phys. 2009;36(11):4920.
3. Hellerhoff K. Digitale Brusttomosynthese. Der Radiologe. 2010;50(11):991–8.
4. Kastanis I, Arridge S, Stewart A, et al. 3D digital breast tomosynthesis using total variation regularization. Proc IWDM. 2008; p. 621–7.
5. Sidky EY, Duchin Y, Reiser I, et al. Optimizing algorithm parameters based on a model observer detection task for image reconstruction in digital breast tomosynthesis. Proc IEEE NSS/MIC. 2011; p. 4230–2.
6. Park JC, Song B, Kim JS, et al. Fast compressed sensing-based CBCT reconstruction using Barzilai-Borwein formulation for application to on-line IGRT. Med Phys. 2012;39(3):1207–17.
7. Gross D, Heil U, Schulze R, et al. GPU-based volume reconstruction from very few arbitrarily aligned X-ray images. SIAM J Sci Comput. 2009;31(6):4204–41.

Freehand Tomographic Nuclear Imaging Using Tracked High-Energy Gamma Probes

Asli Okur[1,2], Dzhoshkun I. Shakir[1,2], Philipp Matthies[1], Alexander Hartl[1,2], Sibylle I. Ziegler[2], Markus Essler[2], Tobias Lasser[1,3], Nassir Navab[1]

[1]Computer Aided Medical Procedures (CAMP), TU München
[2]Dept. of Nuclear Medicine, Klinikum rechts der Isar, TU München
[3]Institute of Biomathematics and Biometry, Helmholtz Zentrum München
okur@cs.tum.edu

Abstract. Systems allowing freehand SPECT imaging inside the operating room have been introduced previously. In this work, we aim to take one step further and enable 3D freehand imaging using positron emitting radio-traces such as [18F]FDG. Our system combines a high-energy gamma probe with an optical tracking system. Detection of the 511keV annihilation gammas from positron-emitting radio-tracers is modeled analytically. The algorithm iteratively reconstructs the radioactivity distribution within a localized volume of interest. Based on the PET/CT data of 7 patients with tumors and lymph node metastases in the head and neck region, we build a neck phantom with [18F]FDG-filled reservoirs representing tumors and lymph nodes. Using this phantom, we investigate the limitations and capabilities of our method. Finally, we discuss possible improvements and requirements needed so that our approach becomes clinically applicable.

1 Introduction

Patients diagnosed with head and neck squamous (epithelial) cell carcinoma (HNSCC) are mostly treated by a surgical procedure where the major aim is to resect the tumor and all lymph node (LN) metastases. Although the metastatic LNs can be identified pre-operatively with high sensitivity and specificity using [18F]FDG positron emission tomography (PET) and computed tomography (CT), in clinical practice all LNs in the region of the suspicious one(s) are resected. The tumor itself is mostly easily accessible for the surgeon, however, the intra-operative detection and resection of the metastatic LNs is very difficult because of the presence of vital anatomic structures such as nerves and vessels in the neck region. In order to detect the metastatic LNs, pre-operative injection of [18F]FDG (e.g. 1 hour before surgery) and intra-operative usage of dedicated high energy gamma radiation detectors are required, since the metastatic LNs cannot be assessed visually. Aesthetic concerns motivate minimally invasive interventions as well.

In this work, we describe freehand PET (fhPET), a system to image and detect PET-positive LNs intra-operatively. The proposed system combines a high-energy gamma probe with a 3D optical tracking system, similar to the freehand SPECT (fhSPECT) system introduced by Wendler et al. [1, 2]. The iterative 3D reconstruction of the radio-tracer distribution within the volume of interest (VOI) is based on analytical models of the detection physics [3].

High-energy gamma probes are used in clinical practice, for example in HNSCC [4] and thyroid cancer applications [5], however without tracking and navigation capabilities. Intra-operative PET scanners [6, 7], combined intra-operative PET and trans-rectal ultrasound [8], or hand-held PET imaging probes with an external detector ring for full tomographic data [9] are also introduced in the literature.

2   Materials and methods

2.1   Freehand imaging with high-energy gamma probes

A high-energy gamma probe is a hand-held radiation counter, typically with a thick shielding around the detector head, that can detect annihilation gamma rays (511 keV) from positron-emitting radio-tracers. In contrast to regular PET systems, which can detect the two simultaneous gamma rays in opposite directions, a high-energy gamma probe can only detect single gamma rays. Furthermore, since these annihilation gammas have a much higher energy (511 keV) compared to the gamma rays emitted by SPECT tracers such as ^{99m}Tc (140keV), a much better and thicker collimation is required for the high-energy gamma probe (Fig. 1).

A gamma probe gives only 1D signal which is proportional to the amount of detected radiation in the field of view. It is by itself not sufficient for generating 3D images. Therefore a model of the physical factors affecting the detection of the radiation is required. Also it needs to be combined with a spatial positioning system so that the acquired probe signals during the scanning phase are mapped to the positions and orientations of the probe with respect to the VOI (discretized into voxels). Each probe measurement is decomposed into a linear combination of the contributions a_{ij} of the unknown activity values x_i in all voxels

$$m_j = \sum_i a_{ij} x_i \qquad (1)$$

All the measurements within a scan can be stacked into a system of linear equations $m = Ax$ using this decomposition. The activity distribution in the VOI can be retrieved using an iterative solver like maximum likelihood expectation maximization (MLEM) [1]. The system matrix A with the contributions a_{ij} is needed for the inversion, so the contributions are computed on-the-fly using an ad-hoc model of the detection physics of the probe [3], since the acquisition geometry is not fix.

2.2   System description

The proposed solution combines a high-energy gamma probe (NodeSeeker 800, Intra Medical Imaging LLC, CA, USA) with an optical tracking system (Polaris

Vicra, Northern Digital Incorporated, ON, Canada). An application workstation (CSS300, SurgicEye GmbH, Munich, Germany) is available for synchronization of the data as well as the computation of the reconstruction and its augmented visualization. The software on this workstation is tuned for supporting the detection model and the characteristics of this specific probe.

Although the introduced fhPET system is similar to the fhSPECT technology, the accurate modeling of the high-energy gamma rays and their detection provoke some additional challenges. First of all, these annihilation gamma rays caused by positron-emitting radio-tracers such as [18F]FDG can penetrate through matter more than e.g. the gamma rays of ^{99m}Tc due to their much higher energies. Even though the high-energy probes are constructed with much thicker shielding, it is not sufficient enough to block all the gammas. Furthermore, the [18F]FDG is injected to the patient systematically, which is distributed via the blood vessels to the whole body and cause also some unspecific [18F]FDG uptake in tissue. In contrast, the radio-tracers used in sentinel LN procedures are injected locally around or close to the tumor and are distributed via the lymphatic system, resulting in almost no unspecific uptake.

2.3   Experiments

We prepared a phantom simulating a tumor and a LN in the neck region, using a plastic cylinder with 125 mm diameter and three rigidly fixed plastic lab reservoirs with 2 ml volume each. (Fig. 1). Using this phantom, we conducted three sets of experiments in total to evaluate fhPET for the localization of tumors and lymph node metastases in HNSCC. For the first set of experiments, we investigated PET/CT images from 7 patients (mean age: 53, 6m/1f). Each patient had one or two PET-positive LNs. Based on these data sets, we derived the radioactivity we needed for the reservoirs in our realistic experiments with [18F]FDG (Tab. 1). The plastic cylinder was then filled with water to simulate human tissue.

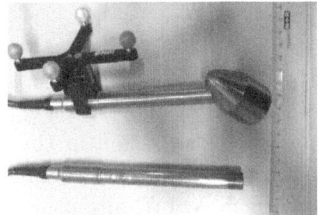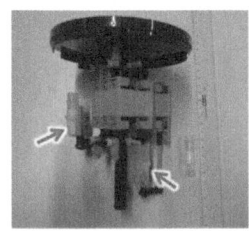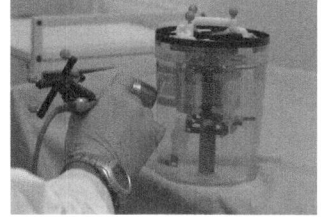

Fig. 1. (High-energy gamma probe has a thicker collimation in contrast to the low-energy gamma probe (left). The neck phantom was constructed by using a plastic cylinder (very close to the human neck in dimension) and three 2 ml laboratory reservoirs: two were rigidly glued to each other for simulating the tumor (middle, blue arrow), and a third one was used for simulating the lymph node (middle, red arrow). A tracking target was attached on top of the phantom, and after preparation with [18F]FDG, the phantom was scanned using our system (right).

Table 1. Geometrical and activity-related parameters calculated from clinical data.

Parameter	Mean ± standard deviation
Tumor depth from the surface	5.3 ± 1.06 cm
Lymph node depth from the surface	2.6 ± 0.99 cm
Tumor-to-background (T/BG) uptake ratio	3.3 ± 1.17
Tumor-to-lymph node (T/LN) uptake ratio	1.5 ± 0.97
Tumor uptake	23.8 ± 9.41 kBq/ml
Lymph node uptake	21.3 ± 12.75 kBq/ml

In order to determine the limits of our current system, we increased the activity proportions in the second set of experiments, where we aimed to determine the activity level which the system can reconstruct both the tumor and the LN.

For comparison of our system with the images of the commercially available fhSPECT system, we conducted a third set of experiments, where we used the same radioactivity proportions as before but used ^{99m}Tc and a conventional gamma probe this time instead of $[^{18}F]$FDG and the high-energy gamma probe.

In all these experiments, two operators scanned each phantom configuration either two or three times each, with an angular coverage of about 120 degrees and with 3000 measurements. In each case the resulting system of linear equations was inverted using MLEM with 20 iterations. On the obtained reconstructions a 4 or 6 mm Gaussian filter was applied to reduce noise due to the highly undersampled acquisition with insufficient statistics as in fhSPECT.

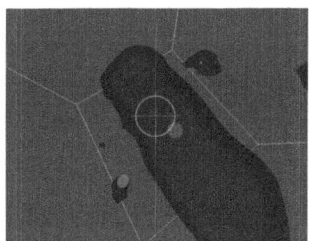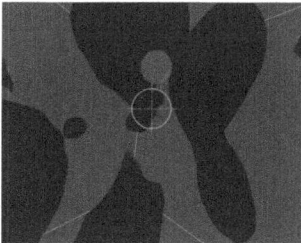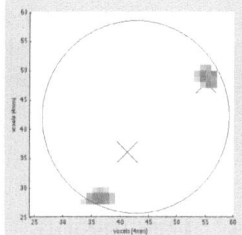

Fig. 2. The shape of the reservoir can be distinguished in the visualization of the reconstruction as seen from the probe tip (left). The two reservoirs next to each other representing the tumor can be seen separately in one reconstruction although they are deeply seated (middle). A transverse slice of one reconstructed image. red: reconstructed LN, blue: reconstructed tumor, circle: an outline of the phantom, crosses: positions obtained from the ground truth (right).

Table 2. Accuracies achieved in experiments with different configurations.

Experiment setup	BG:T:L	Lymph node loc. error	Tumor loc. error
1. [^{18}F]FDG low	0:17:10	12.67 ± 2.48 mm	n/a
2. [^{18}F]FDG high	0:20:20	13.57 ± 4.22 mm	34.79 ± 6.20 mm
	1:20:20	14.41 ± 5.75 mm	47.39 ± 22.28 mm
3. ^{99m}Tc high	0:20:20	11.35 ± 4.26 mm	39.39 ± 10.60 mm
	1:20:20	10.85 ± 4.07 mm	20.42 ± 2.55 mm

3   Results

For evaluating our experiments qualitatively, we checked the visibility of the tumor and the LN in the individual reconstructions. In the first set of experiments, we identified the LN in 3 of the 6 reconstructions. We could not distinguish the tumor visually in any of these 6 reconstructions with realistic activity concentrations.

We could identify the LN in all of the 16 reconstructions in the second set of experiments (Fig. 2, left). Furthermore, we could see the tumor in 6 reconstructions where 3 out of 6 were even with BG activity. In one of the reconstructions we could even identify the two individual reservoirs next to each other, simulating the deeply seated tumor (Fig. 2, middle).

In the third set of experiments using ^{99m}Tc and a conventional gamma probe, we could identify the LN in all of the 12 reconstructions. The tumor was visible in 8 out of 12 reconstructions, 3 out of 6 with BG radioactivity.

For quantitative evaluation, we obtained a CT of our phantom as the ground truth. We registered the CT to the fhPET and fhSPECT images using the phantom tracking target (Fig. 2, right). We manually selected the midpoint of the LN and the tumor in the CT images and computed the distances to the LN and the tumor in the registered images, for the cases where they were clearly identified.

4   Discussion

We were able to reconstruct the reservoir filled with [^{18}F]FDG representing the LN in all cases, however with a localization error between 12.7 and 14.4mm (Tab. 2). At realistic activity concentrations we were not able to detect the tumor site and with higher activities it was detected with high localization errors. Although the detection of the tumor itself is not the primary focus of this clinical application, it still indicates that some improvements are required. The sub-optimal collimation in the currently available high-energy gamma probes limits the accuracy of the detection. Placing a detector block under the patient and detecting the coincidences can be considered to overcome this issue. However, this would require major modification inside the operating room, so our proposed system would be more feasible for the surgery, if it can meet the accuracy requirements of the intervention.

A better physical model of the detection process or inclusion of attenuation correction and scatter effects could improve the image quality of the fhPET system. Registration of pre-operative PET/CT data would provide attenuation correction information for better reconstructions. It would also provide the possibility for acquisition guidance and artifact reduction using prior information. Intra-operative ultrasound can be considered for the registration of the pre-operative clinical data inside the operating room.

In summary, we have shown first results demonstrating feasibility of intra-operative freehand tomographic imaging using high-energy gamma probes on phantom experiments based on clinical data. Furthermore, we discussed possible improvements and requirements needed so that our approach becomes clinically applicable.

Acknowledgement. This research was funded/supported by the Graduate School of Information Science in Health (GSISH), the TUM Graduate School (Munich, Germany) and SFB 824 (DFG, Germany).

References

1. Wendler T, Hartl A, Lasser T, et al. Towards intra-operative 3D nuclear imaging: reconstruction of 3D radioactive distributions using tracked gamma probes. Lect Notes Computer Sci. 2007;4792:909–17.
2. Wendler T, Herrmann K, Schnelzer A, et al. First demonstration of 3-D lymphatic mapping in breast cancer using freehand SPECT. Eur J Nucl Med. 2010;37(8):1452–61.
3. Hartl A, Shakir DI, Kojchev R, et al. Freehand SPECT reconstructions using look up tables. Proc SPIE. 2012;8316:83162H.
4. Meller B, Sommer K, Gerl J, et al. High energy probe for detecting lymph node metastases with 18F-FDG in patients with head and neck cancer. Nuklearmedizin. 2006;45(4):153–9.
5. Kim WW, Kim JS, Hur SM, et al. Radioguided surgery using an intraoperative PET probe for tumor localization and verification of complete resection in differentiated thyroid cancer: a pilot study. Surgery. 2011;149(3):416–24.
6. Stolin AV, Majewski S, Raylman RR, et al. Hand-held SiPM-based PET imagers for surgical applications. Proc IEEE NSS-MIC. 2011.
7. Majewski S, Stolin A, Martone P, et al. Dedicated mobile PET prostate imager. J Nucl Med Meeting Abstracts. 2011;52(1):1945.
8. Huber J, Moses W, Pouliot J, et al. Dual-modality PET/ultrasound imaging of the prostate. IEEE Nucl Sci Symp Conf Rec. 2005;4:2187–90.
9. Huh SS, Rogers WL, Clinthorne NH. An investigation of an intra-operative PET imaging probe. IEEE Nucl Sci Symp Conf Rec. 2007; p. 552–5.

Kategorisierung der Beiträge

Modalität bzw. Datenmaterial
Röntgen, 33, 39, 45, 51, 57, 63, 69, 110, 122, 134, 146, 187, 223, 283, 319, 331, 343, 361
- konventionell, 21, 27, 87, 99, 116, 122, 128, 146, 152, 164, 170, 193, 205, 211, 217, 247, 283, 289, 307, 319, 325, 349
- digital, 128, 175, 355
Endoskopie, 87, 193, 205, 247
Optische Verfahren
- sonstige, 21, 27, 99, 116, 122, 152, 170, 211, 247, 289, 307, 325
Signale (EKG; EEG; etc.), 99, 349
Multimodale Daten, 122, 128, 146, 217, 283, 319
Durchleuchtung, 241
Angiographie, 175, 241, 337
Computertomographie, 3, 9, 69, 93, 104, 128, 134, 140, 158, 175, 181, 223, 229, 253, 259, 265, 277, 295, 313, 319, 349
- hochauflösend, 175, 259
- spiral, 187
Sonographie, 15, 75, 81, 271, 301
Kernspintomographie, 33, 45, 57, 63, 69, 110, 134, 146, 283, 331
- funktionell, 319, 343
- hochauflösend, 33, 39, 51, 122, 187
Positron-Emission-Tomographie, 361
- hochauflösend, 283
Szintigraphie, 223

Dimension der Daten
Signal (1D), 99, 217, 349
Bild (2D), 27, 63, 81, 87, 93, 122, 146, 152, 164, 170, 193, 199, 205, 211, 217, 223, 229, 247, 271, 277, 289, 301, 337, 355
Bildsequenz (2D+t), 15, 21, 27, 99, 116, 128, 205, 241, 247, 301, 325
Volumen (3D), 3, 33, 39, 51, 57, 69, 75, 104, 110, 122, 128, 134, 140, 146, 158, 175, 181, 187, 223, 229, 241, 253, 259, 265, 277, 283, 295, 301, 307, 313, 319, 331, 337, 343, 355, 361
Volumensequenz (3D+t), 9, 45, 75, 134, 301, 349

Pixelwertigkeit
Einkanal, 3, 9, 21, 33, 57, 63, 75, 81, 99, 110, 116, 128, 134, 140, 158, 164, 170, 181, 187, 205, 241, 247, 253, 265, 271, 277, 283, 295, 319, 337, 349, 355, 361
Mehrkanal, 51, 87, 152, 193, 199, 205, 211, 217, 247, 289, 307, 343

Untersuchte Körperregionen
Schädel, 33, 39, 51, 57, 99, 104, 110, 122, 181, 187, 271, 283, 289, 337, 343
Wirbelsäule, 3, 9, 63, 69
Extremitäten
- obere, 81, 164
- untere, 81, 175, 259, 313
Thorax, 9, 75, 134, 187, 235, 241, 247, 253, 295, 331, 349
Mamma, 45, 146, 355
Abdomen, 3, 9, 15, 21, 87, 187, 193, 205, 265, 319
Becken, 205

Betrachtetes Organsystem
Systemübergreifend, 116, 223, 289, 337
Endokrines System, 223
Zentrales Nervensystem, 33, 39, 51, 57, 110, 152, 283
Vegetatives Nervensystem, 3
Kardiovaskuläres System, 75, 99, 175, 181, 187, 235, 241, 247, 331
Respiratorisches System, 9, 134, 187, 253, 295, 349
Gastrointestinales System, 9, 15, 21, 87, 187, 193, 205, 265
Uropoetisches System, 205
Muskoloskeletales System, 3, 27, 81, 158, 313

Primärfunktion des Verfahrens
Bilderzeugung und -rekonstruktion, 69, 93, 104, 134, 205, 223, 343, 355, 361
Bildverbesserung und -darstellung, 21, 69, 181, 187, 301, 337, 343
Bildtransport und -speicherung, 301
Merkmalsextraktion und Segmentierung, 33, 39, 45, 63, 75, 81, 87, 99, 110, 152, 158,

H.-P. Meinzer et al. (Hrsg.), *Bildverarbeitung für die Medizin 2013*, Informatik aktuell,
DOI: 10.1007/978-3-642-36480-8, © Springer-Verlag Berlin Heidelberg 2013

175, 199, 205, 211, 247, 253, 259, 265, 271, 277, 283, 289, 295, 301, 307, 313, 325

Objekterkennung und Szenenanalyse, 27, 69, 116, 170, 193, 247, 271, 301, 319, 325

Quantifizierung von Bildinhalten, 51, 69, 75, 116, 152, 158, 175, 247, 295, 301, 331

Multimodale Aufbereitung, 57, 122, 128, 146, 217, 223, 241, 301, 331

Art des Projektes

Grundlagenforschung, 39, 45, 69, 99, 116, 152, 199, 205, 217, 307, 313, 325, 349

Methodenentwicklung, 9, 15, 21, 27, 33, 39, 45, 51, 57, 63, 69, 87, 93, 99, 104, 110, 116, 122, 128, 134, 146, 152, 164, 170, 181, 211, 217, 223, 235, 247, 253, 271, 277, 283, 289, 295, 301, 313, 319, 325, 331, 343, 355

Anwendungsentwicklung, 3, 33, 87, 93, 110, 116, 158, 164, 170, 187, 205, 247, 259, 265, 271, 349, 355

Klinische Diagnostik, 33, 51, 75, 81, 87, 175, 289, 313, 337

Autorenverzeichnis

Aach T, 87
Al-Maisary S, 75
Al-Zubaidi A, **271**
Angelopoulou E, 27
Astvatsatourov A, 289

Bäuerle T, 313
Bauer S, 331
Bazin P-L, 39
Becker S, 57
Bendl R, 313
Bergen T, 205
Berkels B, **122**
Bier B, **337**
Biesdorf A, 307
Biesterfeld S, 211
Binnig G, 217
Bischof A, 146
Bista SR, **289**
Blendowski M, **349**
Böcking A, 211
Borsdorf A, 128
Bourier F, 241
Brandt C, 63
Bretschi M, 313
Burek P, 116
Burgkart R, 259
Burmester FS, **265**
Buzug TM, 57, 93, 265

Cabrilo I, 122
Chaisaowong K, 253, 295
Chen L, 271
Chitiboi T, **199**
Cobos AL, 211

de Simone R, 75
Dennerlein F, 104
Deserno TM, 164, 289
Dinse J, **39**
Dogan S, 289
Düber C, 355
Duriez C, 235

Eck S, **307**
Egger J, 69

Egli A, 27
Ehrhardt J, 134, 146
Elson DS, **2**
Elter M, 277
Engelke K, 158, 175
Essler M, 361

Faltin P, 253, 295
Fortmeier D, 3, 9, **140**
Fränkel S, **355**
Fränzle A, **313**
Franz AM, 15, **301**
Freisleben B, 69
Fried E, 110, **283**
Friedl S, **247**
Friedrich D, **211**
Fritzsche KH, 51

Gasteiger R, 187
Gayetskyy S, **175**
Gerner B, **158**
Geyer S, 39
Glaßer S, **45**
Glauche I, 116
Goch CJ, **51**
Golembiovský T, 235
Gollmer ST, 265
Graser B, **75**
Graumann R, 27
Groß D, **355**
Gross S, 87
Grossgasteiger M, 75

Haak D, **164**
Haase S, 21
Hachmann H, **295**
Hänler A, 259
Hagenah J, 271
Hahn H, 199
Hahn HK, 181
Haller S, 122
Handels H, 3, 9, 134, 140, 146, 349
Harmsen M, 164
Hartl A, 361
Hecht T, 3, **9**

H.-P. Meinzer et al. (Hrsg.), *Bildverarbeitung für die Medizin 2013*, Informatik aktuell,
DOI: 10.1007/978-3-642-36480-8, © Springer-Verlag Berlin Heidelberg 2013

Heck C, 343
Heil U, 355
Henze R, 51
Hering J, 51
Herre H, 116
Hess A, 175
Heye T, 75
Hoffmann M, **241**
Hofmann HG, 104, 337
Homeier A, 259
Homeyer A, 199
Hornegger J, 21, 27, 104, 128, 170, 229, 241, 331, 337

Iszatt J, 15

Jung F, **319**

Kiencke S, **93**
Kikinis R, **1**, 69
Kirschner M, 319
Kislinskiy S, **235**
Kleinszig G, 27
Koch M, **331**
Köhler T, 21
König S, 247
König T, **81**
Kondruweit M, 247
Koy T, 63
Kraus M, 21
Kraus T, 253, 295
Krüger J, **146**
Kuehne T, 235
Kunze M, 116

Lasser T, 361
Lawonn K, **187**
Leist M, 152
Lempe G, **99**
Levakhina YM, 93
Libuschewski P, **325**
Linsen L, 199
Lipinski H-G, 223

Maass N, 277
März K, **15**, 301
Magaraggia J, **27**
Maier-Hein L, 15, 301
Maier A, 104, 229, 277, 337
Malberg H, 99

Mang A, **57**
Martin P, 39
Marx M, **134**
Mastmeyer A, **3**, 9, 140
Matthies P, 361
Meding S, 217
Meinzer H-P, 15, 51, 75, 235, 301
Merhof D, 33, 152
Mertins A, 271
Meyer-Ebrecht D, 211
Modersitzki J, 343
Mösges R, 289
Mohammadi S, 343
Morariu CA, **87**
Mualla F, **170**
Müller M, 301
Müller-Ott K, 307
Museyko O, 158, 175

Nagarajah J, 223
Navab N, 361
Neumann G, 81
Niemann U, 45
Nimsky C, 69
Nodeln M, 301
Nowack S, **205**
Nzegne PMK, **253**

Okur A, **361**
Özmen D, **193**

Pauli J, 87
Paulus D, 205
Pener I, **181**
Petersik A, 259
Pilz T, **110**, 283
Pohle-Fröhlich R, **63**
Preim B, 45, 187
Preim U, 45

Radeleff B, 15
Rak M, 81
Richter M, **33**
Riesenkampff E, 235
Rippe K, 307
Roeder I, 116
Rohr K, 307
Rumpf M, 122
Ruthotto L, **343**

Schäfer A, 39

Schaller C, 122
Schasiepen I, 277
Scherf N, **116**
Schett G, 175
Schlemmer H-P, 134
Schmidt G, 217
Schmidt M, 181
Schöll S, 170
Schömer E, 355
Schönmeyer R, **217**
Schuetz TA, 57
Schulze R, 355
Schwanecke U, 355
Schwarzenberg R, **69**
Schwemmer C, 337
Seitel A, 15, 301
Seitel M, 75
Shakir DI, 361
Shen M, **152**
Siedhoff D, 325
Simon H, 164
Sommerfeldt B, 170
Spiliopoulou M, 45
Steffen J, 81
Stieltjes B, 15, 51
Stritzel J, 57
Strobel N, 241, 331
Struffert T, 337
Surup T, **259**

Taubmann O, 21
Thierbach K, 116
Thiering B, **223**
Tian M, **277**
Timm C, 325
Tönnies KD, 81
Töpfer D, 158

Toma A, 57
Turner R, 39

van Waasen S, 110, 283
von Oldenburg G, 259
von Rohden L, 81

Wagenknecht G, 110, 283
Walch A, 217
Wald D, 75, 235
Wang J, **128**
Weichert F, 325
Weinheimer O, 355
Weiskopf N, 343
Werner R, 134, 349
Wesarg S, 319
Wetzl J, **21**
Weyand M, 247
Wilms M, 349
Wirthgen T, 99
Wittenberg T, 205, 247
Wörz S, 307
Wolf I, 75
Wu H, **229**
Wunder K, 355

Xia Y, **104**, 337

Yang Q, 277
Yu J, 164

Zahn A, 15
Zaunseder S, 99
Zelzer S, 301
Zerjatke T, 116
Ziegler SI, 361
Zimmer B, 152
Zipser S, 99

Stichwortverzeichnis

Abbildung, 217
Ähnlichkeit, 331
Aktive Kontur, 87, 211
Anatomie, 69, 187, 259
Artefakt, 93, 337, 343
Atlas, 164
Auflösung, 21, 175, 217
Augmented Reality, 361
Ausbildung, 3

B-Spline, 134, 146
Benutzerschnittstelle, 295
Bewegung, 9, 21, 128
Bewegungsanalyse, 134, 247, 349
Bildfusion, 21, 128, 217, 331
Bildgenerierung, 93
Bildqualität, 93, 355
Bioinformatik, 152, 307, 325
Biomechanik, 235, 247

Clusteranalyse, 45
Computer, 158, 301
Computer Aided Diagnosis (CAD), 45, 69, 81, 87, 164, 181, 289, 295, 301
Computer Assisted Radiology (CAR), 69, 301
Computer Assisted Surgery (CAS), 27, 87, 301, 361
Content Based Image Retrieval (CBIR), 164

Datenbank, 199
Deformierbares Modell, 110, 140, 146, 235, 307, 331
Detektion, 69, 87, 253, 319
Diffusion, 211
Diskriminanzanalyse, 33

Echtzeit, 3, 15, 140, 301, 325
Erweiterte Realität, 241, 361
Evaluierung, 15, 93, 187, 205, 259, 295, 355
– klinisch, 289

Farbmodell, 87, 241, 289
Farbnormierung, 289
Filterung, 253, 361

Finite Elemente Modell (FEM), 122, 235
Fourier-Transformation, 211, 247
Fusion, 217
Fuzzy Logik, 325

Gabor-Transformation, 87, 271
Geometrie, 158, 187
Gesichtsbildanalyse, 99, 289
Gradient, 110
Graph Matching, 69, 122
Graphical User Interface (GUI), 301

Haptik, 3, 140
Histogramm-Transformation, 110
Hochgeschwindigkeitskamera, 247
Hough-Transformation, 247, 289, 337

Interpolation, 110, 217, 235

Kalibrierung, 27
Kantendetektion, 158, 337
Karhunen-Loéve-Transformation, 87, 265
Klassifikation
– statistisch, 33, 81, 164, 170, 271
– unscharf, 325
Koordinatentransformation, 170
Korrelation, 33, 93
Kovarianzmatrix, 265
Krümmungsanalyse, 187

Labeling, 181, 253, 283
Landmarke, 289
Lineare Regression, 33, 349
Live Wire, 110, 283
Lokale Adaption, 110, 175, 211
Lokalisation, 39, 87, 289, 319

Marching Cube, 175, 187
Matching, 122
Merkmalskarte, 39, 57
Mikroverkalkung, 355
Minimalinvasive Chirurgie, 9, 15, 361
Modellierung, 57, 75, 122, 134, 158, 265, 331, 349
Morphologie, 175, 181
Multispektral, 217

H.-P. Meinzer et al. (Hrsg.), *Bildverarbeitung für die Medizin 2013*, Informatik aktuell,
DOI: 10.1007/978-3-642-36480-8, © Springer-Verlag Berlin Heidelberg 2013

Navigation, 15, 361
Numerik, 122, 355

Oberfläche, 69, 110, 187, 253
Objekterkennung, 63, 170, 289, 319
Operationsplanung, 3, 9, 235, 361
Optimierung, 57, 93, 158, 229

Partialvolumeneffekt, 158
Perfusion, 45, 99, 175
Plattform, 301
Plug-In Mechanismus, 301
Point-Distribution-Modell, 265

Quantisierung, 158, 175

Radon-Transformation, 355
Region of Interest (ROI), 33, 45, 99, 104, 110, 164, 175, 283, 319, 361
Region-Growing, 175, 199, 247, 283
Registrierung, 122, 128, 134, 146, 217, 241, 343
– elastisch, 33, 331, 349
Regression, 164, 349
Rekonstruktion, 93

– 3D, 69, 104, 259, 355, 361
Relaxation, 235
ROC-Kurve, 33

Schwellwertverfahren, 93, 175, 253, 259
Simulation, 3, 57, 158, 235, 349
Snake
– 2D, 211
Stereoskopie, 69

Template Matching, 69, 181
Textur, 81, 87, 271
Topologie, 21, 235, 253, 283, 295
Tracking, 15, 116, 128, 181, 205
Tumorstaging, 57

Validierung, 3, 93, 158, 259, 349
Video, 99, 247
Virtuelle Realität, 3, 140
Visualisierung, 187, 241
– 3D, 69, 235, 259
Volume Rendering, 128, 140, 241
Volumetrie, 295

Wavelet-Transformation, 81

The manufacturer's authorised representative in the EU is Springer
Nature Customer Service Centre GmbH, Europaplatz 3, 69115 Heidelberg,
Germany. If you have any concerns regarding our products, please
contact ProductSafety@springernature.com

Printed and bound by CPI Group (UK) Ltd, Croydon, CR0 4YY
27/04/2026
02097625-0004